Reducing Inequalities in Health:
A European Perspective

D0217520

Socio-economic inequalities in health are present to a greater or lesser extent in all European countries and the available data suggests that the health gap is increasing. Many studies have been conducted to explain inequalities in health and from them much has been learnt about the different contributory factors. However, in practice it seems hard to translate the knowledge of causes into effective interventions and policies. *Reducing Inequalities in Health: A European Perspective*:

- brings together an unrivalled collection of contemporary data on *successful* policies and interventions
- compares differences in approach by country
- includes the latest evaluation studies
- discusses conceptual issues for research
- provides examples of good and bad practice
- draws out the policy and research implications for the future.

With contributions from leading researchers in 14 different European countries this book provides a comprehensive source of reference for the reader interested in what really works in the field of health promotion and in what sort of policies reduce the health gap.

Johan Mackenbach is chair of the Department of Public Health, Erasmus University Rotterdam and **Martijntje Bakker** at the time of editing the book, worked as a researcher at the Department of Public Health, Erasmus University Rotterdam. She is now working as a policy worker with the Public Health Fund.

The publication of this book was supported by a grant from the European Commission (Health and Consumer Protection Directorate-General, 1998/ PRO/2037). This book reflects the views of its authors only. The European Commission is by no means liable for any use that may be made of the information contained in this book.

Reducing Inequalities in Health: A European Perspective

Edited by

Johan Mackenbach
Martijntje Bakker

Editorial board:

Joan Benach
Bo Burström
Espen Dahl
Ken Judge
Eero Lahelma
Piroska Östlin
Karien Stronks
Margaret Whitehead

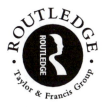

London and New York

First published 2002
by Routledge
11 New Fetter Lane, London EC4P 4EE

Simultaneously published in the USA and Canada
by Routledge
29 West 35th Street, New York, NY 10001

Routledge is an imprint of the Taylor & Francis Group

© 2002 Selection and editorial matter, Johan Mackenbach
and Martijntje Bakker; individual chapters, the contributors

Typeset in 10/12pt Times New Roman by Graphicraft Ltd, Hong Kong
Printed and bound in Great Britain by Antony Rowe Ltd, Chippenham, Wiltshire

British Library Cataloguing in Publication Data
A catalogue record for this book is available
from the British Library

Library of Congress Cataloging in Publication Data
Reducing inequalities in health : a European perspective / edited by
Johan Mackenbach and Martijntje Bakker.
      p.   cm.
   Includes bibliographical references and index.
   1. Medical care—Europe.   2. Health services accessibility—
Europe.   3. Social classes—Health aspects—Europe.
4. Discrimination in medical care—Europe.   5. Medical policy—
Social aspects—Europe.   I. Mackenbach, Johan P.   II. Bakker,
Martijntje, 1969–

RA395.E85 R43 2002
362.1′094—dc21   2001048671

ISBN 0-415-25984-3 (pbk)
ISBN 0-415-25983-5 (hbk)

Contents

Figures

Tables

Boxes

Contributors

Amanda Amos
Public Health Sciences
Department of Community
   Health Sciences
Medical School
University of Edinburgh
Teviot Place
Edinburgh EH8 9AG
United Kingdom

Martijntje J. Bakker
Public Health Fund (Fonds OG2)
PO Box 93064
2509 AB The Hague
The Netherlands

Ruth Barnes
39 Chevening Road
Queens Park NW6 6DB
United Kingdom

Joan Benach
Dept. Experimental and
   Health Sciences
Universitat Pompeu Fabra
C/ Dr. Aiguader, 80
08003 Barcelona
Spain

Michaela Benzeval
Department of Geography
Queen Mary and Westfield College
Mile End Road

London E1 4NS
United Kingdom

Carme Borrell
Municipal Institute of Public
   Health
Pl Lesseps 1
08023 Barcelona
Spain

Sven Bremberg
National Institute of Public Health
SE – 10352 Stockholm
Sweden

M. Teresa Brugal
Municipal Institute of Public Health
Pl Lesseps 1
08023 Barcelona
Spain

Bo Burström
Department of Social Medicine
Norrbacka
Karolinska Institute
17176 Stockholm
Sweden

Giuseppe Costa
Department of Public
Health and Microbiology
University of Turin
Turin

Antonio Daponte
Escuela Andaluza de Salud Pública
Campus Universitario de la Cartuja
Apartado de Correos 2070
Granada 18080
Spain

Finn Diderichsen
Department of Social Medicine
Norrbacka
Karolinska Institute
17176 Stockholm
Sweden

Elia Díez
Municipal Institute of Public Health
Pl Lesseps 1
08023 Barcelona
Spain

Nerina Dirindin
Dipartimento di Scienze
Economiche e Finanziark
 "G. Prato"
Università degli Studi di Torino
Corso Unione Souietica, 218bis
10134 – Torino
Italy

Margaret Douglas
32 Redford Rd
Edinburgh EH13 0AA
Scotland

Didier Fassin
Centre de Recherche sur les Enjeux
 contemporains en Santé Publique
Université Paris 13
74, rue Marcel Cachin
93017 Bobigny
France

Wendy Gnich
Research Unit in Health, Behaviour
 and Change
University of Edinburgh Medical
 School
Teviot Place
Edinburgh EH8 9AG
United Kingdom

Vilius Grabauskas
Kaunas University of Medicine
Mickevicius str. 9
3000 Kaunas
Lithuania

Hilary Graham
Department of Applied Social
 Science
Cartmel College
Lancaster University
Lancaster LA1 4YL
United Kingdom

Hélène Grandjean
INSERM U558,
Faculté de Médecine Purpan
37, Av J Guesde
31073 Toulouse
France

Christer Hogstedt
National Institute of Public Health
10352 Stockholm
Sweden

Philippa Howden-Chapman
Wellington School of Medicine and
 Health Sciences
Department of Public Health
Main Street, Newtown
PO Box 7343
Wellington South
New Zealand

Karin F. A. M. Hulshof
TNO Nutrition and Food Research
Department of Nutritional
 Epidemiology

P.O. Box 360
3700 AJ Zeist
The Netherlands

Ken Judge
Department of Public Health
University of Glasgow
1, Lilybank Gardens
Glasgow G12 8RZ
United Kingdom

Monique Kaminski
INSERM Unité 149
16 Avenue Paul Vaillant Couturier
94807 Villejuif Cedex
France

Panagiota Karnaki
University of Athens Medical
   School
Department of Hygiene and
   Epidemiology
Center for Health Services Research
25, Alexandroupoleos Street
11527 Athens
Greece

Ichiro Kawachi
Department of Health and Social
   Behavior
Harvard School of Public Health
677 Huntington Avenue
Boston MA 02115
USA

Ilmo Keskimäki
STAKES, Outcome and Equity
   Research
PO Box 220
00531 Helsinki
Finland

Anton E. Kunst
Erasmus University Rotterdam
Department of Public Health

PO Box 1738
3000 DR Rotterdam
The Netherlands

Eero Lahelma
Department of Public Health
P.O. Box 41
00014 University of Helsinki
Finland

Thierry Lang
Département d'Epidémiologie et de
   Santé Publique
INSERM U558
Faculté de Médecine Purpan
37, Av J Guesde
31073 Toulouse
France

Annette Leclerc
INSERM U88
Hôpital National
14, rue du Val d'Osne
94415 Saint-Maurice
France

Fred Louckx
Free University of Brussels
Department of Medical Sociology
   and Health Sciences
103 Laarbeeklaan
1090 Brussels
Belgium

Ingvar Lundberg
Department of Occupational
   Health
Norrbacka
17176 Stockholm
Sweden

Johan P. Mackenbach
Erasmus University Rotterdam
Department of Public Health
PO Box 1738

3000 DR Rotterdam
The Netherlands

Mhairi Mackenzie
Department of Public Health
University of Glasgow
1, Lilybank Gardens
Glasgow G12 8RZ
United Kingdom

Andreas Mielck
GSF-Gesundheitsöhonomie
Institut für und Management im
   Gesundheitswesen
Postfach 1129
85758 Neuherberg
Germany

Per-Olof Östergren
Department of Community
   Medicine, Lund University
Malmö University Hospital
20502 Malmö
Sweden

Piroska Östlin
Dept. of Public Health Sciences
Karolinska Institute
Norrbacka
17176 Stockholm
Sweden

Zilvinas Padaiga
Department of Preventive Medicine
Faculty of Public Health
Kaunas Medical University
Eiveniu str. 2, LT-3007
Kaunas
Lithuania

Odette Parry
Research Unit in Health,
   Behaviour and Change
University of Edinburgh Medical
   School

Teviot Place
Edinburgh EH8 9AG
United Kingdom

Iain Paterson
Department of Public Health
University of Glasgow
1, Lilybank Gardens
Glasgow G12 8RZ
United Kingdom

Stephen Platt
Research Unit in Health,
   Behaviour and Change
University of Edinburgh Medical
   School
Teviot Place
Edinburgh EH8 9AG
United Kingdom

Ritva Prättälä
Department of Epidemiology and
   Health Promotion
National Public Health Institute
Mannerheimintie 166
00300 Helsinki
Finland

Ossi Rahkonen
Department of Social Policy
P.O. Box 18
00014 University of Helsinki
Finland

Anna Ritsatakis
World Health Organization,
   European Centre for Health
   Policy
Ministère des Affaires Sociales,
   de la Santé Publique et de
   l'Environnement
Cité administrative de l'Etat
Bd. Pacheco 19, bte 5, room 3.02
1010 Brussels
Belgium

Gun Roos
SIFO/ National Institute for
    Consumer Research
P.O. Box 173
1325 Lysaker
Norway

Alex Scott-Samuel
EQUAL, Department of Public
    Health
University of Liverpool
Whelan Building, Quadrangle
L659 3GB Liverpool
United Kingdom

Marita Sihto
STAKES, Outcome and Equity
    Research
PO Box 220
00531 Helsinki
Finland

Teresa Spadea
Servizio di Epidemiologia
Regione Piemonte – ASL 5
Via Sabaudia, 164
10095 – Grugliasco (TO)
Italy

Karien Stronks
Academic Medical Center
Department of Social Medicine

Meibergdreef 15
1105 AZ Amsterdam
The Netherlands

Yannis Tountas
University of Athens Medical
    School
Department of Hygiene and
    Epidemiology
Center for Health Services
    Research
25, Alexandroupoleos Street
11527 Athens
Greece

Dimitra Triantafyllou
University of Athens Medical
    School
Department of Hygiene and
    Epidemiology
Center for Health Services
    Research
25, Alexandroupoleos Street
11527 Athens
Greece

Joan R. Villalbí
Municipal Institute of Public
    Health
Pl Lesseps 1
08023 Barcelona
Spain

Foreword

In 1995 the King's Fund published a report titled 'Tackling inequalities in health. An agenda for action'. Following this publication Ken Judge (one of the editors of the report), Sven-Olof Isacsson and Johan Mackenbach developed the idea that international collaboration would be useful for exchanging experiences in this area. Based on these discussions they took the initiative to found the European Network on Interventions and Policies to Reduce Socioeconomic Inequalities in Health. At the beginning, most members of the Network originated from the United Kingdom, Sweden and The Netherlands, but today the Network has over 40 members who cover almost all European countries and some non-European countries (New Zealand, United States).

The Network has two purposes:

- to exchange the various national experiences with interventions and policies to reduce socioeconomic inequalities in health;
- to explore opportunities for developing comparative or collaborative research to evaluate such interventions and policies.

Meetings of the Network have been organized yearly since 1996. The first two meetings were organized by members of the Network in Sweden and England, during which mainly conceptual issues were discussed. In 1998 the third meeting was organized in The Netherlands where it was decided to pursue four subjects of interest to the Network in small so-called cross-national 'homework groups' to increase international collaboration. Additionally, it was decided to write a grant application to the European Commission to be able to include new members of European countries not yet included in the Network and to obtain financial support for the publication of a book on Interventions and Policies to Reduce Socioeconomic Inequalities in Health in Europe. In 1999 the European Commission decided to support the Network financially, which has resulted in this publication.

Until now, most publications about socioeconomic inequalities in health have focused on the description of socioeconomic inequalities in health in countries, comparisons between countries and the explanation of these inequalities. From these studies we have learnt much about the different factors which influence socioeconomic inequalities in health. However, in practice it seems hard to translate these factors into interventions and policies which can effectively reduce socioeconomic inequalities in health. The main purpose of this book is, therefore, to describe available evidence of interventions and policies which have been successful in the reduction of socioeconomic inequalities in health.

For this purpose several sections have been incorporated in this book. In the section about interventions and policies (Part II) the relationships between specific topics such as income maintenance policies, nutrition and smoking policies and healthcare and socioeconomic inequalities in health are described, together with an overview of effective interventions and policies to reduce those inequalities. Specific policies or interventions are highlighted to provide a more in-depth description of effective measurements.

In the national experiences section (Part III) detailed country reports provide the opportunity to compare how different countries within Europe deal with socioeconomic inequalities in health at the research and policy level. Countries are selected to cover both the north and south of Europe as well as the accession countries in Eastern Europe.

In the section about evaluation (Part IV) two new promising approaches are presented, health impact assessment and theory-based evaluation, which might solve some of the problems related to the lack of a good evidence base of effective interventions and policies which might reduce socioeconomic inequalities.

The final sections reflect on the information presented in the book and deal with the gender perspective of socioeconomic inequalities in health, an outsider's perspective on the situation in Europe by two non-European members of the Network and a concluding chapter with key messages.

The editing of this book has been a very interesting experience for us. We have learnt a lot from the different ways countries deal with socioeconomic inequalities in health and how, for instance, politicization of the topic can both stimulate as well as hamper dealing with the issue in an effective way. Additionally, we have gained more insight into effective interventions and policies to tackle socioeconomic inequalities in health. At the same time it is important to realize that most of the literature about interventions and policies originates from the United States. Only a few studies in Europe have been published and many studies do not use methodologically sound evaluation designs. Therefore, it will be very important to pay more attention to the evaluation of interventions and policies aimed at the reduction of socioeconomic inequalities in health. Additionally, it is essential that the results of these studies be translated into concrete recommendations for policy-makers to make optimal use of the findings.

Johan Mackenbach and Martijntje Bakker

Acknowledgements

Between the first idea of writing a book about policies and interventions to reduce socioeconomic inequalities in health in Europe and the final publication of this book, a lot of time has past. During this period many people and organizations have been essential for the realization of this project.

First we would like to thank the Health and Consumer Protection Directorate-General of the European Commission for providing a grant to realize the writing of this book and the extension of the Network on Interventions and Policies to Reduce Socioeconomic Inequalities in Health to almost all countries in Europe. As a representative of the Commission, Wilfried Kamphausen has shown great interest in our work, for which we would like to thank him.

As editors of this book we were very lucky to be able to use the expertise of many well known experts in the field of socioeconomic inequalities in health, most of whom are members of the Network. On a voluntary basis many contributed to this book as authors of one or more chapters and the following members were willing to take a seat on the editorial board: Joan Benach, Bo Burström, Espen Dahl, Ken Judge, Eero Lahelma, Piroska Östlin, Karien Stronks and Margaret Whitehead. We would like to thank the authors and editorial board members for making time in their busy schedules to contribute to this book. We especially would like to thank Ken Judge for hosting a meeting of the editorial board in London where important steps were taken towards the finalization of the content of the chapters.

The Network meeting in 1999 was hosted by STAKES, the Finnish national research and development centre for welfare and health, and organized by Ilmo Keskimäki and Kristiina Manderbacka. In 2000 the meeting was hosted by the Municipal Institute of Public Health of Barcelona and organized by Carme Borrell and Joan Benach. During these meetings we had the opportunity to discuss the realization of the book in great detail. We would like to thank the organisers for hosting the meetings and creating such a pleasant environment to work in.

We would finally like to thank Jennifer Bew for her careful editing of the manuscript.

Part I
Introduction

1 Socioeconomic inequalities in health in Europe

An overview

Johan P. Mackenbach, Martijntje J. Bakker, Anton E. Kunst and Finn Diderichsen

Introduction

At the start of the twenty-first century all European countries are faced with substantial socioeconomic inequalities in health, and it is the purpose of this chapter to briefly review the empirical evidence from around Europe. Such evidence relates to both the size and the nature of these inequalities and to their explanation, and is intended to lay the foundation for later chapters in this book.

Historical evidence suggests that socioeconomic inequalities in health are not a recent phenomenon, but it is only relatively recently, during the nineteenth century, and on the basis of mortality statistics, that socioeconomic inequalities in health were 'discovered'. Before that time socioeconomic inequalities in morbidity and mortality went unrecognized, and there was even a general perception that all human beings were equal before death (1). In the nineteenth century, however, great figures in public health, such as Villermé in France, Chadwick in England and Virchow in Germany, devoted a large part of their scientific and practical work to the issue of socioeconomic inequalities in health (2–4). This was made possible by the availability of national population statistics, which permitted the calculation of, for example, mortality rates by occupation or by city district.

Since the nineteenth century the magnitude of socioeconomic inequalities in mortality has certainly declined in absolute terms: owing to the general decline in mortality the absolute difference in mortality rates between those with a high and those with a low socioeconomic position has become much smaller. It is less clear whether relative inequalities in mortality have also declined over time: relative risks of dying for those in a low rather than a high socioeconomic position have remained remarkably stable. During the past few decades there has even been a clear increase of relative inequalities in mortality in many developed countries (5–11). As a consequence, at the end of the twentieth century socioeconomic inequalities in health were seen by some as the biggest public health issue (12).

In the meantime, the emphasis of research in the area of socioeconomic inequalities in health has gradually shifted from description to explanation, and although the number of countries for which the results of explanatory studies are available is still limited, a general understanding of the factors involved has emerged. Childhood circumstances, material factors, health-related behaviours and psychosocial factors have all been shown to contribute significantly to the explanation of socioeconomic inequalities in health (13–17). A better understanding of this explanation has also laid the foundation for a systematic development of strategies to reduce such inequalities (18–20).

For the purpose of this book, socioeconomic inequalities in health will be defined as systematic differences in morbidity and mortality rates between individual people of higher and lower socioeconomic status to the extent that these are perceived to be unfair. In the literature on health inequality there is, unfortunately, no agreement about the way to conceptualize socio-economic position. As in the sociological literature the choice is mainly between concepts of 'class' and 'status'. Concepts of social class are based on theories of society, such as the Marxist theory of exploitation or the Weberian theory of market mechanisms creating inequality in access to resources. Concepts of socioeconomic status try to capture overall welfare along several dimensions of inequality but generally have no theory of the political and economic forces generating inequality attached to them (21). Measures of socioeconomic status might therefore be better predictors of health, as they better describe the material and behavioural conditions of individuals that are important causes of disease. For purposes of health inequality analysis it might nevertheless be more useful to think about socioeconomic position as defined by a theory of society rather than a theory of disease causation. The reason for this is that through such a definition, inequality in health is explicitly linked to a theoretical understanding of the societal mechanisms 'upstream' in the causal pathways.

Positions in a social structure should be distinguished from the individuals occupying those positions (21). Socioeconomic positions are defined by their function in that specific society's division of labour, and have attached to them a number of characteristics of importance for health, such as power, working conditions and income. The health effects attached to a given socioeconomic position can be understood, however, only when they are analysed together with the biological, mental and behavioural characteristics of the individual who occupies it. The allocation of individuals to socioeconomic positions is strongly selective with regard to education, age, gender, race and health. The health distribution we observe across socioeconomic positions is the final outcome of all those effects and processes on health.

Socioeconomic inequalities in morbidity and mortality in Europe

Before we present some summary data on socioeconomic inequalities in health, it is useful to look at some general indicators of health and socio-economic development in Europe.

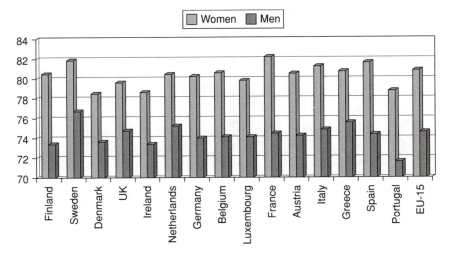

Figure 1.1 Life expectancy (in years) at birth: women and men (1997)

Source: Eurostat Yearbook 2000 (96)

In 1997, life expectancy for women living in the European Union (EU) was 81 years and for men approximately 5 years less (Figure 1.1). There were no clear differences between countries in the north and the south with regard to life expectancy. Life expectancy for women was highest in France and Sweden and lowest in Denmark, Ireland and Portugal.

In 1998 the average unemployment rate was 12 per cent for women and 9 per cent for men (Figure 1.2). Unemployment rates for women were particularly high in Spain, Italy and Greece, and for men in Spain, Finland and France. In general, gross domestic product was higher in countries in the north of Europe than in those in the south (Figure 1.3), indicating more prosperity in the north of Europe. Furthermore, income is generally more unequally distributed in countries in the south of Europe (Table 1.1).

Socioeconomic inequalities in morbidity

Many countries have health interview, level of living or multipurpose surveys with questions on both socioeconomic status (education, occupation, income) and self-reported morbidity (for example, self-assessed health, chronic conditions, disability). Analysis of these data shows that inequalities in self-reported morbidity are substantial everywhere, and nearly always in the same direction: persons with a lower socioeconomic status have higher morbidity rates (22–25).

A comparative study covering 11 countries in Western Europe showed that in the mid- and late 1980s the risk of ill-health was 1.5–2.5 times higher in the lower half of the socioeconomic distribution than in the upper half.

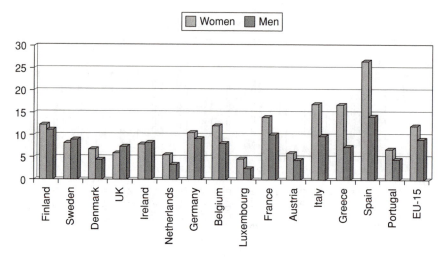

Figure 1.2 Unemployment rate (in percentages) of women and men (1998)

Source: Eurostat Yearbook 2000 (96)

Note: The Eurostat unemployment rates are calculated according to the recommendations of the 13th international Conference of Labour Statisticians organized by the International Labour Office (ILO) in 1982. Unemployed persons are those persons aged 15 years and over who are without work, are available to start work within the next two weeks and have actively sought employment at some time during the previous four weeks.

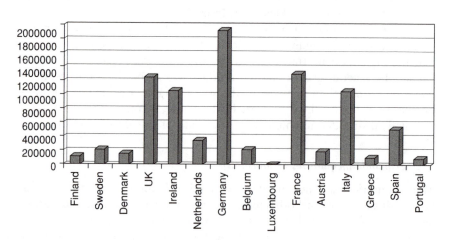

Figure 1.3 Gross domestic product at market prices current series in million ECU (1998)

Source: Eurostat Yearbook 2000 (96)

Table 1.1 Indicators of income distribution[a] in the EU, 1994

	P90/P10[b]	*Gini coefficient*[c]
Belgium	3.9	0.296
Denmark	2.6	0.227
Germany	3.9	0.296
Greece	5.3	0.351
Spain	4.9	0.340
France	3.7	0.290
Ireland	4.6	0.357
Italy	4.4	0.314
Luxembourg	4.0	0.304
Netherlands	3.0	0.247
Austria	4.1	0.297
Portugal	5.6	0.368
Finland[d]	2.5	0.212
Sweden[e]	2.5	0.242
United Kingdom	4.5	0.345
EU-15	4.5	0.322

Notes:

a The income distribution data refer to the distribution of persons arranged according to increasing level of their equivalized household income. Deciles of equivalized income distribution are defined in terms of number of persons rather than of households.

b The top decile group (P90) is the 10 per cent of individuals/households with the highest income. The bottom decile group (P10) is the 10 per cent of individuals/households with the lowest income. The decile ratio is P90/P10.

c Summary measure of inequality in the income shares. It is defined in terms of the relationship of cumulative shares of the population arranged according to the level of equivalized income (bottom 10 per cent, bottom 20 per cent, etc.) to cumulative share of the total income received by them.

d Source: Statistics Finland, Income Distribution Survey 1994.

e Source: Jansson K. Inkomstfördelningen under 1990-talet (Income distribution in the 1990s), in Bergmark, Å (ed.) *Välfärd och forsorjning* (Stockholm: Fritzes, 2000). Because of changes in taxation, the indicators were slightly higher in 1994 because people with certain properties and shares sold these to benefit from the rules in 1994. Adjusted figures excluding these effects are P90/P10: 2.4 and Gini coefficient: 0.208.

Source: Eurostat 1998 (97)

Substantial inequalities in health were found in all countries participating in this study, from Spain to Finland and from Great Britain to Italy. Surprisingly, substantial inequalities in self-reported morbidity were also found in the Nordic countries, despite their long histories of egalitarian socioeconomic and healthcare policies (26, 27). During the mid- and late 1980s, similar results were found in Central and Eastern Europe: for example, in the Czech Republic, Estonia and Hungary socioeconomic inequalities in self-reported morbidity are about equal to those in most Western European countries (28).

It is unclear whether socioeconomic inequalities in self-reported morbidity are increasing, stable or decreasing. Some studies have reported increasing inequalities, but a recent comparative overview of the situation in six Western

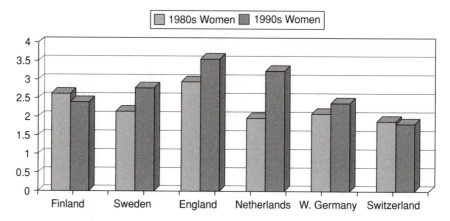

Figure 1.4a Odds ratio for prevalence of 'less than good health' comparing
the lowest income quintile to the highest income quintile, women
25–69 years in two periods

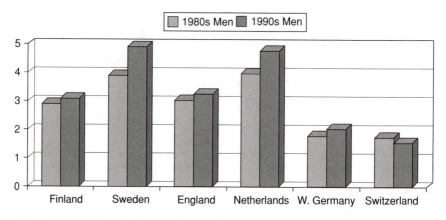

Figure 1.4b Odds ratio for prevalence of 'less than good health' comparing
the lowest income quintile to the highest income quintile,
men 25–69 years in two periods

Source: Kunst *et al.* 2000 (29)

European countries has shown that the picture is far from clear. The
direction and magnitude of the changes seem to vary by country, socioeconomic indicator and type of health problem (29). The clearest patterns
were seen for self-reported morbidity by income level, which has increased
in a number of countries (Figure 1.4a and Figure 1.4b). Trends in the prevalence of 'less-than-good' perceived general health have been more favourable
in the higher than in the lower income groups, and as a result inequalities
have increased, adding to the urgency of the problem. Whether this rise

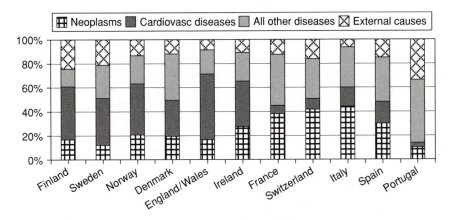

Figure 1.5 Contribution of four broad causes-of-death groups to the difference between manual and non-manual classes in all-cause mortality. Men 45–59 years at death

Source: Kunst 1997 (40)

reflects increasing income inequalities or the increasing economic consequences of illness due to changes in insurance systems, is unclear.

Socioeconomic inequalities in mortality

For mortality, a harder but rarer outcome measure, similar findings have been reported. Socioeconomic inequalities in mortality of considerable magnitude are found in all countries with available data. For example, the excess risk of premature mortality among middle-aged men in manual occupations compared to those in non-manual occupations ranged between 33 and 71 per cent in a comparative study of the situation in the 1980s (30). The results of this study have given rise to an interesting discussion on the interpretation of 'relative' inequalities in health, such as those just cited, and 'absolute' inequalities in health. On the basis of 'relative' differences, such as rate ratios of dying for the lower compared to the upper social groups, there is no evidence for smaller inequalities in mortality in the Nordic countries. On the other hand, if 'absolute' differences are determined, such as rate differences between the lower and the upper social groups, a country such as Sweden does have rather small socioeconomic inequalities in mortality. It has been argued that these smaller absolute inequalities are an effect of egalitarian social and healthcare policies in this 'universalist' welfare state (31).

Mortality data permit a classification by cause of death, which may help in exploring possible explanations of inequalities in mortality. An analysis by cause of death reveals a striking north–south pattern within Western Europe (Figure 1.5). In the Nordic countries and in England/Wales and Ireland, half or more of the socioeconomic gap in total mortality is due to an excess risk of cardiovascular disease in the lower socioeconomic groups. In France, Switzerland, Italy, Spain and Portugal cardiovascular diseases account for a small fraction of the higher risks of premature mortality in the lower socioeconomic groups only, whereas cancers (but not lung cancer) and gastrointestinal diseases (such as liver cirrhosis) do have a large share in the excess risks (32, 33). These data suggest that explanations for socio-economic inequalities in mortality are likely to be partly different between the north and the south of Europe: currently, cardiovascular risk factors such as smoking and intake of animal fats are likely to be important in the north, excessive alcohol consumption in the south (34).

This international pattern can also be interpreted as an expression of different stages of epidemiological development. In the north of Western Europe (and also in the United States) mortality from cardiovascular disease has not always been higher in the lower socioeconomic groups. In the 1950s and 1960s ischaemic heart disease mortality was still higher in the higher socioeconomic groups, and it was only during the late 1960s and 1970s that a reversal occurred (35–39). It is possible that the situation in the south of Western Europe represents an earlier stage of epidemiological development, and that the smaller size of inequalities in cardiovascular disease mortality will prove to be a temporary phenomenon.

In Central and Eastern Europe socioeconomic inequalities in mortality are as large as or larger than in Western Europe. The real outlier seems to be Hungary, which had by far the largest inequalities in mortality among the countries included in a recent comparative study (40, 41). Among middle-aged men the risk of dying was 165 per cent higher in manual than in non-manual occupations. These very large relative differences combine with the high average death rates in Hungary to form extremely large absolute differences in mortality between the higher and lower socioeconomic groups.

Studies of trends in socioeconomic inequalities in mortality during the last decades of the twentieth century have generally shown a widening of the gap (5–11). Trends in mortality have been more favourable in the upper than in the lower socioeconomic groups, and as a consequence relative differences in total mortality have increased in all countries with available data (Figure 1.6). This is due to a large extent to a faster decline in cardiovascular disease mortality in the upper than in the lower socioeconomic groups (29).

Socioeconomic inequalities in health expectancy

As was shown in the previous two sections, both morbidity and mortality rates are higher in the lower socioeconomic groups. These two aspects combine to create even larger inequalities in health expectancy, because people in the lower socioeconomic groups not only live shorter lives but also spend a larger proportion of their life in poor health. Whereas socioeconomic inequalities in life expectancy usually amount to 3–7 years, differences in,

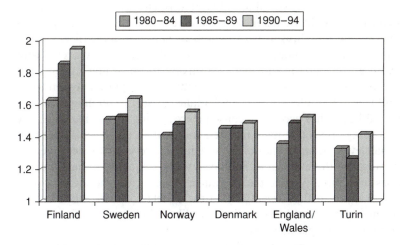

Figure 1.6 Relative risk of dying comparing manual classes to non-manual classes, men 30–59, in three periods (rate ratio)

Source: Kunst *et al.* 2000 (29)

for example, disability-free life expectancy amount to more than 10 years between the highest and the lowest socioeconomic groups (42, 43).

Explanatory perspectives on socioeconomic inequalities in health

Research into socioeconomic inequalities in health has given us many clues about the precipitating factors and mechanisms in populations. These can be grouped into a number of complementary perspectives on the explanation for socioeconomic inequalities in health: the 'selection versus causation' perspective, the 'specific determinants' perspective, and the 'life-course' perspective. We will briefly review some of the evidence supporting each of these, and then discuss some general models for the explanation of socioeconomic inequalities in health that have been proposed in the literature.

As we have mentioned earlier, it is important to acknowledge the fact that this explanation may be partly different in different European countries. The fact that the size of socioeconomic inequalities in health is similar in different countries might conceal the fact that the mechanisms generating them are different, and that social context interacts with these mechanisms (33, 44).

The 'selection versus causation' perspective

Social selection explanations imply that health determines socioeconomic position, instead of socioeconomic position determining health. There is some evidence that during social mobility, that is, changes in socioeconomic position during an individual's life, compared either with his or her parents (intergenerational mobility) or with himself or herself at an earlier point in time (intragenerational mobility), selection on (ill) health may occur, with people who are in poor health being less likely to move upward or more likely to move downward (45–49). Here one might distinguish between when illness influences the allocation of individuals to socioeconomic positions and when ill-health has economic consequences owing to varying eligibility for and coverage by social insurance schemes and so on. Because people's educational level, occupational class and income level are determined at different stages of the life course, and because the frequency of health problems varies substantially across the life course, these socioeconomic indicators are likely to differ in their sensitivity to the effects of health-related selection. Income-related health inequalities are likely to be more affected, and education-related inequalities less so.

Although the occurrence of health-related selection as such is undisputed, it is less clear what its contribution to the explanation of socioeconomic inequalities in health is. Only a few studies have investigated this directly, and these have shown that the contribution to inequalities in health by occupational class is small (45, 49, 50). Moreover, it is not at all clear that health-selective social mobility always increases socioeconomic inequalities in health: there is some evidence that it may actually constrain such inequalities. Those who are downwardly mobile have worse health than others in their class of origin, but better health than others in their class of destination (51).

A different form of selection has been proposed which may have a stronger impact: 'indirect selection'. Indirect selection implies that social mobility is selective on the determinants of health, not on health itself (52). There is very little empirical evidence so far on the occurrence and importance of indirect selection, so it is difficult to assess its importance for the explanation of socioeconomic inequalities in health. A few studies have, however, indicated that it might have an important role (53). It is also important to take into account the fact that health determinants on which indirect selection takes place could themselves be related to living circumstances during earlier stages of life. Indirect selection would then be part of a mechanism of accumulation of disadvantage over the life course (54).

The 'specific determinants' perspective

Longitudinal studies in which socioeconomic status has been measured before health problems are present, and in which the incidence of health problems has been measured during follow-up, show higher risks of developing health problems in the lower socioeconomic groups, and suggest 'causation' instead of 'selection' as the main explanation for socioeconomic inequalities in health (50, 55–57). This 'causal' effect of socioeconomic status on health is likely to be mainly indirect, through a number of more specific health determinants which are differentially distributed across socioeconomic groups.

Material factors

There is no doubt that 'material' factors, for example, exposure to low income and to health risks in the physical environment, contribute to the explanation of socioeconomic inequalities in health. Despite the fact that low income is such a fundamental aspect of low socioeconomic status, however, the evidence for its role in generating health inequalities is far from complete. Income-related indicators of socioeconomic status, such as level of household income, house and car ownership, or area-based measures of deprivation, have been demonstrated to be relatively strong predictors of ill-health (54, 58–60). How low income affects health, and what the relative importance of pathways related to low income is, however, are far from clear. It is obvious that income may affect exposure to a wide range of health determinants, either directly or indirectly, but there has been surprisingly little empirical research into these mechanisms.

Most of the recent research into the health effects of income inequality has focused on the aggregate relationship between the extent of income inequality in a population and its average mortality level or life expectancy (61–63). This has shown that after accounting for differences between populations in average income level, a wider disparity in income within a population is associated with a higher mortality level and a lower life expectancy. Although this suggests that reducing income inequalities may not only reduce health inequalities but also improve the overall health of a population, it is not yet clear how the association is to be explained. It may be due to the psychosocial effects of income inequality (more relative deprivation, less social cohesion) or to the lack of investment in human resources that is usually found in regions with more income inequality (64, 65).

Psychosocial factors

The recent interest in psychosocial pathways between low socioeconomic status and ill-health has been stimulated by the observation that socioeconomic inequalities in morbidity or mortality cannot be explained entirely by well known behavioural or material risk factors for disease. This is particularly true for cardiovascular disease outcomes, where risk factors such as smoking, high serum cholesterol and high blood pressure explain less than half of the socioeconomic gradient in mortality (56, 66, 67). Together with the observation that inequalities in health have a generalized character, in the sense that the risks for diseases with widely different aetiologies are similarly socially patterned, this has given rise to the hypothesis that a lower socioeconomic status may be associated with a higher 'generalized susceptibility' to disease (68). This could be due to psychosocial factors: being in a

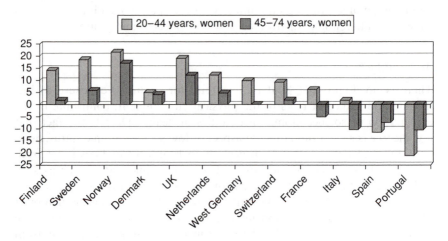

Figure 1.7a Absolute differences between low and high educated persons in current smoking, women

Source: Cavelaars *et al.* 1998 (26)

low socioeconomic position may be a psychosocial stressor which, through biological or behavioural pathways, could lead to ill-health (69). Psychosocial factors related to work organization, such as job strain, have indeed been shown to play an important role in the explanation of socioeconomic inequalities in health (70, 71).

Health-related behaviour

Health-related behaviours, such as smoking, diet, alcohol consumption and physical exercise, are certainly important 'proximal' determinants of socioeconomic inequalities in health. In most European countries smoking is more prevalent in the lower socioeconomic groups (72–74). There are some exceptions, however, particularly in southern Europe, where smoking seems to be more prevalent in the higher socioeconomic groups, particularly among women (Figure 1.7a and Figure 1.7b). These patterns are likely to be related to differences between countries in the progression of the smoking epidemic. This started in northern Europe, among men and in the higher socioeconomic groups, and then diffused into southern Europe, to women and to the lower socioeconomic groups. The cessation of smoking followed a similar pattern, and the 'reverse' patterns for women in southern Europe are probably due to the fact that southern Europe is at an earlier stage of the smoking epidemic. Unfortunately, the situation in younger cohorts suggests that countries in southern Europe are rapidly catching up. Because of the strong impact of smoking on health, socioeconomic differences in smoking contribute importantly to socioeconomic inequalities in health, at least in some countries.

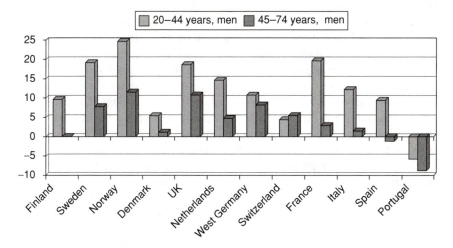

Figure 1.7b Absolute differences between low and high educated persons in current smoking, men

Source: Cavelaars *et al.* 1998 (26)

The contribution of diet to inequalities in health is less clear. In many countries people in lower socioeconomic groups consume fewer fresh vegetables and fruits (75, 76), but data on fat consumption do not suggest consistent differences between socioeconomic groups (77, 78). On the other hand, obesity is very strongly associated with socioeconomic status, with much higher prevalence rates of obesity in the lower socioeconomic groups, particularly in richer countries (34, 79).

Data on socioeconomic differences in alcohol consumption are also not always consistent, but frequently lower socioeconomic groups have higher rates of both abstinence and excessive alcohol consumption (34, 80, 81). Cause-of-death patterns suggest a substantial contribution of excessive alcohol consumption to inequalities in mortality in at least some countries, such as Finland (82) and countries in southern Europe (32).

Finally, lack of leisure-time physical activity is more prevalent in the lower socioeconomic groups (83–85), but it is unclear to what extent this is compensated for by higher rates of work-related physical activity. It is unlikely that such compensation is substantial in the rich service economies of northern Europe, but it may still be in poorer countries.

The 'life-course' perspective

This discussion of the explanation of socioeconomic inequalities in health has so far largely ignored the importance of time: disease usually occurs as a result of prolonged exposure to these risk factors, and exposure may be the result of long individual life histories. Socioeconomic status in childhood (for example, father's occupational class) determines socioeconomic status in adulthood (despite social mobility, many adults are in the same occupational class as their parents), and it has been shown that lifelong exposure to low socioeconomic status carries higher risks of ill-health than exposure during one stage of life only (86). Many health-related behaviours (for example, smoking) are formed in adolescence, that is, under the influence of socioeconomic status in childhood, and it has been shown that socioeconomic inequalities in health-related behaviour are partly the result of different exposures to low socioeconomic status in childhood (87). The same is likely to apply to other intermediary factors, such as coping style, locus of control and other psychosocial factors (88). Health may have a certain continuity across the life course, with ill-health in adulthood tracking back to ill-health in childhood and therefore to determinants acting in earlier stages of life (89–90). Socioeconomic inequalities in health may thus be due to the cumulative effect of disadvantage across the life course.

Health during one stage of the life course may also affect socioeconomic status at a later stage, owing to processes of health-related selection. The life-course perspective enables us to see more clearly the iterative nature of some of these processes, and suggests a 'co-evolution' of social position and health, taking away the sharp contradiction between 'selection' and 'causation' explanations (14, 91). It also makes it possible to think in terms of 'windows of susceptibility', that is, in certain periods of life the individual is more susceptible to the effects of certain exposures – malnutrition and infections during the fetal period, emotional attachment during infancy, and so on.

Integrated models for the explanation of socioeconomic inequalities in health

In order to synthesize all these insights into the explanation of socioeconomic inequalities in health, many authors have tried to sketch integrated models (92–95) (see Box 1.1).

These models, although different in degree of complexity and detail, are all based on a 'layered' or 'chain-like' view of the causation of health inequalities: a low socioeconomic status leads to ill-health through a number of other factors, which are represented as 'layers' or 'links' between socioeconomic status and health. The different layers and links, as well as the arrows between socioeconomic status, layers/links and health, all represent potential entry points for policies and interventions to reduce health inequalities.

The main differences between the models relate to:

* The extent to which a life-course perspective is taken into account. Some of the models are restricted to what happens during adult life; others try to incorporate explicitly what happens during childhood.
* The extent to which biological pathways are represented. Some of the models only or mainly represent determinants that are external to the

Box 1.1   Some integrated models for the explanation of socioeconomic inequalities in health

Model Diderichsen

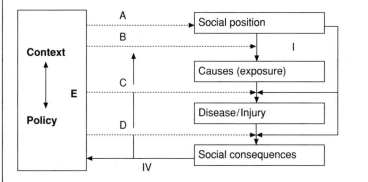

Model Whitehead

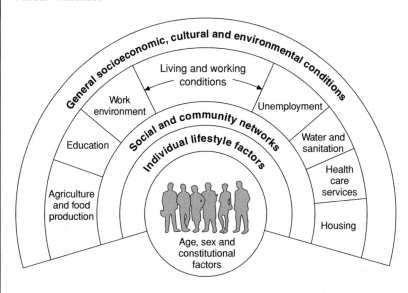

Source: Dahlgren and Whitehead 1991 (93)

Model Mackenbach

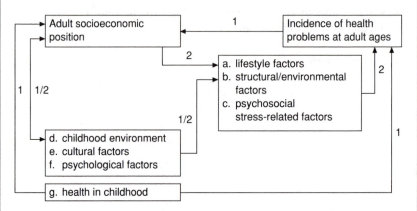

Note: The 'selection' processes (1) are represented by an effect of health problems at adult ages on adult socioeconomic position, and by an effect of health in childhood on both adult socioeconomic position and health problems at adult ages. The 'causation' mechanism (2) is represented by the three groups of risk factors which are 'intermediary' between socioeconomic position and health problems. Childhood environment, cultural factors and psychological factors are included in the model, which acknowledges their contribution to inequalities in health through both 'selection' and 'causation' (1/2).

Source: Mackenbach *et al.* 1994 (94)

Model Marmot and Wilkinson

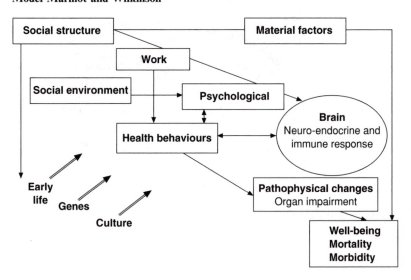

Note: Social determinants of health. The model links social structure to health and disease via material, psychosocial and behavioural pathways. Genetic, early life, and cultural factors are further important influences on population health.

Source: Marmot and Wilkinson 1999 (95)

individual; others show how social inequalities 'get under the skin' and have biological effects which in the end lead to ill-health.

- The extent to which macrosocial factors and policies are represented. Some of the models are limited to what happens at the individual level; others try to represent the macrosocial environment or policies that cause the social inequalities as well.
- The representation, or not, of 'reverse' effects of health on socioeconomic status. Some of the models ignore these effects, whereas others incorporate them explicitly.

If the models are to be useful for policy-making, conflicting requirements have to be met: they must contain all the relevant entry points, and must not be too complex for policy-makers to understand. Perhaps one could argue that biological pathways are more relevant for clinical intervention and less relevant for policy-making (it is unlikely that we will want to reduce health inequalities by direct intervention in the biological pathways), but all the other aspects do seem to be relevant.

Conclusions

The international patterns highlighted in this chapter not only suggest that explanations of socioeconomic inequalities in health are partly different in different countries, but also that interventions and policies to reduce socioeconomic inequalities in health may be partly different. Although the basic socioeconomic structures are similar, the pathways through which low socioeconomic status affects health are partly different, and interventions targeting more proximal determinants of socioeconomic inequalities in health should therefore be adapted to the situation prevailing in a country.

References

1. Mackenbach JP. Social inequality and death as illustrated in late-medieval death dances. *Am J Public Health* 1995: 85: 1285–92.
2. Coleman W. Death is a social disease; *Public Health and Political Economy in Early Industrial France.* Madison: University of Wisconsin, 1982.
3. Chave SPW. The origins and development of public health. In: Holland WW, Detels R, Knox G, eds. *Oxford Textbook of Public Health.* Oxford: Oxford University Press, 1984.
4. Ackerknecht EH, Virchow R. *Doctor, Statesman, Anthropologist.* Madison: University of Wisconsin Press, 1953.
5. Drever F, Bunting J. Patterns and trends in male mortality. In: Drever F, Whitehead M, eds. *Health Inequalities.* London: The Stationery Office, 1997.
6. Vågerö D, Lundberg O. 1995 Socioeconomic mortality differentials among adults in Sweden. In: Lopez AD, Casselli GTV, eds. *Adult Mortality in Developed Countries: From Description to Explanation.* Oxford: Clarendon Press, 223–42.

7. Valkonen T. Trends in regional and socio economic mortality differentials in Finland. *Int J Health Sci* 1993: 3: 157–66.

8. Lang T, Ducimetiere P. Premature cardiovascular mortality in France: divergent evolution between social categories from 1970 to 1990. *Int J Epidemiol* 1995: 24: 331–9.

9. Regidor E, Gutierrez-Fisac JL, Rodriguez C. Increased socioeconomic differences in mortality in eight Spanish provinces. *Soc Sci Med* 1995: 41: 801–7.

10. van de Mheen H, Reijneveld SA, Mackenbach JP. Socioeconomic inequalities in perinatal and infant mortality from 1854 till 1990 in Amsterdam, The Netherlands. *Eur J Public Health* 1996: 6: 166–74.

11. Diderichsen F, Hallqvist J. Trends in occupational mortality among middle-aged men in Sweden 1961–1990. *Int J Epidemiol* 1997: 26: 782–7.

12. Mackenbach JP. Tackling inequalities in health. *Br Med J* 1995: 310: 1152–3.

13. Smith GD, Blane D, Bartley M. Explanations for socioeconomic differentials in mortality. Evidence from Britain and elsewhere. *Eur J Public Health* 1994: 4: 131–44.

14. Vågerö D, Illsley R. Explaining health inequalities: beyond Black and Barker. *Eur Sociol Rev* 1995: 3: 1–23.

15. Macintyre S. The Black Report and beyond: what are the issues? *Soc Sci Med* 1997: 44: 723–45.

16. Kaplan GA, Keil JE. Socioeconomic factors and cardiovascular disease: a review of the literature. *Circulation* 1993: 88: 1973–98.

17. Carroll D, Bennett P, Smith GD. Socioeconomic health inequalities: their origins and implications. *Psychology Health* 1993: 8: 295–316.

18. Whitehead M, Dahlgren G. What can be done about inequalities in health? *Lancet* 1991: 338: 1059–63.

19. Dahlgren G, Whitehead M. *Policies and Strategies to Promote Equity in Health.* Copenhagen: World Health Organization, 1992.

20. Benzeval M, Judge K, Whitehead M. *Tackling Inequalities in Health; An Agenda For Action.* London: King's Fund, 1995.

21. Sorensen AB. The basic concepts of stratification research: class, status and power. In: Grusky DB, ed. *Social Stratification.* Boulder, CO: Westview Press, 1994.

22. Illsley R, Svensson PG. Social inequalities in health. *Soc Sci Med* 1990: 31 (special issue): 223–40.

23. Mielck A, do Rosario Giraldes M. *Inequalities in Health and Healthcare. Review of Selected Publications From 18 Western European Countries.* Münster: Waxmann, 1993.

24. Kunst AE, Geurts JJ, van den Berg J. International variation in socioeconomic inequalities in self reported health. *J Epidemiol Commun Health* 1995: 49: 117–23.

25. Lahelma E, Arber S. Health inequalities among men and women in contrasting welfare states. Britain and three Nordic countries compared. *Eur J Public Health* 1994: 4: 213–26.

26. Cavelaars AE, Kunst AE, Geurts JJ, Crialesi R, Grotvedt L, Helmert U *et al.* Differences in self reported morbidity by educational level: a comparison of 11 Western European countries. *J Epidemiol Commun Health* 1998: 52: 219–27.

27. Cavelaars AE, Kunst AE, Geurts JJ, Helmert U, Lundberg O, Mielck A *et al.* Morbidity differences by occupational class among men in seven European

countries: an application of the Erikson–Goldthorpe social class scheme. *Int J Epidemiol* 1998: 27: 222–30.

28. Groenhof F, Kunst AE, Holub J, Józan P, Leinsalu M, Rychtariková J *et al. Socioeconomic Inequalities in Morbidity and Mortality in Central and Eastern Europe: A Comparison To Some Western European Countries.* Rotterdam: Department of Public Health, Erasmus University, 1996.

29. Kunst AE, Bos V, Mackenbach JP. *Monitoring Socioeconomic Inequalities in Health in the European Union: Guidelines and Illustrations.* Rotterdam: Department of Public Health, Erasmus University, 2000.

30. Mackenbach JP, Kunst AE, Cavelaars AE, Groenhof F, Geurts JJ. Socioeconomic inequalities in morbidity and mortality in Western Europe. The EU Working Group on Socioeconomic Inequalities in Health. *Lancet* 1997: 349: 1655–9.

31. Vagero D, Erikson R. Socioeconomic inequalities in morbidity and mortality in Western Europe. *Lancet* 1997: 350(9076): 516; discussion 517–18.

32. Kunst AE, Groenhof F, Mackenbach JP, Health EW. Occupational class and cause specific mortality in middle aged men in 11 European countries: comparison of population based studies. EU Working Group on Socioeconomic Inequalities in Health. *Br Med J* 1998: 316: 1636–42.

33. Kunst AE, Groenhof F, Andersen O, Borgan JK, Costa G, Desplanques G *et al.* Occupational class and ischemic heart disease mortality in the United States and 11 European countries. *Am J Public Health* 1999: 89: 47–53.

34. Cavelaars AEJM, Kunst AE, Mackenbach JP. Socioeconomic differences in risk factors for morbidity and mortality in the European Community: an international comparison. *J Health Psychol* 1997: 2: 353–72.

35. Marmot MG, Adelstein AM, Robinson N, Rose GA. Changing social-class distribution of heart disease. *Br Med J* 1978: 2: 1109–12.

36. Marmot MG, McDowall ME. Mortality decline and widening social inequalities. *Lancet* 1986: 2: 274–6.

37. Stallones RA. The rise and fall of ischemic heart disease. *Sci Am* 1980: 243: 53–9.

38. Wing S, Hayes C, Heiss G, John E, Knowles M, Riggan W *et al.* Geographic variation in the onset of decline of ischemic heart disease mortality in the United States. *Am J Public Health* 1986: 76: 1404–8.

39. Mackenbach JP, Looman CW, Kunst AE. Geographic variation in the onset of decline of male ischemic heart disease mortality in The Netherlands. *Am J Public Health* 1989: 79: 1621–7.

40. Kunst AE. 1997 *Cross-National Comparisons of Socioeconomic Differences in Mortality.* PhD thesis, Erasmus University, Rotterdam.

41. Mackenbach JP, Kunst AE, Groenhof F, Borgan JK, Costa G, Faggiano F *et al.* Socioeconomic inequalities in mortality among women and among men: an international study. *Am J Public Health* 1999: 89: 1800–6.

42. Valkonen T, Sihvonen AP, Lahelma E. Health expectancy by level of education in Finland. *Soc Sci Med* 1997: 44: 801–8.

43. Sihvonen AP, Kunst AE, Lahelma E, Valkonen T, Mackenbach JP. Socioeconomic inequalities in health expectancy in Finland and Norway in the late 1980s. *Soc Sci Med* 1998: 47: 303–15.

44. Whitehead M, Burstrom B, Diderichsen F. Social policies and the pathways to inequalities in health: a comparative analysis of lone mothers in Britain and Sweden. *Soc Sci Med* 2000: 50: 255–70.

45. Stern J. Social mobility and the interpretation of social class mortality differentials. *J Soc Policy* 1983: 12: 27–49.

46. Illsley R. Social class selection and class differences in relation to stillbirths and infant deaths. *Br Med J* 1955: 2: 1520–4.

47. Wadsworth MEJ. Serious illness in childhood and its association with later-life achievement. In: Wilkinson RG, ed. *Class and Health, Research and Longitudinal Data.* London: Tavistock, 1986.

48. Luft HS. The impact of poor health on earnings. *Rev Econ Statistics* 1974: 65: 43–57.

49. van de Mheen H, Stronks K, Schrijvers CT, Mackenbach JP. The influence of adult ill-health on occupational class mobility and mobility out of and into employment in The Netherlands. *Soc Sci Med* 1999: 49: 509–18.

50. Fox AJ, Goldblatt PO, Adelstein AM. Selection and mortality differentials. *J Epidemiol Commun Health* 1982: 36: 69–79.

51. Bartley M, Plewis I. Does health-selective mobility account for socioeconomic differences in health? Evidence from England and Wales, 1971 to 1991. *J Health Soc Behav* 1997: 38: 376–86.

52. West P. Rethinking the health selection explanation for health inequalities. *Soc Sci Med* 1991: 32: 373–84.

53. Hemmingsson T, Lundberg I, Diderichsen F, Allebeck P. Explanations of social class differences in alcoholism among young men. *Soc Sci Med* 1998: 47: 1399–405.

54. Smith GD, Blane D, Bartley M. Explanations for socioeconomic differentials in mortality. Evidence from Britain and elsewhere. *Eur J Public Health* 1994: 4: 131–44.

55. Fox AJ, Goldblatt PO, Jones DR. Social class mortality differentials: artefact, selection or life circumstances? *J Epidemiol Commun Health* 1985: 39: 1–8.

56. Rose G, Marmot MG. Social class and coronary heart disease. *Br Heart J* 1981: 145: 13–19.

57. Marmot MG, Smith GD, Stansfeld S, Patel C, North F, Head J *et al.* Health inequalities among British civil servants: the Whitehall II study. *Lancet* 1991: 337: 1387–93.

58. Goldblatt P. 1990 Mortality and alternative social classifications. In: Goldblatt P, ed. *Longitudinal Study: Mortality and Social Organisation.* London: HMSO: 163–92.

59. Townsend P, Phillimore P, Beattie A. *Health and Deprivation: Inequality and the North.* London: Croom Helm, 1988.

60. Carstairs V, Morris R. Deprivation and mortality: an alternative to social class? *Commun Med* 1989: 11: 210–19.

61. Wilkinson RG. Income distribution and life expectancy. *Br Med J* 1992: 304: 165–8.

62. Kaplan GA, Pamuk ER, Lynch JW, Cohen RD, Balfour JL. Inequality in income and mortality in the United States: analysis of mortality and potential pathways. *Br Med J* 1996: 312: 999–1003.

63. Kennedy BP, Kawachi I, Prothrow-Stith D. Income distribution and mortality: cross sectional ecological study of the Robin Hood index in the United States. *Br Med J* 1996: 312: 1004–7.

64. Wilkinson RG. *Unhealthy Societies: The Afflictions of Inequality.* London: Routledge, 1996.

65. Lynch JW, Kaplan GA. Understanding how inequality in the distribution of income affects health. *J Health Psychol* 1997: 2: 297–314.

66. Lynch JW, Kaplan GA, Cohen RD, Tuomilehto J, Salonen JT. Do cardiovascular risk factors explain the relation between socioeconomic status, risk of all-cause mortality, cardiovascular mortality, and acute myocardial infarction? *Am J Epidemiol* 1996: 144: 934–42.

67. Smith GD, Shipley MJ, Rose G. Magnitude and causes of socioeconomic differentials in mortality: further evidence from the Whitehall Study. *J Epidemiol Commun Health* 1990: 44: 265–70.

68. Marmot MG, Shipley MJ, Rose G. Inequalities in death – specific explanations of a general pattern? *Lancet* 1984: 1: 1003–6.

69. Brunner E, Marmot M. Social organization, stress, and health. In: Marmot M, Wilkinson RG, eds. *Social Determinants of Health*. Oxford: Oxford University Press, 1999.

70. Marmot M, Theorell T. Social class and cardiovascular disease: the contribution of work. *Int J Health Serv* 1988: 18: 659–74.

71. Hallqvist J, Diderichsen F, Theorell T, Reuterwall C, Ahlbom A. Is the effect of job strain on myocardial infarction risk due to interaction between high psychological demands and low decision latitude? Results from Stockholm Heart Epidemiology Program (SHEEP). *Soc Sci Med* 1998: 46: 1405–15.

72. Cavelaars AEJM, Kunst AE, Geurts JJM, Crialesi R, Grötvedt L, Helmert U et al. Educational differences in smoking: an international comparison. *Br Med J* 2000: 320: 1102–7.

73. van Reek J, Adriaanse H. Cigarette smoking cessation rates by level of education in five western countries. *Int J Epidemiol* 1988: 17: 474–5.

74. Pierce JP. International comparisons of trends in cigarette smoking prevalence. *Am J Public Health* 1989: 79: 152–7.

75. Bolton-Smith C, Smith WC, Woodward M, Tunstall-Pedoe H. Nutrient intakes of different social-class groups: results from the Scottish Heart Health Study (SHHS). *Br J Nutrition* 1991: 65: 321–35.

76. Osler M. Social class and health behaviour in Danish adults: a longitudinal study. *Public Health* 1993: 107: 251–60.

77. Smith GD, Brunner E. Socioeconomic differentials in health: the role of nutrition. *Proc Nutrition Soc* 1997: 56: 75–90.

78. Hoeymans N, Smit HA, Verkleij H, Kromhout D. Cardiovascular risk factors in relation to educational level in 36,000 men and women in The Netherlands. *Eur Heart J* 1996: 17: 518–25.

79. Sobal J, Stunkard AJ. Socioeconomic status and obesity: a review of the literature. *Psychl Bull* 1989: 105: 260–75.

80. Hupkens CL, Knibbe RA, Drop MJ. 1993 Alcohol consumption in the European community: uniformity and diversity in drinking patterns. *Addiction* 88: 1391–404.

81. Cummins RO, Shaper AG, Walker M, Wale CJ. Smoking and drinking by middle-aged British men: effects of social class and town of residence. *Br Med Jl (Clin Res Ed)* 1981: 283: 1497–502.

82. Mäkelä P, Valkonen T, Martelin T. Contribution of deaths related to alcohol use of socioeconomic variation in mortality: register based follow up study. *Br Med J* 1997: 315: 211–16.

83. Lynch JW, Kaplan GA, Salonen JT. Why do poor people behave poorly? Variation in adult health behaviours and psychosocial characteristics by stages of the socioeconomic lifecourse. *Soc Sci Med* 1997: 44: 809–19.

84. Holme I, Helgeland A, Hjermann I, Leren P, Lund-Larsen PG. Physical activity at work and at leisure in relation to coronary risk factors and social class. A 4-year mortality follow-up. The Oslo study. *Acta Med Scand* 1981: 209: 277–83.

85. Tenconi MT, Romanelli C, Gigli F, Sottocornola F, Laddomada MS, Roggi C *et al.* The relationship between education and risk factors for coronary heart disease. Epidemiological analysis from the nine communities study. The Research Group ATS-OB43 of CNR. *Eur J Epidemiol* 1992: 8: 763–9.

86. Smith GD, Hart C, Blane D, Gillis C, Hawthorne V. Lifetime socioeconomic position and mortality: prospective observational study. *Br Med J* 1997: 314: 547–52.

87. van de Mheen H, Stronks K, Looman CW, Mackenbach JP. Does childhood socioeconomic status influence adult health through behavioural factors? *Int J Epidemiol* 1998: 27: 431–7.

88. Bosma H, van de Mheen HD, Mackenbach JP. Social class in childhood and general health in adulthood: questionnaire study of contribution of psychological attributes. *Br Med J* 1999: 318: 18–22.

89. van de Mheen H, Stronks K, Looman CW, Mackenbach JP. Role of childhood health in the explanation of socioeconomic inequalities in early adult health. *J Epidemiol Commun Health* 1998: 52: 15–19.

90. Wadsworth ME. Health inequalities in the life course perspective. *Soc Sci Med* 1997: 44: 859–69.

91. van de Mheen H, Stronks K, Mackenbach JP. A lifecourse perspective on socioeconomic inequalities in health: the influence of childhood socioeconomic conditions and selection processes. *Sociol Health Illness* 1998: 20: 754–77.

92. Whitehead M, Diderichsen F, Burström B. Researching the impact of public policy on inequalities in health. In: Graham H, ed. *Understanding Health Inequalities.* London: Open University Press, 2000.

93. Dahlgren G, Whitehead M. *Policies and Strategies to Promote Social Equity in Health.* Stockholm: Institute for Future Studies, 1991.

94. Mackenbach JP, van de Mheen H, Stronks K. A prospective cohort study investigating the explanation of socioeconomic inequalities in health in The Netherlands. *Soc Sci Med* 1994: 38: 299–308.

95. Marmot M, Wilkinson RG. *Social Determinants of Health.* Oxford: Oxford University Press, 1999.

96. Eurostat Yearbook 2000. *A Statistical Eye on Europe.* Data 1988–98. © European Communities, 1995–2001.

97. Eurostat. *Social Portrait of Europe.* Luxembourg: Office for Official Publications of the European Communities, 1998.

2 Strategies to reduce socioeconomic inequalities in health

Johan P. Mackenbach, Martijntje J. Bakker,
Marita Sihto and Finn Diderichsen

Introduction

Socioeconomic inequalities in health have been with us for years and we cannot expect to be able to reduce them without a powerful, sustained and systematic effort. This chapter deals with some of the 'systematic' aspects of this effort: the elements that any strategy to reduce socioeconomic inequalities in health must have in order to be effective.

In this chapter we build upon several reports published in Europe during the 1990s which mark the search for new strategies to reduce socioeconomic inequalities in health. These include Whitehead's paper on *The Concepts and Principles of Equality in Health* (1), Whitehead and Dahlgren's paper on *Policies and Strategies to Promote Equality in Health* (2), the King's Fund report on *Tackling Inequalities in Health* (3), and *The Independent Inquiry into Inequalities in Health* (4).

The first two of these were part of a series commissioned by the European Office of the World Health Organization (WHO). After the adoption by all WHO member states of the 38 targets of the Health for All by the year 2000 strategy, including the important equality target (5), it was felt necessary to help countries develop strategies to achieve this target. The first report dealt with the normative justification of policies to reduce inequalities in health, arguing effectively that socioeconomic inequalities in health are at least partly unjust (1). The second developed a first outline for a systematic strategy to reduce inequalities in health, and was illustrated with examples from around Europe (2).

In several European countries initiatives were taken to develop these strategies further. Many of these national experiences will be documented in later chapters of this book, and we will restrict ourselves here to mentioning only two important reports from the United Kingdom, which have served as a source of inspiration for many. The King's Fund report, of which Whitehead was a co-author, looked in detail at four policy areas: housing, social security, smoking and healthcare. An attempt was made to synthesize the available scientific evidence on the role of these factors in generating socioeconomic inequalities in health, and on the effectiveness of interventions in these areas (3). This development culminated in the report of *The Independent Inquiry into Inequalities in Health*, written at the request of a newly elected Labour government, which contains an immense list of 'recommendations for further policy development' (4).

Our digest of these and other publications, to be cited later, is reflected in this chapter. A systematic approach to reducing socioeconomic inequalities in health requires a great deal of strategic thinking in order to develop effectively each of the main phases of the policy process: initiation, implementation, evaluation and reformulation of the policy. Although we cannot cover all relevant aspects of each of these phases, we will deal with the following:

- Justification, objectives and use of evidence
- Strategic options
- Selected implementation and evaluation aspects.

Justification, objectives and use of evidence

Justification

Why should socioeconomic inequalities in health be reduced? Basically, there are two possible justifications:

- Because inequalities in health contradict values of fairness and justice;
- Because reducing inequalities in health may lead to better average health in the population as a whole.

The second of these two arguments is relatively straightforward, although it assumes that policies will lead to a differential improvement in the health of the lower socioeconomic groups, and not to a worsening of the health of the higher. The first argument, however, puts specific demands on how we describe and analyse health distributions in a population. We need to decide what distributions are unfair – in other words: what health differences are health inequalities (or, in a stronger phrasing which we do not use in this book, health inequities). Whitehead, in an early analysis, defined inequitable distributions of health as those that are avoidable, unnecessary and unfair. Differences in health which arise as a result of natural, biological variation, or of freely chosen health-damaging behaviour, will not commonly be perceived as 'unfair'. On the other hand, differences in health resulting from health-damaging behaviour not freely chosen, or from exposure to health hazards in the environment, or from impaired access to healthcare services, will be perceived as 'unfair' and are also potentially avoidable (1). Table 2.1 summarizes this reasoning.

However, as medical technologies advance, the borderline between avoidable and unavoidable inequalities is moving, and, as we increasingly find

Table 2.1 Whitehead's scheme for judging the (un)fairness of socioeconomic inequalities in health

Which health differences are inequitable? *Determinants of health* *differentials*	*Potentially* *avoidable*	*Commonly viewed* *as unacceptable*
1. Natural, biological variation	No	No
2. Health-damaging behaviour is freely chosen	Yes	No
3. Transient health advantage of groups who take up health-promoting behaviour first (if other groups can easily catch up)	Yes	No
4. Health-damaging behaviour where choice of lifestyle is restricted by socioeconomic factors	Yes	Yes
5. Exposure to excessive health hazards in physical and social environment	Yes	Yes
6. Restricted access to essential healthcare	Yes	Yes
7. Health-related downward social mobility (sick people move down social scale)	Low income – yes	Low income – yes

Source: Adapted from Whitehead 1990 (1)

that health behaviours such as smoking are concentrated in groups with adverse social conditions, the question of what is freely chosen and what not is becoming less clear. Ethical theories may help us in further developing our arguments.

Every plausibly defensible ethical theory of social arrangements tends, as Sen (5, 6) has pointed out, to demand equality in some respect – such as liberties, rights, opportunities, income or wealth. Sen (5) argues that the 'space' in which equality is demanded is important, as human diversity means that equality in one space will result in inequality in another. If only liberties are equal, income and wealth will not be, whereas if we argue for equality in terms of income, liberties will have to be restricted for some. Sen then proposes as the ultimate criterion for development in society that we try to maximize people's freedom to live the lives they have reason to value, or, in other words, to choose their own 'life plan' (6). Because health problems may constitute an obstacle to that freedom, it is important to try to achieve an equal distribution of the circumstances that influence an individual's probability of being healthy. Clearly, this provides a powerful argument to reduce certain variations in health, particularly those that have consequences in terms of premature mortality, disability and social participation.

One of the most influential theories of justice in the twentieth century has been John Rawls's 'justice as fairness'. This states that social and economic differences will be fair only if they satisfy two conditions: 'First, they must be attached to offices and positions open to all under conditions of fair equality of opportunity; and second they must be to the great benefit of the least advantaged members of society.' Advantage is judged by resources in terms of 'primary social goods' – including 'rights, liberties and opportunities, income and wealth, and the social base for self-respect' (7).

It is difficult to see how differences in health could be justified on the basis of Rawls's theory. Socioeconomic differences in health are not to the benefit of the lower socioeconomic groups. One could, however, argue that certain variations in health determinants are the result of arrangements or developments that ultimately benefit the least advantaged groups. For example, it is difficult to imagine an efficient society without inequalities in working conditions and income, with a concomitant impact on health. On the whole, however, Rawls's principle of justice identifies as unjust those variations in health that are the result of a division of labour which benefits the better-off at the expense of the worse-off. Our evaluation of the social order of a society will thus depend on the social distribution of health in that society, and vice versa: our evaluation of the social distribution of health will depend on how we evaluate the fairness of the causally related social arrangements. As it would be difficult to argue that healthy social 'positions are open to all under conditions of fair equality of opportunity', this again reinforces the idea that variations in health between socioeconomic groups are at least partly unfair.

We have emphasized the need to explicitly justify policies to reduce socio-economic inequalities in health, not only because it is important to convince policy-makers of different political convictions that something needs to be done, but also because one's choice of justification will partly determine which policies should receive priority. For example, if the main purpose is to remove differences in the freedom to choose one's 'life plan', then one might wish to emphasize reducing health inequalities in children. Health problems in children which are caused by living in unfavourable socio-economic circumstances cannot be blamed on their own choices, but do limit their opportunities to lead productive and happy lives. One might then also wish to give priority to reducing the consequences of illness in terms of disability and participation, rather than in terms of well-being (6).

Objectives

The obvious objective of the policies discussed in this chapter (and in the rest of this book) is to reduce socioeconomic inequalities in health, but it is not immediately clear what this means. This becomes apparent as soon as we try to make the objective operative in measurable terms. Do we intend to reduce relative or absolute inequalities in health? To redistribute health from the higher to the lower socioeconomic groups? Or to differentially improve the health of the lower socioeconomic groups? Does 'health' refer to the occurrence of specific health problems or to integrated health measures such as health expectancy? Although some answers are perhaps obvious, others are not, and in any case we think that explicit and operational objectives are an important element of strategies to reduce socioeconomic inequalities in health. Explicit and operational objectives help to focus policies and interventions and provide a yardstick with which eventually to measure our success.

Although this does not necessarily imply that these objectives should be phrased in quantitative terms, it is useful briefly to discuss the experience with quantitative health equality targets. The target agreed in 1984 by the member states of the World Health Organization (European region) was that 'by the year 2000, the actual differences in health status . . . should be reduced by at least 25 per cent, by improving the level of health of disadvantaged . . . groups' (8). Although it is easy to criticize this target, for example for its vagueness, it has in fact helped in putting inequalities in health on the policy agenda in many European countries. Also, it specified that inequalities in health must be reduced by improving the health of the worst off, thereby reassuring those policy-makers who would otherwise fear that health should somehow be redistributed, as one would redistribute income. Finally, it proposed a seemingly reasonable level of ambition: reducing health inequalities by a quarter, not abolishing them altogether.

Many aspects are left unspecified, however. There are many ways to measure the size of socioeconomic inequalities in health, as shown by a systematic analysis of measures used in the literature (9). One of the most important distinctions is that between relative measures, such as rate ratios, and absolute measures such as rate differences (see Chapter 1). It can be argued that absolute inequalities are more relevant for public health policy and for the individuals involved: it is the absolute inequalities that directly influence a person's life chances, and the aim should therefore be primarily to reduce absolute inequalities in health. If one accepts this line of reasoning, the number of available policy options increases substantially. Any policy or intervention that reduces average rates of mortality or morbidity, without changing the size of the relative inequalities, will help in achieving this objective. Investing in overall improvements of population health, while taking care to achieve similar relative rates of improvement in higher and lower socioeconomic groups, is a potentially powerful way of reducing inequalites in health, and may not even require an explicit commitment to do so.

The WHO equality target was agreed upon in 1984 and has not been reached. In reality, socioeconomic inequalities in health have mostly increased on a relative scale, and have at best remained stable on an absolute scale

(10). Is this because national governments have not made serious efforts, or because the target was too ambitious? Probably both. A review by WHO (Europe) of progress in achieving the Health for All by the year 2000 targets in all 51 member countries showed that, although many countries reported they had done something to reduce inequalities in health, in reality policies and interventions were mainly limited to achieving equal access to healthcare (11). Similarly, a review of policies and interventions to reduce socio-economic inequalities in health in Finland, The Netherlands, Spain, Sweden and the United Kingdom showed that, despite good intentions in some countries, the scale and intensity of the efforts have been very modest, at least until 1998 (12). But one could also rightly argue that the target was far too ambitious. In many countries there is evidence of a largely unexplained widening of socioeconomic inequalities in health (see Chapter 1). It is likely that these 'ideopathic' trends would have counteracted any beneficial effect of serious efforts to implement health equality targets.

What can realistically be achieved is a function of, first, underlying trends, and second, the potential effect of the interventions and policies that will be implemented. Until recently, few systematic attempts have been made to develop methods for realistic target setting in this area. What is needed is:

- an assessment of the current size and recent trends in inequalities in health, including an evaluation of their causes;
- an exploration of possible future trends in inequalities in health;
- an inventory of possible policies and interventions to reduce inequalities in health;
- an estimation of the potential impact of these policies and interventions;
- and finally, the formulation of realistic health equality targets.

This is certainly a difficult exercise, and there is a great need for method development in this area.

Recently, the World Health Organization renewed its health targets for inclusion in the Health 21 strategy. Although the total number of targets has been reduced from 38 to 21, the first two are still devoted to equality: one relates to health inequalities between countries and the other to health inequalities within countries (13) (Box 2.1). The latter has become more specific but is still rather ambitious – apparently more an aspiration than an aim that might realistically be achieved. For policy-makers, another and perhaps more useful approach could be to formulate targets in terms of intermediate outcomes or process measures, such as a degree of reduction in the prevalence of smoking or unfavourable working conditions in the lower socioeconomic groups. This is the approach adopted in two sets of quantitative health policy targets recently developed in Sweden and The Netherlands (see Chapters 17 and 19).

Box 2.1   Examples of quantitative health policy targets relating to inequalities in health

Health for all by the year 2000

By the year 2000, the actual differences in health status between countries and between groups within countries should be reduced by at least 25 per cent, by improving the level of health of disadvantaged nations and groups.

This target could be achieved if the basic prerequisites for health were provided for all; if the risks related to lifestyles were reduced; if the health aspects of living and working conditions were improved; and if good primary healthcare were made accessible to all.

Health 21

Target 2 – Equality in health

By the year 2020, the health gap between socioeconomic groups within countries should be reduced by at least one fourth in all Member States, by substantially improving the level of health of disadvantaged groups.

In particular:

2.1 the gap in life expectancy between socioeconomic groups should be reduced by at least 25 per cent;
2.2 the values for major indicators of morbidity, disability and mortality in groups across the socioeconomic gradients should be more equally distributed;
2.3 socioeconomic conditions that produce adverse health effects, notably differences in income, educational achievement and access to the labour market, should be substantially improved;
2.4 the proportion of the population living in poverty should be greatly reduced;
2.5 people having special needs as a result of their health, social or economic circumstances should be protected from exclusion and given easy access to appropriate care.

Use of evidence

If possible, one should try to prioritize interventions and policies on the basis of their potential effectiveness in reducing inequalities in health. For this, two types of evidence are required:

- evidence that the determinant addressed by the intervention or policy plays a key role in the causation of socioeconomic inequalities in health;
- evidence that the proposed intervention or policy can be expected to effectively reduce exposure to that determinant in the lower socio-economic groups (or to reduce socioeconomic inequalities in exposure to that determinant).

The first type is usually easier to obtain than the second. In recent years there has been an abundance of observational studies trying to understand how socioeconomic inequalities in health arise; these have even produced quantitative estimates of the contribution of specific determinants to the explanation of inequalities in health. If we can be reasonably certain that a particular determinant makes a substantial contribution to the explanation of socioeconomic inequalities in an important health problem, then there is a good reason for prioritizing interventions or policies targeting the prevalence of that determinant in the lower socioeconomic groups.

This is not enough, however: we must also have good reason to think that the proposed intervention or policy will actually reduce exposure to the determinant in the lower socioeconomic groups, and consequently reduce inequalities in health. This second type of evidence is more difficult to collect. There have been very few methodologically sound studies of the effectiveness of interventions and policies to reduce socioeconomic inequalities in the determinants of health. This may be partly because this has never been seen as a research priority, but it is also because the evaluation of these interventions and policies is faced with a number of methodological and practical difficulties.

Interventions and policies targeting downstream determinants at the individual level may lend themselves to conventional evaluation designs such as the randomized controlled trial, but this is generally not true for determinants at the group (school, company, neighbourhood, etc.) level or for upstream determinants. In the case of relatively straightforward interventions and policies aiming at determinants at the group level, experimentation may still be feasible, for example in the form of a community intervention trial. In the case of more complex interventions that depend on active cooperation from different actors and institutions, and in the case of policies implemented at the national level, experimentation may be altogether impossible, and quasi-experimental or completely observational designs may be the highest achievable. If the aim of the intervention or policy is not only to reduce health problems in the lower socioeconomic groups, but also to reduce socioeconomic health inequalities, then the design will need to be even more complex, because one will have to look separately at the lower and higher socioeconomic groups within both the 'experimental' and the 'control' groups (14).

Several reviews have shown the relative scarcity of methodologically sound evaluation studies of interventions and policies to reduce socioeconomic inequalities in health (15–17). It is easy to adopt a sceptical attitude, and to wait until sound evidence on effectiveness is available before these interventions and policies are implemented on a larger scale. Given the many different policy options and the difficulty of evaluation, however, it may take decades to build up a reasonably extensive evidence base. It is therefore better to be pragmatic and to be prepared to decide for the implementation of policies and interventions in the absence of full documentation of their effectiveness. Sometimes, effectiveness can reasonably be expected on the basis of experience in another setting, or evidence of effects on intermediate outcomes. In such cases it is all the more important that while the policies or interventions are being implemented, evaluations are carried out so that their effectiveness can be determined at a later stage, and changes made if effectiveness remains below expectations.

In reality, all this implies that it will usually be difficult to prioritize policies and interventions on the basis of scientific evidence only. Other considerations, for example, on the (political) feasibility of certain strategic options, are likely to have a profound influence on priority setting in this area.

Strategic options

Entry points

Any attempt to reduce socioeconomic inequalities in health should be based on an understanding of their causes. The explanatory models discussed in the previous chapter suggest a number of different 'entry points' for intervention and policy, including:

- reducing inequalities in power, prestige, income and wealth linked to different socioeconomic positions;
- reducing the effect of health on socioeconomic position, and reducing the economic consequences of ill-health;
- reducing the effect of socioeconomic position on the risk of being exposed to specific health determinants ('intermediary' material, psychosocial and behavioural factors), or reducing the effect of these determinants in the lower socioeconomic groups;
- reducing the health effects (including the consequences of illness) of being in a lower socioeconomic position through healthcare.

Finally, one could consider modifying the entire social context in a way that would be protective against some of the individual level effects. We will briefly discuss each of these options, but refer the reader to other chapters for more detailed examples.

Social inequality is the root cause of socioeconomic inequalities in health, and therefore the most fundamental approach to reducing such inequalities is to address directly inequalities in education, occupation and income. Depending on what is already in place in a particular country, investments in the educational and social security systems, and labour market policies that strengthen the position of those at greatest risk, may be necessary to achieve these goals. In addition to generic measures that reduce inequalities in society as a whole, targeted measures may be necessary to increase socio-economic opportunities for the most disadvantaged groups, for example, preschool education for ethnic minority children, or income support for families in poverty.

Although social selection is less important than social causation for the explanation of socioeconomic inequalities in health, those who are in poor health generally face higher risks of downward social mobility, through lower educational achievement, problems in finding and keeping a job, and fewer opportunities for upward mobility within a job. Depending on the levels and coverage of social insurance, the economic effects (even without changing social position) might be substantial and could contribute to the perpetuation and cumulation of health disadvantage. Policies directed towards improving the labour market position and job opportunities for the chronically sick, and adequate social security systems that protect them against a drop in income, may therefore help reduce inequalities in health.

As discussed in Chapter 1, the effect of socioeconomic status on health goes through a number of more specific health determinants, and these material, psychosocial and behavioural factors therefore provide important entry points for interventions and policies to reduce socioeconomic inequalities in health. Relevant interventions and policies include: housing policies and community development programmes in disadvantaged neighbourhoods; workplace interventions and health and safety regulations; school-based programmes to help children develop adequate coping skills; and health promotion strategies which are sensitive to the situation of disadvantaged groups, and which address incentives and barriers to behavioural change in these groups.

Healthcare interventions and policies may also be used to reduce socio-economic inequalities in health. Over the past 50 years healthcare has become increasingly effective, and providing equal access to it will help to alleviate some of the excess health burden in lower socioeconomic groups. This is partly a matter of securing equal financial access through adequate healthcare finance policies, for example avoiding upfront payments. It is also a matter of securing equal cultural access, because communication between providers and patients is likely to be less effective in lower socioeconomic groups. In addition to securing equal access, specific healthcare programmes, particularly in a primary care setting, can be offered to improve the health situation in disadvantaged groups.

Finally, social context interventions might be important, to the extent that social context may modify the effects of individual-level determinants. As a result of studies showing that unequal income distributions go together with lower average life expectancy, and suggesting that part of this effect may be due to the erosion of social cohesion, a great deal of attention has recently been paid to the possible effect of 'social capital' on health (18). Earlier studies had shown that social networks may protect against health problems (19), but the concept of 'social capital' emphasizes the structural and material aspects of the connections between individuals in a community. If further studies confirm an independent effect of social capital on health, this would open up an entirely new entry point for interventions and policies to reduce socioeconomic inequalities in health.

'Upstream' versus 'downstream' solutions

Changing the basic socioeconomic distributions addresses the root causes of inequalities in health and is very much an upstream solution. This is likely to have more leverage than downstream solutions, because each fundamental cause is linked to a range of more immediate causes and, through these, to an even larger range of health effects, as is illustrated by the fact that practically all diseases have higher death rates in the low-income groups. By addressing the fundamental causes of inequalities in health one also avoids the possibility that after one of the more immediate causes has been eliminated, other immediate causes take its place because the same fundamental causes are still in operation. On the other hand, health policy-makers do not usually take decisions about basic socioeconomic distributions, and because of the long causal chain between low socioeconomic status and ill-health we cannot be certain that reducing the inequalities in power and wealth between social positions will invariably lead to reduced inequalities in health.

At the other end of the spectrum, healthcare interventions are very much a downstream solution. They are usually expensive and can never totally eliminate the problem, because people will have to fall ill before extra healthcare can repair the damage. Consequently, interventions have only limited potential for reducing inequalities in health. On the other hand, decisions about healthcare are at least partly under the control of health policy-makers, and although the health effects may be limited they are at least relatively well documented. Involving healthcare personnel can also lead to important advocacy for reducing inequalities in health with other policy sectors.

In between these upstream and downstream solutions we can distinguish a number of midstream solutions: for example, reducing exposure to unfavourable specific material living conditions, psychosocial factors and behavioural risk factors in the lower socioeconomic groups. These combine some of the advantages and disadvantages of both upstream and downstream solutions: the leverage and decision-making power of health policy-makers may be limited, but the health effects of changing the socioeconomic distribution of some of the more powerful determinants, such as smoking and work environment, can be expected to be substantial.

This comparison of upstream, midstream and downstream solutions actually suggests that we should not so much wish to make a choice between them, but that we should try to build strategies that contain elements from all three. We must address the root causes, but doing so will not necessarily eliminate inequalities in health. We cannot ignore the possible contributions of the healthcare system, because this is the only policy instrument that is entirely within the power of health policy-makers, but healthcare interventions will never eliminate inequalities in health. We therefore need midstream solutions in the context of a broader strategy.

Universalist versus selectivist approaches

Another important strategic choice is that between universalist and selectivist approaches. These terms originally refer to two different approaches to welfare provision. Universalism implies that social benefits and social services are provided to all individuals according to the same standards. Selectivism, that is, individual means-tested selectivity, implies that different benefits and services are provided to people with different needs (20).

Historically, universalist welfare states can be seen as the result of the struggle of the working class against the stigmatizing effect of means-tested benefits and services (21). Another argument in favour of universalism relates to welfare state legitimacy: if well-off people are given a role only as sponsors and not as recipients of benefits, this can cause criticism and rebellion against taxation (20). Universalism has also been criticized, however. The assumption that everyone should be treated equally ignores already existing inequalities (22, 23). Different socioeconomic groups approach the welfare state in different ways on the basis of their particular social characteristics and culture (24). Some have even argued that, following the Matthew principle,[1] the middle class has been the primary beneficiary of the welfare state (25, 26). Actually, international comparisons have shown that universal welfare states are the most redistributing (27), partly because in the long term they have been politically more sustainable.

The universalist versus selectivist debate is also relevant to the discussion on how to reduce socioeconomic inequalities in health: can these inequalities best be reduced by universalist or by selectivist policies, or perhaps by a combination of the two? Within the health policy field so far there has not been much debate on this question. An example would be the discussion on targeting lifestyle interventions to lower socioeconomic groups: 'that might be described in terms of dominant social groups claiming the right to crack cognitive, aesthetical and moral codes of dominated social groups' (28).

There is a clear link here with discussions on the usefulness of a 'high risk' versus a 'population approach' to prevention (29, 30). Health inequalities do not just exist between the poor and the non-poor, but across the entire socioeconomic gradient. Therefore, selective targeting of people with the highest risks, that is, the lowest socioeconomic status, is inappropriate. The 'challenge of the gradient' implies that health policy measures should aim at improving the health of the whole population (or at least very large segments of it) (31, 32). The question remains, however, whether, on top of universalist health policy measures, selectivist measures are needed to improve the health situation of people in the lowest socioeconomic groups.

Can universalist policies and interventions sufficiently reduce socio-economic inequalities in health (33)? It is interesting to note that even in countries such as Finland, where social welfare provision is firmly based on universalism, it is seen to be important to pay 'extra' attention to those most in need or those at high risk (34).

In Great Britain too, examples can be found of combinations of universalist and selectivist measures. Health Action Zones are specifically targeted towards disadvantaged areas, and aim to reduce inequalities by improving the health of the most disadvantaged (see Chapters 12 and 21). Later chapters of this book contain examples of both universalist and selectivist approaches.

It is obvious that more research is needed to determine the relative effectiveness of universalist and selectivist approaches to reducing socioeconomic inequalities in health. Until the results of such studies are available it seems safe to conclude that a combination of the two is probably necessary.

Comprehensive packages

As it is unlikely that any single policy or intervention will significantly reduce socioeconomic inequalities in health, what we need are 'packages' of policies and interventions of a comprehensive nature. As indicated in the previous paragraphs, there are many entry points and we may need combinations of upstream, midstream and downstream policies, as well as of universalist and selectivist approaches. Since 1980 a number of proposals for such packages have been formulated, some of which are summarized in Box 2.2.

The Black Report (35) contained a number of specific and radical recommendations on income, housing, tobacco, school meals, healthcare, screening programmes and so on. Although it is remembered primarily for its recommendations on reducing income inequality and alleviating poverty, it was actually much broader than that and, in contrast to any of the other policy documents mentioned in Box 2.2, even contained a cost estimate for its recommendations.

The Black Report was received coolly and largely ignored by the Conservative government that was in power when it was issued. In anticipation of an imminent change in government, the King's Fund revisited the area and made a systematic attempt to review the scientific evidence for effective policies and interventions to reduce socioeconomic inequalities in health. It focused on four different policy areas: physical environment, social and economic influences, 'barriers to adopting a healthier personal lifestyle', and 'access to appropriate and effective health and social services' (3). In a way,

Box 2.2   Overview of recommendations in five major policy documents

A summary of the recommendations of the Black report
THE WORKING GROUP ON INEQUALITIES IN HEALTH
Chair Sir Douglas Black
Report November 1980

37   RECOMMENDATIONS

Basis of recommendations:

- multicausal nature of inequalities in health
- early childhood is the period of life at which intervention could most hopefully weaken the continuing association between health and class

Specific recommendations for:

- Monitoring (for example, school health statistics, nutritional surveillance in relation to health)
- Health and welfare of mothers and preschool and school children
- The care of elderly and disabled people in their own homes
- Prevention: the role of the government
- Additional funding for ten special areas
- Measures to be taken outside the health services

A summary of the recommendations of the WHO report
POLICIES AND STRATEGIES TO PROMOTE EQUITY IN HEALTH
Authors: Dahlgren and Whitehead
Report: 1992

RECOMMENDATIONS

- Action on low income
- Action on unhealthy living conditions
- Action on working conditions
- Action on unemployment
- Action on personal lifestyle factors
- Action on restricted access to health care
  - economic access
  - geographical access
  - cultural access
- The crucial role of education

A summary of the recommendations of the King's Fund report
TACKLING INEQUALITIES IN HEALTH
Authors: Benzeval, Judge and Whitehead
Report: 1995

RECOMMENDATIONS

What could be done?

- strengthen individuals
- strengthen communities
- improve access to essential facilities and services
- encourage macroeconomic and cultural change

What should be done?
Important factors:

- *The physical environment*, such as adequacy of housing, working conditions and pollution
- *social and economic influences* such as income and wealth, levels of unemployment, and the quality of social relationships and social support
- *barriers to adopting a healthier personal lifestyle*
- *access to appropriate and effective health and social services*

A summary of the recommendations of the Acheson report
INDEPENDENT INQUIRY INTO INEQUALITIES IN HEALTH
Chair: Sir Donald Acheson

Report: 1998
RECOMMENDATIONS

I.   General recommendations

II. Areas for future policy development
     1. Poverty, income tax and benefits
     2. Education
     3. Employment
     4. Housing and environment
     5. Mobility, transport and pollution
     6. Nutrition and the common agricultural policy
     7. Mothers, children and families
     8. Young people and adults of working age
     9. Older people
     10. Ethnicity
     11. Gender

III. The National Health Service

A summary of the recommendations of the Dutch programme committee
THE DUTCH PROGRAMME COMMITTEE ON SOCIO-
ECONOMIC INEQUALITIES IN HEALTH second phase
Chair: Prof. Dr W. Albeda
Report: 2001

RECOMMENDATIONS

Objective: Reduction of socio-economic inequalities in health by
25 per cent by the year 2020

Strategies

1. Reduction of inequalities in education, income and other socioeconomic factors
2. Reduction of the negative effects of health problems on socioeconomic position
3. Reduction of the negative effects of socioeconomic position on
   health
4. Improve access and effectiveness of healthcare for low socioeconomic groups

26 specific recommendations

In general, continuation of research, development, monitoring and
evaluation is necessary.

it paved the way for the Independent Inquiry into Inequalities in Health,
held by the Acheson Committee (4). This again, with the help of a large
number of experts, reviewed all the evidence, without limitation to a few
policy areas, and came up with 123 recommendations in eleven areas for
'future policy development'. Without a doubt this is the most comprehensive set of recommendations ever prepared – to the extent that it has been
criticized for its resemblance to a shopping list (36). The British Government in 1999 published its official response to these recommendations, and
this 'action report' focuses very much on the upstream determinants, listing
policies in the areas of low income, education, housing, community development and so on, with relatively few specific health-related policies (37).

    There are also some examples of comprehensive packages that have been
developed outside the UK. In The Netherlands the national Programme
Committee on Socioeconomic Inequalities in Health has recently issued a
set of 26 recommendations which cover most of the entry points mentioned
earlier (38). These deal with economic and social policies (for example,
no further increase in income inequality, reductions in poverty, no cuts in
disability benefits), work and employment policies (increase labour participation of the chronically ill, reduce physically demanding work, increase job

control), health promotion policies (increase tobacco taxation, implement school health policies), healthcare policies (no reductions in insurance entitlements, more and better equipped primary care in deprived areas) and research policies (more research and development to increase availability of effective instruments to reduce socioeconomic inequalities in health). The Programme Committee has also developed quantitative targets for many of these recommendations (Box 2.3).

In Sweden a parliamentary committee recently suggested targets and strategies for a new policy to reduce inequalities in health, 'Health on equal terms' (described in (39)). The committee gave priority to more than a dozen determinants, ranging from contextual factors such as housing segregation (with effects on children's opportunities and health) and work organization (with effects on job strain) to vulnerability to the addictive effects of alcohol and smoking. Targets were set for these determinants, and in some cases specific target groups of those who are particularly exposed or susceptible to the health effects of those determinants were defined (Box 2.4).

The policy developments in England, The Netherlands and Sweden are reviewed more extensively in Chapters 12, 17 and 19.

Box 2.3   Health policy targets, Dutch Programme Committee on Socioeconomic Inequalities in Health, 2001

4 Strategies:

1. Reduction of inequalities in education, income and other socio-economic factors
   1.1 Further increase in percentage of children of (un)skilled workers, who decide to follow secondary or higher education, with 12 per cent in 1989 to 25 per cent in 2020
   1.2 Maintenance of income inequalities in The Netherlands at the level of 1996
   1.3 Reduction of the percentage of households with an income up to 105 per cent of the social minimum with 10.6 per cent in 1998 to 8 per cent in 2020

2. Reduction of the negative effects of health problems on socio-economic position
   2.1 Maintenance of the average benefit level (as a percentage of the last earned wage) at complete incapacity for work and/or incapacity for work due to work-related complaints at the level of 2000
   2.2 Increase of the percentage of chronically ill people in the age group of 25–64 years with paid employment with 48 per cent in 1995 to 57 per cent in 2020

3. Reduction of the negative effects of socioeconomic position on health

    3.1 Reduction of the difference between lower and higher educated people in the percentage of smokers with 25 per cent, through a decrease in the percentage of lower educated smokers with 38 per cent in 1998 to 35 per cent or less in 2020

    3.2 Reduction in the difference between lower and higher educated people in the percentage of leisure time physical activity with 25 per cent, through a reduction in the percentage of physical inactivity of lower educated people with 57 per cent in 1994 to 53 per cent or less in 2020

    3.3 Reduction of the difference between lower and higher educated people in the percentage of serious overweight with 25 per cent, through a reduction in the percentage of serious over-weight of lower educated people with 15 per cent in 1998 to 12 per cent or less in 2020

    3.4 Reduction of the difference between lower and higher educated people in the percentage of complaints due to physical load with 25 per cent, through a reduction in the percentage of high physical load of lower educated people with 53 per cent in 1999 to 48 per cent or less in 2020

    3.5 Reduction of the difference between lower and higher educated people in the percentage of people who can decide themselves about the execution of work with 25 per cent, through an increase in the percentage of lower educated people with 58 per cent in 1999 to 63 per cent in 2020

4. Improve access and effectiveness of healthcare for low socio-economic groups

    4.1 Maintenance of the differences between lower and higher educated people in healthcare utilization (visit to GP, specialist and dentist, hospital admission, use of prescription drugs) at the level of 1998

Selected implementation and evaluation aspects

Multiple settings, intersectoral policies

The implementation of policies and interventions to reduce socioeconomic inequalities in health requires the involvement of many different players. Progress in achieving greater equality in health depends very much on decisions and actions in sectors other than healthcare, for example, education, finance, social security and so on. Structures will need to be set up to mobilize these other sectors and to coordinate their efforts. A promising approach which has recently been chosen in the United Kingdom involves the formation

Box 2.4 The 19 health policy objectives of the Swedish National Public Health Commision, 2000

1. Gini coefficient under 0.25
2. Proportion of people living in poverty according to EU norms under 4 per cent
   Proportion of people with income below the social welfare poverty line under 7 per cent
   Proportion of households with children with long-term dependency on social assistance reduced to half
3. Proportion of people with long-term dependency on social welfare reduced to less than 1 per cent
4. Proportion of voters in general elections increased by 5 per cent in districts where fewer than 60 per cent voted in 1998; voter participation among people with foreign citizenship increased by 10 per cent
5. Number of suicides reduced by 25 per cent by 2010
6. Increase in employment from 78 per cent to 85 per cent; long-term unemployment reduced from 1.4 per cent to 0.5 per cent
7. 40 per cent of the labour force over the age of 25 with access to at least 5 working days of education every year
8. Proportion of people involved in making decisions about the form and content of their own work increased from 73 per cent to 90 per cent
   Proportion allowed to learn new skills and develop on the job increased from 53 per cent to 75 per cent
   Proportion of people engaging in heavy lifting declined from 25 per cent to 15 per cent
   Proportion of parents of small children working overtime reduced to 20 per cent for both sexes and the proportion of people with flexible working hours increased to 75 per cent
9. Proportion of children growing up in vulnerable neighbourhoods reduced to less than 10 per cent; allocation of resources to pre-schools, schools, primary care, police and recreation sector complies with indicators of needs
10. No child leaves compulsory school or secondary school with incomplete final marks
11. Employment among people aged 20–64 with long-term illness and impaired capacity to work increased from 53 per cent to 70 per cent
12. Increased proportion of senior citizens and people with long-term illness visited at home at least once a year by social services or healthcare personnel for the purpose of promoting health

13. Nobody subjected to environmental tobacco smoke in public premises by 2010; no homes with radon levels over 400 Bq/m^3; 75 per cent of all homes with satisfactory ventilation
14. Disease burden for injuries sustained in traffic calculated as DALYs reduced by 5 per cent per year
15. Proportion of the population that smokes daily reduced by 1 per cent per year; smoking reduced to zero among pregnant women and people under the age of 19 by 2010
16. Total average consumption of alcohol declined by 25 per cent, from 8 to 6 litres of 100 per cent alcohol per person per year
17. Fat content of the diet reduced to 30 per cent of energy intake, with a maximum of 1/3 saturated fat; percentage of energy from carbohydrates increased to 55 per cent; intake of fruit and vegetables increased to 600 grams per person per day
18. Proportion of people taking exercise once a week increased from 50 per cent to 70 per cent
19. Proportion of adults severely overweight reduced from 8 per cent to 5 per cent; proportion of children under 16 moderately overweight reduced from 7 per cent to less than 5 per cent

of 'policy action teams' – groups of representatives from various ministries operating from the Prime Minister's office and aiming to develop intersectoral policies to reduce social exclusion.

Another approach that may help to more actively involve other policy sectors is that of 'health impact assessment', the analysis of the possible health effects of policies outside the health policy field. Including an equality focus in health impact assessment is likely to be instrumental in signalling policies that will enlarge or reduce socioeconomic inequalities in health (see Chapter 20).

In order to achieve these goals it is necessary for policies and interventions to reach large sections of the population, and this will be possible only if we use multiple 'settings' for their implementation. Children spend a large proportion of their waking hours at school, so reaching children may be easiest in the school setting. Similarly, reaching working-age adults may require the use of the workplace or the local community. These settings can sometimes be used for health promotion interventions, although improving health is not their intrinsic purpose – the increasing popularity of the concept of the 'health-promoting school' in different European countries illustrates this.

Monitoring and evaluation

Within each strategy for reducing socioeconomic inequalities in health, monitoring should occupy an important position. Routine monitoring of socioeconomic inequalities in health, for example within national systems of health monitoring or health statistics, is important for several reasons:

- The routine production and publication of data on socioeconomic inequalities in health will keep these inequalities on the policy agenda. Many countries have long been unaware of the existence of health inequalities, and this is due partly to the fact that information on health inequalities was (and sometimes is) not routinely published.
- Socioeconomic inequalities in health are a dynamic phenomenon. During recent decades there has been a general widening of the disparities, at least of relative inequalities in mortality. It is important that up-to-date information be available to policy-makers, so that adequate counter-measures can be taken.
- Monitoring socioeconomic inequalities in health will enable assessment of the success of policies and interventions to reduce health inequalities at the population level. Even if separate policies and interventions are evaluated carefully, the effect on health inequalities in the population as a whole will be difficult to infer. If targets have been formulated, it will be useful to assess regularly whether the strategy is on the right track to achieve its aims.

As pointed out earlier, policies and interventions will frequently address determinants that mediate the effect of social position on health, and targets may actually have been set for these determinants. Monitoring the level and socioeconomic distribution of health determinants may therefore often be instrumental.

Many countries routinely collect information by which health inequalities can be monitored. A recent inventory for the European Commission has shown that many member countries of the European Union have regular health interview or multipurpose surveys with questions on socioeconomic status, by which inequalities in self-reported health can be monitored. The majority of countries also have mortality data classified by socioeconomic status (mainly through linkage to a census), by which inequalities in mortality by cause of death can be monitored (11) (see Chapter 1 for some results). Further improvement of health inequalities monitoring is necessary, however, because not all countries have these data and many countries do not routinely analyse and regularly publish data on socioeconomic inequalities in health.

Conclusions

As this chapter has documented, in recent years major progress has been made in developing strategies to reduce socioeconomic inequalities in health. Arguments to support the need for these strategies have been refined. Quantitative targets have been developed, and the instrument of target setting has been improved by including health determinants in the targets. We have learned to live with insufficient evidence on effectiveness of interventions and policies, and there is a great awareness of the need to carefully evaluate all ongoing and future efforts in this area. Entry points for policies and interventions to reduce socioeconomic inequalities in health have been defined, and a wide range of possibilities has been defined. Finally, there seems to be a consensus that we need comprehensive packages consisting of upstream, midstream and downstream policies and interventions, and including universalist and selectivist approaches.

The rest of this book is divided into three main parts. Part II focuses on a number of policies and interventions that have been proposed to reduce socioeconomic inequalities in health. It reviews the rationale for these in terms of the evidence that the determinants to be addressed do indeed play a key role in health inequalities. It also reviews the evidence for the effectiveness of specific policies and interventions in terms of reducing the exposure to these determinants in the lower socioeconomic groups.

Part III analyses the way in which different European countries have dealt with the issue of socioeconomic inequalities in health during the past two decades. National policy-makers in the countries described in this book are in different phases of awareness of, and willingness to take action on, socioeconomic inequalities in health. Margaret Whitehead has proposed a schematic 'action spectrum' to characterize the stage of diffusion of ideas on this subject. Starting with a primordial stage in which socioeconomic inequalities in health are not even measured, the spectrum covers the stages of 'measurement', 'recognition', 'awareness', 'denial/indifference', 'concern', 'will to take action', 'isolated initiatives', 'more structured developments' and 'comprehensive coordinated policy' (40). The action spectrum should not be regarded as a linear progress and countries will not necessarily go through all stages of it (Figure 2.1).

There has been a remarkable increase in the awareness of socioeconomic inequalities in health, partly through a substantial increase in research efforts in this area. Several countries have had national research programmes, and our increased understanding of the causes of health inequalities has laid a basis for policies and interventions by which several countries have made serious attempts to develop reduction strategies. This part takes stock of these developments.

Part IV deals with evaluation issues. Health impact assessment is discussed, as well as a number of new developments in research methodology with relevance to evaluating interventions to reduce health inequalities.

The book concludes with three reflective chapters. The first looks at the information provided in this book through a gender lens. The second provides an outside perspective from two non-European authors on the situation in Europe. The final chapter provides key messages for policy-makers.

No single country has the capacity to contribute more than a fraction of the knowledge necessary to support strategies for reducing inequalities in

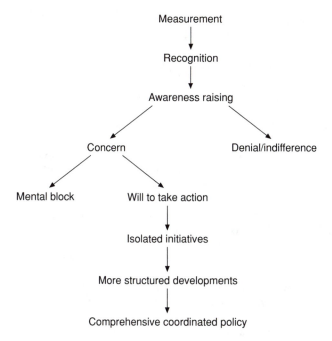

Figure 2.1 Action spectrum on inequalities in health (Whitehead 1998) (40)

health. This is a matter not only of restricted manpower or financial resources for research, but also of restricted opportunities for implementing policies and interventions. Some policies can be implemented in some countries and not in others, either because they have already been implemented or because they are politically unfeasible. Different countries present different opportunities for evaluation, and international exchange and perhaps coordination is therefore necessary. There is an important role for international agencies, such as the European Union, to support this development.

Note

1. The gospel text goes: 'For unto every one that hath shall be given, and he shall have abundance; but from him that hath not shall be taken away even that which he hath' (Matthew 13: 12).

References

1. Whitehead M. *The Concepts and Principles of Equality and Health*. Copenhagen: World Health Organization, 1990.
2. Dahlgren G, Whitehead M. *Policies and Strategies to Promote Equality in Health*. Copenhagen: World Health Organization, 1992.

3.   Benzeval M, Judge K, Whitehead M. *Tackling Inequalities in Health; An Agenda for Action.* London: King's Fund, 1995.

4.   Anon. *Independent Inquiry into Inequalities in Health.* London: The Stationery Office, 1998.

5.   Sen A. *Inequality Re-examined.* Cambridge MA: Harvard University Press, 1992.

6.   Sen A. *Development as Freedom.* New York: Oxford University Press, 1999.

7.   Rawls J. *A Theory of Justice.* Cambridge MA: Harvard University Press, 1971.

8.   World Health Organization. *Targets for Health for All.* Copenhagen: World Health Organization, 1985.

9.   Mackenbach JP, Kunst AE. Measuring the magnitude of socioeconomic inequalities in health: an overview of available measures illustrated with two examples from Europe. *Soc Sci Med* 1997: 44: 757–71.

10. Kunst AE, Bos V, Mackenbach JP. *Monitoring Socioeconomic Inequalities in Health in the European Union: Guidelines and Illustrations.* Rotterdam: Erasmus University Department of Public Health, 2000.

11. van de Water HPA, van Herten LM. *Health policies on target? Review of Health Target and Priority Setting in 18 European Countries.* Leiden: TNO Prevention and Health, 1998.

12. Mackenbach JP, Droomers PCA. *Interventions and Policies to Reduce Socioeconomic Inequalities in Health.* Rotterdam: Erasmus University Department of Public Health, 1999.

13. World Health Organization. *Health 21 – Health for All in the 21st Century.* Copenhagen: World Health Organization, 1999.

14. Mackenbach JP, Gunning-Schepers LJ. How should interventions to reduce inequalities in health be evaluated? *J Epidemiol Commun Health* 1997: 51: 359–64.

15. Gepkens A, Gunning-Schepers LJ. Interventions to reduce socioeconomic health differences: a review of the international literature. *Eur J Public Health* 1996: 6: 218–26.

16. Arblaster L, Entwistle V, Lambert M, Forster M, Sheldon T, Watt I. *Review of the Research on the Effectiveness of Health Service Interventions to Reduce Variations in Health*, CRD report no. 3. York: NHS Centre for Reviews and Dissemination, 1995.

17. Macintyre S, Chalmers I, Horton R, Smith R. Using evidence to inform health policy: case study. *Br Med J* 2001: 27: 222–5.

18. Berkman LF, Kawachi I. *Social Epidemiology.* New York: Oxford University Press, 2000.

19. Berkman LF, Glass T, Brissette I, Seeman TE. From social integration to health: Durkheim in the new millennium. *Soc Sci Med* 2000: 51: 843–57.

20. Forma P. Alhaalta ylös vai päinvastoin? Sosiaalipoliittisten intressien välittyminen mielipidekyselyn valossa. (From bottom up or from top downwards? Social political interest – mediation in the light of opinion – data). *Hallinnon Tutkimus* 1998: 1: 25–35.

21. Esping-Andersen G. *The Three Worlds of Welfare Capitalism.* Oxford: Polity Press, 1990.

22. Williams F. Somewhere over the rainbow: universality and diversity in social policy. *Socl Policy Rev* 1992: 4: 200–19.

23. Pratt A. Universalism or selectivism? The provision of services in the modern welfare states. In: Lavalette M, Pratt A, eds. *Social Policy, A Conceptual and Theoretical Introduction.* London: Sage, 1997.

24. Deleeck H. The Mattheus effect in healthcare. A proposed explanation of social inequalities. In: Gunning-Schepers LJ, Spruit IP, Krijnen JH, eds. *Socio-economic Inequalities in Health: questions on trends and explanations.* The Hague: Ministry of Welfare, Health and Cultural Affairs, 1989.

25. Powell M. The strategy of equality revisited. *J Soc Policy* 1995: 24: 163–85.

26. Gal J. Formulating the Matthew principle: on the role of the middle classes in the welfare state. *Scand J Soc Welfare* 1998: 7: 42–55.

27. Korpi W, Palme J. The paradox of redistribution and strategies of equality: welfare state institutions, inequality and poverty in western countries. *Am Sociol Rev* 1998: 63: 661–87.

28. Lindbladh E, Lyttkens CH, Hanson BS, Östergren P-O. Equality is out of fashion? An essay on autonomy and health policy in the individualized society. *Soc Sci Med* 1998: 46: 1017–25.

29. Hayes MV. The risk approach: unassailable logic? *Soc Sci Med* 1991: 33: 55–70.

30. Rose G. Sick individuals and sick population. *Int J Epidemiol* 1985: 14: 32–8.

31. Marmot M, Fuhrer R, Ettner S, Marks N, Bumpass LL, Ryff CD. Contribution of psychosocial factors to socioeconomic differences in health. *Milbank Quarterly* 1998: 76: 403–48.

32. Marmot M. Acting on the evidence to reduce inequalities in health. *Health Affairs* 1999: 18: 42–4.

33. Östergren P-O. Life style interventions and health inequality – the Swedish scene. In: Mackenbach JP, Droomers M, eds. *Interventions and Policies to Reduce Socioeconomic Inequalities in Health. Proceedings of the Third Workshop of the European Network on Interventions and Policies to Reduce Socioeconomic Inequalities in Health.* Rotterdam: Erasmus University Department of Public Health, 1999.

34. Ministry of Social Affairs and Health (MSAH). *Health for All by the Year 2000, A Revised Strategy for Co-operation.* Painatuskeskus, 1993.

35. Townsend P, Davidson N, Whitehead M. *Inequalities in Health (The Black Report and the Health Divide).* London: Penguin, 1988.

36. Davey Smith G, Morris JN, Shaw M. The Independent Inquiry into Inequalities in Health. *Br Med J* 1998: 317: 1465–6.

37. Department of Health. Reducing health inequalities: an action report. London: The Stationery Office, 1999.

38. Programmacommissie Sociaal-economische gezondheidsverschillen Tweede Fase. *Sociaal-economische Gezondheidsverschillen Verkleinen.* (Reducing socioeconomic inequalities in health). The Hague: Zorgonderzoek Nederland, 2001.

39. Ostlin P, Diderichsen F. *Equality-Oriented National Strategy for Public Health in Sweden. A Case Study.* Policy Learning Curve Series, 1. Brussels: European Centre for Health Policy, 2000.

40. Whitehead M. Diffusion of ideas on social inequalities in health: a European perspective. *Millbank Quarterly* 1998: 76: 469–92.

Part II

Interventions and policies to reduce socioeconomic inequalities in health

3 Income maintenance policies

Determining their potential impact on socioeconomic inequalities in health

Finn Diderichsen

Introduction

Income maintenance policy is not a set of interventions designed to prevent social and medical problems. The idea of and demand for income maintenance policy originates from the industrial and political changes of the nineteenth century and was a conscious effort to deal with the destitution of the poor, uprooted and landless on their transition from working the land to entering the market as 'free' industrial workers. All societies need forms for reproduction in terms of mechanisms to sustain the physical and mental capacity of the workforce and their families, including the sick, children and the elderly (1). In rural society, production and reproduction were closely interwoven in units of the family, the farm and the system of craft guilds. This link needed to be broken, as industrialization needed an ever-increasing free mobile workforce. New institutional arrangements were needed to ensure the material and economical reproduction of the workforce when the integration of production and reproduction in the rural society was broken. At the same time the perceived threat from the growing masses of the poor led to explicit efforts to integrate them into society. In most European countries social insurance became the predominant response to this, and was one of many possible routes to the modern welfare state. Others could have been more democracy with universal suffrage, better public education or policies for full employment, but these policies came much later (2).

As these policies are not a set of evaluated interventions, and as the majority of observational studies on social policies hardly have studied health and health inequalities as outcomes, it is not possible to write this chapter as a presentation of best practice. We will, rather, bring five areas together and draw some major conclusions about the potential effects on health equality of social security systems.

This chapter will first describe the four main functions all types of income maintenance policies have in common, and second how these functions might be associated with some of the established aetiological mechanisms linking income to health. Third, we will describe the three main principles according to which income maintenance policies are organized, and, fourth, how they work in relation to different social strata created by the changing labour market in a globalized world. Finally, we will describe how these principles are mixed in the three main types of welfare state that have developed in Europe during the twentieth century, and draw some conclusions as to how different income maintenance policies may affect the social distribution of health. In Chapter 4 an example will be provided of how income maintenance policies have buffered the negative effects of a major economic recession on socioeconomic inequalities in health in Finland, an example of a social democratic welfare state.

Income maintenance policies

The functions of income maintenance policies

Different social forces have conflicting but also to a large extent common interests in developing social insurance, and different abilities to articulate them. The actual alliances created and the period of industrial development during which they were possible differ throughout Europe, and the various systems differ in important respects, but they all have in common the fact that they explicitly or implicitly serve the following four important functions:

1. To protect the basic economic and material survival of those unable to sell their labour owing to unemployment, sickness, old age or childhood. These policies have gradually developed to protect against major income loss, not only absolute poverty. The degree to which people are forced unconditionally to accept any work for their own and their family's maintenance has a major influence on their control over their life circumstances.
2. To enhance the mobility of the workforce by making it less dependent on reproduction organized within the family or the employer. These aims have been achieved in one of two ways: by implementing strict limitations on the protective policies mentioned above, thereby forcing workers to move to other jobs or places when labour demand was changing, or through extensive safety nets and retraining programmes to make people more inclined to risk moving to a new job (3).
3. To integrate the increasing number of marginalized individuals into society. Although initially this was done primarily through ideological means by the churches and schools, other institutions of social policy, such as universal social insurance and services, have become increasingly important. Systems where all strata of society both benefit and contribute will tend to create a vertical cohesion, even if they have been criticized for eroding horizontal cohesion within families and other structures of society (4).
4. To implement principles of equity and justice through redistributive mechanisms. All societies are built on ethical principles that demand

equality in some respect, such as basic liberties, rights, opportunities or capabilities (5). Even if the actual emphasis placed on these different dimensions is very different across countries, social insurance policies have been important tools to implement them. Child allowances have thus served to give children more equal opportunities at the beginning of their lives, and health insurance systems have served to reduce the handicap and increase the capabilities of the disabled.

The basic source of income is of course gainful employment, but labour market policies aiming at high employment rates are usually not included in what are called income maintenance policies. Welfare regimes differ, however, according to their impact on overall levels of employment and the distribution across both class and gender. Female employment rates are particularly sensitive to social policies, and therefore poverty rates in female-headed households are dependent not only on social insurance but also on employment policies, including the expansion of services that provide care for children and the elderly, thereby making employment possible for mothers and daughters and at the same time providing jobs for them (6).

The degrees to which various regimes have fulfilled these functions are, however, conspicuously different. Even if only the first of these functions initially had an explicit health purpose we now have evidence that all of them might have implications for the level and distribution of health in the population.

The aetiological role of income

A basic assumption is that income mediates the effect of social position on health. The protective functions of income maintenance policies influence the incidence and duration of poverty in both the absolute and relative sense of the word, and serve to protect against income loss due to age, sickness, disability, unemployment and so on.

Recent reviews and studies from both Britain and Germany have shown a strong relationship between income and nutritional behaviour (7, 8). Low income is associated with poor nutrition at all stages of life, from lower rates of breastfeeding to higher intakes of saturated fatty acids and lower intakes of antioxidant nutrients. Reduced growth in fetal life is associated with increased risk of morbidity during childhood and increased risk of cardiovascular disease later in life (9). There is also increasing evidence that poor nutrition in childhood is associated with both short- and long-term adverse consequences, such as poorer immune status, higher caries rates and poorer cognitive function and learning ability (7). Low income is also strongly related to lack of physical activity and obesity.

Income also has a strong impact on housing, not only through the obvious health effects, but because poor housing is a major health risk. As social segregation in most cities is considerable, the location of housing can have a profound effect on the young, particularly if resources allocated to daycare and schools are not proportional to their needs. Income is also important in regard to recreation, transportation, healthcare, childcare and so on. Recent studies from Britain have shown that levels of means-tested benefits are clearly below what is needed for healthy living (10).

It is reasonable to assume that increasing income will yield diminishing returns in terms of health, but the relationship between income and health exists across all income strata (11). The strength of this relationship is not, however, the same in all countries. It seems that the national social context, possibly including income maintenance policy, might modify the effect of income on health (12), and not only by modifying the effect of ill-health on income.

Several psychosocial mechanisms have also been suggested. Some studies indicate that the income levels of others in the same society modify the effect of individual income (13). Disparities in income might result in poor health through psychological pathways, for example, frustration engendered by comparison with other individuals. These mechanisms have also been discussed as explanations for the relationship between income distribution and average mortality.

It is also well known from research on working life that high demand interacts with low control in the causal pathways of cardiovascular disease (14). Similar mechanisms may operate outside the workplace, even if empirical evidence is weak. Inadequate income increases a range of daily life demands and reduces the possibility of meeting those demands. Income might therefore buffer the stress generated by life events. It is also known that an imbalance between the demands of the job and the rewards increases the risk of cardiovascular disease. Lynch *et al.* (15) have shown that high demand at work combined with low financial reward is associated with a greater progression of atherosclerosis. This points to the importance of income as a means of control or as a reward, not so much in relation to others' income but to the demands of work and daily life. Several studies have indicated that one of the important pathways through which un-employment affects health is through economic threat or the actual income loss it creates (16).

There is increasing evidence that study of the accumulated exposure to adverse socioeconomic conditions over the life course increases our under-standing of socioeconomic inequalities in health (17). The social position of the parents determines educational opportunities, which in turn determine occupation, employment and income. Employment determines the risk of disability and social exclusion. The extent to which poverty and income loss accumulate over the life course is thus determined by the possibility of an individual breaking the vicious circle with retraining, rehabilitation, etc. Social policies others than income maintenance are crucial here.

More generally, many studies confirm that long-term income levels are more important for health than current or short-term income and income changes. Therefore, persistent poverty is more harmful for health than shorter periods or occasional episodes. It has also been found that the negative effects of income reduction are stronger than the positive effects of increasing income (18).

Types of income maintenance

The potential for income maintenance policies to influence health differ according to the system in operation. These tend to comprise combinations of the following three principles (19):

1. Systems based on universal entitlement if specific demographic, social or health criteria are fulfilled (age, unemployment, disability) without reference to earlier contributions or means tests. In these systems both nationals and, in some cases, even immigrants without national citizenship, are covered. One example of this, which exists in many countries, is the provision of flat-rate cash support for all households with a child, regardless of the parents' income. Often these benefits are at a low level that hardly covers the real cost of a child (usually less than €75 per month). What usually makes a much bigger difference for families is the degree to which costs for daycare are covered. This will determine the carer's ability to participate in the labour market and thereby earn enough to support themselves. Another example is the basic flat-rate pension for the elderly provided to everyone over a certain age. Usually such schemes are combined with additional benefits based on earlier contributions (discussed later). Benefits for sickness or disability pensions are universal, with the limitation that claimants must be certified, usually by a doctor, according to disability in relation to the demands of the job or the local labour market. This interaction between disability and demand makes the eligibility rules more flexible but also more unpredictable. The flat-rate benefits might prevent absolute poverty, but their redistributive power is limited in the sense that they only 'raise the floor'.

2. Social insurance with entitlements to benefit depending on previous contributions exists in all European countries, and is quantitatively the predominant system for income maintenance. Many countries have schemes for pensions, sickness absence, unemployment, and some even for maternity benefits and parental leave based on earlier income. Commercial insurance has to calculate contributions in relation to expected claims, and sometimes even to exclude individuals with particularly high risks. Social insurance, on the other hand, usually allows contributions to be flat or related to income, and benefits to be related to earlier contributions and sometimes even to the duration of contributions. In many countries participation in the schemes is compulsory, to prevent 'good risks' opting out. In many countries in Europe social insurance

dominates the market, crowding out commercial insurance. The systems differ according to occupation, employer, region and so on, and because of this they may contribute to the maintenance of social stratification, rather than to removing it. Systems with high levels of income maintenance in all strata have, however, paradoxically been shown to be more redistributive than other systems (20).

3. Means-tested social assistance might look rather efficient as it aims to concentrate help on those most in need, and at the same time keeps down costs. Benefits are not related to citizenship or previous contributions, but they are usually not given before the individual has exhausted their own resources, and they look carefully at how the money is spent. Means-tested systems often create 'poverty traps' because they are withdrawn when the individual obtains a job, even though this might be low paid and just above the limit. This tends to keep considerable segments of the population on incomes only just above the level guaranteed to the unemployed. The administrative surveillance needed for these systems tends to make the process of obtaining and retaining assistance rather stigmatizing to the clients and leaves them subject to constant suspicion of fraud. Some authors have argued that the shame of being poor is an important mechanism linking poverty and unemployment to ill-health (21).

Differential effects of income maintenance policies

Different social strata are dependent on income maintenance policies to very different degrees, and the three types of policies just discussed act differentially across different strata. This is why income maintenance policies might mitigate poverty and income inequality but at the same time have the potential to aggravate social stratification. One of the reasons why social policies influence not only overall health but also the social distribution of health in the population is the fact that most income maintenance policy regimes act differentially for different groups (19). Traditionally social policies were different for manual and non-manual workers, coverage and eligibility being more favourable for the non-manual classes. These differences are less pronounced today, but globalization, increased female participation and increased labour mobility have generated new cleavages that might be more relevant for the understanding of how income maintenance policies affect health equality.

The post-war welfare states were created typically to insure a male breadwinner who had lifelong stable employment and family life, with the need for protection against the relatively small risks of unemployment and illness and with the need for a decent pension (6). For the core group of qualified non-manual and skilled manual workers with long-term stable employment these systems still work well. Their relationship to income maintenance policy is mainly through their participation in social insurance systems, sometimes combined with private schemes which, in some countries, are only complementary whereas in others they predominate for this group. Such people need hardly any contact with unemployment or means-tested benefits. They will usually use the public healthcare system and their loyalty to the welfare state might depend strongly on how they evaluate the efficiency and quality of such care (22). As these systems have developed in male-dominated labour markets, widowhood and particularly divorce are likely to make women very vulnerable, as these events terminate their access to their husbands' private or employer-driven pensions and so on. In such situations women tend to become much more dependent on the provision of public systems (discussed later).

This traditional corporatist social insurance model, found in much of continental Europe, is, however, under severe strain. The international economy presses for fewer standardized secure employment relationships and more just-in-time jobs, with precarious temporary contracts, greater wage differentiation and increased self-employment – often disguised as franchise working. Workers will of course protect the security of their jobs and wages as much as possible, as they and their families are so dependent on them. The lack of low-skilled jobs, low wages, part-time jobs and so on keeps women and young people out of the labour market. Also, the lack of public care services creates obstacles for women wishing to take employment, and as more women actually do work outside the home the birth rate goes down. The declining number of employed persons, the growing number of pensioners and the declining birth rate increase dependency rates and hence the costs to be covered by the employed population. Their contributions to the welfare state increase labour costs, and so an increasing number of employers and employees opt out. Even if this policy system has so far been able to prevent strong tendencies to social and health inequalities, the lack of flexibility in the labour market tends to hinder the integration of women, young people and immigrants into the economy, which in the long run may have detrimental health effects in these groups.

For a second, rather large group of usually manual workers or low-level non-manual employees – often female – the risk of unemployment, sickness, disability and early retirement is much higher. As their bonds with employers and the labour market are looser than those of the first group they are very dependent on systems with more universal entitlements or universal social insurance systems. The potentially impoverishing effects of unemployment and disability are highly dependent on the degree of income maintenance these systems provide, including the degree to which healthcare is subsidized. Even maternity benefits and parental leave are important for women, as because of childbearing and different social assumptions about their other caring roles, their link to the labour market may become somewhat fragmented over time. Systems that have moved away from a rigid insurance system towards more public responsibility are beneficial for women (23). As globalization increases the pressure on national economies, the constant changes and restructuring of production and organizations increase mobility between employers and make these groups increasingly dependent on the public systems not linked to employers and previous contributions.

As the labour market changes, a third group of unskilled workers will be living with very low levels of job security and low wages that will undermine their entitlements in a social insurance system. They are often immigrants and might even be outside more universal entitlements linked to citizenship. They will often be dependent on means-tested benefits, as their wage levels bring them very close to poverty limits. Many are locked in poverty traps with very low incomes that are difficult to escape from, as increased earnings will immediately deprive them of benefits, leaving them with no net benefit. Countries that have been able to meet the declining demand for low-skilled labour with adequate labour market policies and universal social policies, have been able to keep this group small. Policies with public care services, part-time jobs and parenthood allowances, enabling women, including single mothers, to combine children and work, have been crucial for women's economic independence, helping them to escape their otherwise marginal position in the labour market.

The foregoing illustrates that, as globalization forces change on the labour market, social policies tend to work differentially for different groups, thereby not only influencing their relative size but also modifying the differential impact of those changes on their economic standard and their health. In some societies and for some groups the impact will be mitigated, but social policies might also tend to aggravate the stratification of the labour market. As the divisions in the labour market tend to be more and more related to cleavage between the secure and the insecure, and to the extent that social policies are built on stable relationships between employer and employee for some and means-tested benefits for others, social policies play a central role in reproducing this dynamic. Strong inclusive schemes with universal entitlements will, on the other hand, mitigate the growth of the last group and the incidence of poverty.

Different social policies also tend to work differentially in different stages of the life cycle. Traditionally, poverty cycles were linked to individual life cycles. Improvements in social policies have had an effect on poverty cycles in all countries (24). In most counties, poverty among the elderly has declined and the young have replaced the old as the lowest income group. High poverty rates among families with children remain a major problem in the liberal welfare states, whereas poverty among children is lowest in countries that have combined cash benefits with public childcare services that facilitate parents' participation in the labour market.

Challenges of income-maintenance policies

The macroeconomic and cultural changes in Europe have increased occupational and family mobility and generated new cleavages in the labour force, whereby growing proportions of the population have a more and more fragmented relationship with employers. Social insurance systems based on a stable labour market do not meet the need for poverty protection in these groups if they have no access to commercial insurance. This problem is particularly relevant for women, immigrants and young people, as they have often either been out of work for longer or have not yet established a stable position in the market.

The fact that young people and women in particular are facing poverty because of unstable labour markets, often in combination with unstable marriages, is serious, not only because it keeps down birth rates (important for the long-term survival of the welfare state), but also because we know that children are particularly susceptible to the negative health effects of poverty. Poverty in early childhood is an important cause of health inequalities in later life (25).

Those running the greatest risk of disability and social exclusion later in life are those least likely to have accumulated sufficient social insurance contributions to finance the welfare benefits they require (26). Policies to break this vicious circle need to be able to repair past problems in terms of insufficient education by retraining, and in terms of disability by rehabilitation. Simple income maintenance will be insufficient. Labour market policies geared to raising employment rates among the poorly educated and the disabled are important for reducing both social exclusion and health inequalities over the life course.

In countries where means-tested benefits predominate, the prevalence and effects of poverty are high and the impact on inequalities in health particularly strong, being typically most pronounced among children and their families. Policies that provide more universal entitlements for young parents, including benefits during unemployment, maternity and so on, that keep them well over any poverty lines, are important. Access to affordable daycare will increase their ability to obtain and keep employment.

In those countries where social insurance predominates, poverty among children and families is less pronounced, but the strain placed on them shows up in very low birth rates. As social insurance keeps wage costs high there are other structural hindrances for young people and women to enter employment. Affordable daycare, more opportunities for employment in social services, and ways to reduce wage costs for these groups might be more important.

Even countries with more universal systems have faced a relative increase (from a very low level) in poverty rates among young families and lone mothers, and their generous systems of benefits tend to prioritize the middle-aged and elderly, where the poverty risk is low and the impact on health inequality less. Reallocating some of these benefits in the direction of young families with children, including those with unstable positions in the labour market, might be crucial.

Typology of European welfare states

Based on the seminal work of Esping-Andersen (4) and later developments by Korpi and Palme (20), the following classification of national social policies has proved useful.

Social democratic welfare states with encompassing systems of income maintenance, where universal flat-rate benefits are combined with benefits related to past income and labour market participation. In these countries the principles of universalism and decommodification are extended to the middle classes, ensuring a broad political majority to sustain the high costs they demand. Denmark, Finland, Norway and Sweden are the countries in this category, with high levels of female labour market participation (75– 80 per cent). Such systems prevent the incidence of poverty relatively well and are strongly redistributive. Poverty rates among children are kept particularly low (3–5 per cent). Systems that pursue egalitarian goals and at the same time extend their services to the middle and upper classes are necessarily extremely costly, which in turn demands very high employment rates to make the tax rate acceptable. Public care services have both employed many women and allowed more women to work, as services for children and elderly parents have been provided.

Liberal welfare states, where means-tested benefits and low flat-rate or social insurance plans predominate. The welfare states target their responsibility to the poor. This means lower levels of decommodification, higher poverty rates and larger income inequalities than in the first group. The declining demand for unqualified labour has been met with deregulation and low wages. The United Kingdom is in this group, as well as some countries outside Europe, for example, the United States and Australia. It should be noted that most of these comparative classifications are based on income maintenance systems rather than on service systems: hence the British universal National Health Service (NHS) does not influence the grouping. As demand for low-skilled labour has dwindled, the solution in these countries has often been to make unqualified labour cheaper through labour market deregulation, removing minimum-wage rules, reducing unionism and increasing wage differentiation. When the demand for unqualified workers is reduced, the typical market solution will lower its price until demand increases again. As the demand for workers in industry declines, the new jobs are created mostly in private service, and attract both men and women in the younger age groups as well as ethnic minorities. Their labour market participation may counteract segregation, but this effect is blocked by another tendency: the reduced numbers of unemployed 'welfare poor' have been counteracted by increased numbers of 'working poor'. The most serious effect of this is the poverty trap. As wages decline, welfare benefits will also have to be reduced to ensure the supply of labour, and with declining welfare benefits it is possible to force wages even lower. The result is widespread poverty and large inequalities. Poverty rates among children are 20–25 per cent and thus dramatically higher than in the earlier group.

Corporatist welfare states with high levels of welfare spending. Social insurance is based mainly on corporatist solutions that depend on occupational category and labour market participation, rather than citizenship or proven need. Retrenchment of the labour supply has been the most usual way of handling the declining demand for low-skilled labour; consequently, employment among women and the young is low and rates of labour market exclusion are high. Female employment rates are usually in the range 40–55 per cent and thus much lower than in the first group. France, Germany, Austria, Belgium and The Netherlands are usually classified in this category. Reduced labour supply has been a dominant strategy in these welfare models. In continental Europe the labour supply has been reduced through the extensive early retirement of elderly, predominantly male, workers within the existing social insurance programmes, combined with various disincentives for female labour market participation. Even reductions in working hours and the limited re-export of foreign guest workers have operated along the same lines. At first the labour supply reduction model may seem reasonable in the sense that it increases productivity in what is left of the domestic industry. In so far as the insurance schemes covering the early retired and unemployed are relatively generous (as has been the case in most European countries), it may also avoid widespread poverty and inequalities. Poverty rates among children have usually been kept below 10 per cent. However, it creates a sharp insider/outsider cleavage in the community, whereby one part of the population, during a relative short working life, has to cover the social costs of all the rest. In continental Europe this means that primarily men aged 25–55 must, during this period, earn enough to ensure the survival of their families and to contribute to the increasing number of pensioners. As these countries have built up generous pension schemes, the economic pressures on young families are increasing because of the lack of day-care and the limitations this places on female employment. Some of the southern European countries in this group might be called *late female mobilization welfare states*, where the Church is strong and Catholic social theory still prevails. There is a strong family orientation, together with the principle of 'subsidiarity', that is, that the state should limit its intervention to cases where the resources of the family and community are exhausted. Female labour market participation came about relatively late and is still low (usually around or below 40 per cent). As in the corporatist group, social insurance tends to preserve status differential across occupational classes (Greece, Ireland, Italy, Portugal and Spain belong to this category).

Conclusions

The area dealt with in this chapter does not lend itself to clear conclusions about interventions that will effectively prevent inequalities in health. We are rather left with the possibility of combining some of the observational evidence described above, linking the characteristics of different income maintenance systems to evidence about the impact of income on health and on groups particularly susceptible to this effect.

From this starting point there is no doubt that long-term poverty among families with children is particularly important for socioeconomic inequalities in health, both in childhood and later in life. The effect of income on nutrition, housing and education has far-reaching effects on health development in children. From this point of view it is obvious that systems that rely on targeted means-tested benefits are much less successful in keeping down poverty and income inequality than are other systems. But even those based on social insurance are facing a growing problem, as the pension schemes work quite well to protect income levels among the elderly and disabled but leave young families, and particularly female-headed households, more vulnerable to the effects of macroeconomic change. The provision of daycare and employment opportunities for mothers is an essential way of preventing poverty and its effects on children. Paradoxically, therefore, targeted programmes seem to be much less efficient in reducing poverty and its health effects than are more universal systems. This might prove even more true when mobility in the labour market and the 'marriage market' grows.

Among adults the role of income seems to relate much more to psychosocial mechanisms, where income loss or long-term low income means a relative lack of control and rewards in relation to the demands of work and daily life. Much less is known about the exact mechanisms here, and recommendations should therefore be cautious. Several behavioural patterns of importance for cardiovascular disease are affected negatively by low income, as well as raising the risk of depression through economic hardship. The evidence on whether the health effects of income are modified by the distribution of income in the surrounding society comes primarily from contexts with much larger income inequalities than those found in most European countries with social insurance (27). In countries that rely on means-tested benefits the stigmatizing effect of poverty is particularly strong, and maybe therefore even the health effects. Income and poverty therefore seem to have much less potential to reduce inequalities in health among adults, at least in those countries that already have universal entitlements or social insurance (28). As the demands for flexibility and mobility of labour increase, the earlier well functioning social insurance systems might prove inadequate, leaving growing segments out of the system and hindering employment opportunities, and thereby the prevention of poverty among those with a less stable relationship with the labour market. Systems with universal entitlements might therefore not only increase flexibility and employment, but also prevent income loss and poverty and their health effects. Women, immigrants, the poorly educated and the young may be particularly sensitive to these changes.

References

1. Marklund S. Klass, *Stat och Socialpolitik*. Lund: Arkiv, 1982.
2. Olsson SE. *Social Policy and the Welfare State*. Lund: Arkiv, 1990.
3. van den Berg A, Furåker B, Johansson L. *Labour Market Regimes and Patterns of Flexibility. A Sweden–Canada comparison*. Lund: Arkiv Förlag, 1997.
4. Esping-Andersen G. *The Three Worlds of Welfare Capitalism*. Cambridge: Polity Press, 1990.
5. Sen A. *Reconsidering Inequality*. Cambridge MA: Harvard University Press, 1992.
6. Esping-Andersen G, ed. Welfare states in transition. London: Sage, 1996.
7. Nelson M. Childhood nutrition and poverty. *Proc Nutr Soc* 2000: 59: 307–15.
8. Helmert U, Mielck A, Shea S. Poverty, health, and nutrition in Germany. *Rev Environ Health* 1997: 12: 159–70.
9. Barker DJP. *Mothers, Babies and Health Later in Life*. Edinburgh: Churchill Livingstone, 1998.
10. Morris JN, Donkin AJ, Wonderling D, Wilkinson P, Dowler EA. A minimum income for healthy living. *J Epidemiol Commun Health* 2000: 54: 885–9.
11. Davey Smith G *et al.* Magnitude and causes of socioeconomic differentials of mortality. *J Epidemiol Commun Health* 1990: 44: 265–70.
12. van Doorslaer E, Wagstaff A, Bleichrodt H, Calonge S, Gerdtham UG, Gerfin M, Geurts J, Gross L, Hakkinen U, Leu RE, O'Donnell O, Propper C, Puffer F, Rodriguez M, Sundberg G, Winkelhake O. Income-related inequalities in health: some international comparisons. *J Health Econ* 1997 Feb: 16(1): 93–112.
13. Wilkinson RG. Unhealthy societies – the affliction of inequality. London: Routledge, 1996.
14. Karasek R, Theorell T. *Healthy Work*. New York: Basic Books, 1990.
15. Lynch J *et al.* Workplace demands, economic reward and progression of carotid atherosclerosis. *Circulation* 1997: 96: 302–8.
16. Bartley M, Ferrie J, Montgomery SM. Living in a high unemployment economy: understanding the health consequences. In: Marmot M, Wilkinson RG, eds. *Social Determinants of Health*. London: Oxford University Press, 1999.
17. Kuh D, Ben-Shlomo Y, eds. *A Life Course Approach to Chronic Disease Epidemiology*. Oxford: Oxford University Press, 1997.
18. Benzeval M, Judge K. Income and health: the time dimension. *Soc Sci Med* 2001: 52: 1371–90.
19. Hill M. *Social Policy – a Comparative Perspective*. London: Prentice Hall, 1996.
20. Korpi W, Palme J. The paradox of redistribution and strategies for equality: welfare state institutions, inequality and poverty in the western countries. *Am Sociol Rev* 1998: 63: 661–87.
21. Starrin B, Rantakeisu U, Hagquist C. In the wake of recession – economic hardship, shame and social disintegration. *Scand J Work Environ Health* 1997: 23 Suppl 4: 47–54.
22. Diderichsen F. Market reforms in healthcare and sustainability of the welfare state. *Health Policy* 1995: 32: 141–53.
23. Sainsbury D. *Gender, Equality and Welfare States*. New York: Cambridge University Press, 1996.
24. Kangas O, Palme J. Does social policy matter? Poverty cycles in OECD countries. *Int J Health Serv* 2000: 30: 335–52.

25. Leon D. Common threads: underlying components of inequalities in mortality between and within countries. In: Leon D, Walt G, eds. *Poverty, Inequality and Health*. New York: Oxford University Press, 2001.
26. Blane D. The life course, the social gradient, and health. In: Marmot M, Wilkinson RG, eds. *Social Determinants of Health*. New York: Oxford University Press, 1999.
27. Berkman LF, Kawachi I. *Social Epidemiology*. Oxford: Oxford University Press, 2000.
28. Whitehead M, Diderichsen F, Burström B. Social policies and the pathways to inequalities in health: a comparative analysis of lone mothers in Britain and Sweden. *Soc Sci Med* 2000: 50: 255–70.

4   Income maintenance policies

The example of Finland

*Eero Lahelma, Ilmo Keskimäki and
Ossi Rahkonen*

Introduction

Income is a basic material resource which in all societies is more or less
unequally distributed between individuals and households. Income inequalities are a potential source of other forms of inequalities, including socioeconomic inequalities in health. As income inequalities vary between countries
and change over time, they may give rise to a widening or narrowing of
health inequalities.

In Finland and the other Nordic countries income inequalities have during
the past few decades been smaller than elsewhere (1). However, socioeconomic inequalities in health in these countries are as large as or even larger
than elsewhere in Europe (2, 3). In order to improve our understanding
of the production of socioeconomic inequalities, 'natural experimental' situations, such as large and rapid social and economic transformations, can be
examined.

A Finnish natural experiment is taken as a case study by looking at
socioeconomic inequalities in health by income from the mid-1980s to the
mid-1990s, that is, during a period when the country's economy moved from
economic boom to deep recession. We ask, how did the country cope with
such adverse economic developments in terms of socioeconomic inequalities
in health? What happened to income inequalities *per se* and, in particular, what
happened to socioeconomic inequalities in health as measured by income?

Associations between income and health

Examining socioeconomic inequalities in health by income is a key area of
current research (4–8). For example, it is argued that health inequalities in
society are a reflection of socioeconomic inequalities in general. Thus societies with large income, educational or class inequalities are likely also to
have a poor overall level of health and large health inequalities. An association with high mortality and morbidity has been suggested (5, 7). However,
countries vary in terms of the pattern and magnitude of the association of
income and other socioeconomic inequalities with health (9).

Finland's welfare system

Policies to promote health may aim both at improving the general level of health and at reducing inequalities between population groups. In Finland, a number of major policies, programmes and interventions to promote health and tackle health inequalities can be identified (10). Finnish health policies have traditionally been predominantly universalistic, aiming at a better level of health among the population in general. There was no major reorientation of health policies during the 1990s' adverse economic situation.

In addition, national programmes have also addressed socioeconomic inequalities in mortality and morbidity (11). However, it has been particularly difficult to implement these broad national programmes both within diverse administrative sectors and at the municipal level. Sectoral as well as local programmes typically fail to include socioeconomic inequalities in health. As a result, programmes and policies aiming to reduce health inequalities have not been systematically implemented (12).

Although health policies may be relatively independent of the economic situation, as in Finland, the economic constraints nevertheless influence health policy options and access to financial resources. The type of response to adverse economic development varies depending on the political forces and the broader social structural characteristics of society. First, a *laissez-faire* response is likely to have unequal consequences, as stronger socioeconomic groups cope better with adverse economic developments. Vulnerable groups, such as the unemployed, depend on the social welfare system and benefits to survive during a recession. Second, residual social policies, including safety nets to prevent absolute need among the most vulnerable groups, also give way to deepening inequalities under economic pressures. Third, a broader, welfare state type of response can be expected to have the potential to prevent the consequences of adverse economic development through universal benefits covering all socioeconomic groups. Finland is an example of the social democratic welfare state model, and we examine whether the Finnish welfare state might have helped buffer against the adverse consequences of the early 1990s' economic recession, such as widening health inequalities by income.

The recession and its consequences

From the late 1980s' boom, the Finnish economy moved into a sudden recession in the early 1990s, of a magnitude not seen since the 1930s' Great Depression. In fact, Finland is the only OECD (Organization for Economic Co-operation and Development) country in which the early 1990s' recession was deeper than that in the 1930s (13). Therefore, its consequences need to be assessed at the societal as well as the grass-roots level, including income and health inequalities.

Changes in the economy and income inequalities

As the recession hit in 1991, gross domestic product (GDP) declined by over 10 per cent during 1991–3 (Table 4.1). The average household disposable income declined and was still, in 1996, after the peak recession years, lower than that before the recession in 1990. Similarly, household spending in 1996 remained at a lower level than it was in 1990.

A major consequence of the recession was a very high unemployment level, which peaked at 17 per cent in 1994 (Table 4.1). Finland's unemployment figures were then among the highest in Western Europe. Unemployment hit disproportionately more manual than non-manual workers, but nevertheless, previously well-off regions as well as higher socioeconomic groups also suffered. The national economy started to recover in 1994, but the adverse consequences lasted much longer.

In terms of disposable income, households were affected fairly equally by the recession. Income inequalities measured by the Gini coefficient remained both stable and low throughout the recession years. In 1986 the Gini coefficient was 0.201 and in the peak recession year 1994 it was 0.208 (Figure 4.1). Another major consequence of the recession was that people's incomes declined across the whole socioeconomic spectrum, not just among the poorest.

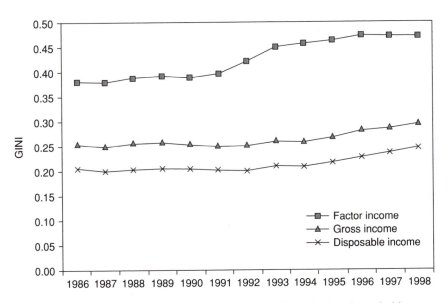

Figure 4.1 Distribution of factor, gross and disposable equivalent household income between persons, 1986–98

Source: Statistics Finland, Income Distribution Statistics 1992, 1998

Table 4.1 National and public economy in Finland in 1986–98

	1986	1987	1988	1989	1990	1991	1992	1993	1994	1995	1996	1997	1998
Change in GDP, %	2.5	4.2	4.7	5.1	0.0	-6.3	-3.3	-1.1	4.0	3.8	4.0	6.3	5.5
Unemployment rate[a]	5.4	5.1	4.5	3.1	3.2	6.6	11.7	16.3	16.6	15.4	14.6	12.7	11.4
Consumer prices, change %	3.6	3.7	4.9	6.6	6.1	4.1	2.6	2.2	1.1	1	0.6	1.2	1.4
Social expenditure as % of GDP	24.5	24.7	23.7	23.4	25.1	29.8	33.6	34.6	33.8	31.8	31.6	29.3	27.2
Tax rate, %	41.6	39.6	42.3	42.6	44.7	46.1	45.9	44.6	46.6	44.9	47.3	46.1	46.0
State debt, EURO billion	8.7	9.8	9.8	8.9	9.6	15.5	29.5	43.0	51.7	60.4	66.5	70.3	70.7
State debt as % of GDP	14.4	14.9	13.1	10.7	10.9	18.4	36.0	51.9	58.9	63.6	67.5	65.8	60.8

Notes:
a From 1989, according to ILO/EU definition.
The Eurostat employment rates are calculated according to the recommendations of the 13th International Conference of Labour Statisticians organized by the International Labour Office (ILO) in 1982. Unemployed persons are those persons aged 15 years and over who are:
– without work
– available to start work within the next two weeks
– and have actively sought employment at some time during the previous four weeks

Source: Statistics Finland, Statistical Yearbooks of Finland 1993 and 2000

The Finnish social security system was also hit by the recession. Financing of the welfare state is very much dependent on taxes paid by employed people. However, this changed drastically as the number of taxpayers and their incomes declined. Instead of focusing cutbacks on particular areas, relatively small cutbacks were introduced across a full range of the social security system, including unemployment benefits, sickness benefits, pensions, family allowances, housing and income support (14). This led to lower benefit levels, restricted eligibility and a shorter duration of benefits.

As the cutbacks were relatively small they did not cause serious financial problems for most beneficiaries. The level of social expenditure was not only maintained, but increased substantially owing to the increasing costs of unemployment and other social benefits. The cost of maintaining the basic welfare state system was covered by increasing the state's indebtedness, whereas the tax rate remained broadly stable throughout the recession (Table 4.1).

Although the adaptation to the recession may seem to have been under political and administrative control, the reality was much more complex. The result was not necessarily due to intentional policies, but rather to a mixture of policies accompanied by constraints related to the political and economic system. The government and politicians were overwhelmed by the sudden economic difficulties and there were no ready-made strategies. Major policy changes were not feasible, partly because of the political system based on broad political coalitions, and partly because of the legal basis of the funding of the welfare. It has even been suggested that the welfare state system may be largely irreversible and therefore does not decline, but works for stability against adverse economic change (13).

Changes in health inequality by income

In order to assess the impacts of the Finnish recession on health inequalities by income, the results of a study repeated in 1986 and 1994 by Rahkonen *et al.* (15) are summarized, during periods when the country's economy was booming and when the recession peaked, with unemployment reaching its highest levels.

Health was measured by using a broad indicator of self-perceived health. Respondents were asked to rate their health on a 5-point scale ranging from excellent to very poor. 'Average', 'poor' and 'very poor' were combined to yield 'less than good' perceived health. This perceived health measure has proved to be a reliable and valid instrument, suitable for populations surveys (16).

Data on income derive from national taxation registers and were linked to the surveys. We analysed net household disposable income per consumption unit ('household income' for short). Income was adjusted for household size using the OECD equivalence scale: the first adult is given the weight of 1.0, other adults 0.7 and children 0.5. Individual members of households

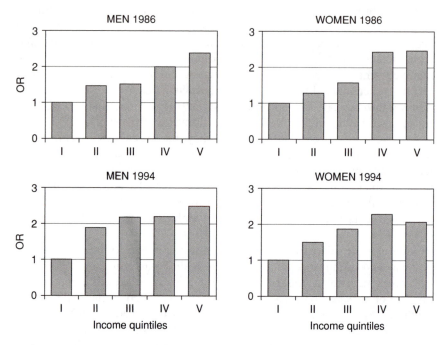

Figure 4.2 Perceived health by equivalent household disposable income quintiles. Age-adjusted odds ratios for Finnish men and women aged 25–64 in 1986 and 1994 (highest income quintile I OR = 1.00)

Source: Adapted from Rahkonen *et al.* 2001 (15)

were classified into five quintiles of equal size according to their adjusted household income, that is, relative income inequalities were examined. This income measure indicates the household's material resources and capacity for consumption.

The association between income and health was examined by using logistic regression analysis separately for men and women. The results are presented as odds ratios (OR) for less than good perceived health. The highest income group is used as the reference category and health in this group is marked by OR = 1.00. Odds ratios for less than good perceived health in the other income groups are compared to the reference category. As age structures in the income groups are likely to vary, the effect of this is eliminated by adjusting for age in the analysis.

The age-adjusted association between perceived health and household income among Finnish men and women in 1986 and 1994 is shown in Figure 4.2 (15). Among men this association was steep and linear. Our main interest was in the changes over time in health inequalities by income. However, the changes from the booming economy in 1986 to the recession in 1994 were minor, and suggest a stable development of health inequalities by income among men.

Among Finnish women, the association between perceived health and income was equally strong and linear as for men in the 1980s. Looking at changes over time from 1986 to 1994 among women we find only minor changes, and these suggest a stable or slightly narrowing development of health inequalities by income.

Thus socioeconomic inequalities in health as measured by income proved to be very stable from the mid-1980s to the mid-1990s among Finnish men and women, with no signs of widening.

Conclusions

The Finnish case study from the mid-1980s to the mid-1990s shows that socioeconomic inequalities in health by income did not change in response to the early 1990s' deep economic recession. Such a stable development has also been found for educational and occupational class health inequalities (17, 18). Comparing Finland with Sweden, a country that underwent a simultaneous economic recession, shows a similar stability (18). In contrast, a comparison between Britain and Finland over the same period suggests that health inequalities in Britain tended to widen (17).

In Finland and Sweden the strategies to cope with the recession were broadly similar, that is, in both countries the welfare state system weakened but the basic structures were not dismantled (19). Social expenditure increased as the number of beneficiaries multiplied. However, there were differences between the countries as well, the main difference being that the Finnish recession was deeper than that in Sweden. Both countries covered the increasing costs of social welfare by increasing state indebtedness, but Sweden collected more taxes in addition. The Finnish taxation level remained broadly static and larger cutbacks were made than in Sweden.

Britain had already undergone a recession in the 1980s, but with the legacy of Thatcherism the country then moved further away from a broad welfare state model. For example, high unemployment levels in Britain were accompanied by widening income inequalities, which may have contributed to widening health inequalities as well (17).

The Finnish case study suggests that, regarding the depth of the recession, the welfare state worked surprisingly well in the way it is expected to do, that is, safeguarding people's well-being and buffering against a major widening in socioeconomic inequalities. Previously, the Finnish universalistic welfare state system had been tested only against relatively small fluctuations of the trade cycle. The 1990s' recession was a test of the welfare state arrangements when economic growth was negative and large segments of the population were in need of social assistance. The system was extremely burdened and its basic structures were shaken.

Maintaining the welfare state structures is likely to have contributed to the stability of health inequalities by income, as the universalistic system provided safety nets not only for those who ran the risk of absolute poverty, but for all those whose well-being was challenged. The piecemeal strategy, including a large number of fairly small cutbacks across the whole social welfare system, instead of major cutbacks in one or more areas, proved to be successful. As a result, most people suffered from the recession, but the amount of suffering was widely spread and therefore usually relatively modest.

So far the Finnish case has shown a reassuring adaptation to a deep economic recession in terms of socioeconomic inequalities in health and other areas of well-being. However, it must be stressed that this was as much the result of fortunate coincidences combined with legal, economic and political constraints than an intentional policy.

Looking at the post-recession development in Finland, signs of widening inequalities can be found. For example, income inequalities have widened from the mid-1990s onward (13). However, this has not been because of poor economic prospects, for example related to the high state indebtedness after the recession, but rather owing to the strong economic growth during the second half of the 1990s. In such favourable economic conditions those at the top of the income ladder have succeeded in increasing their incomes quickly, whereas those at the bottom have remained at their previous income level. A further reason for widening income inequalities relates to the stagnation of the social benefits at the recession level. Nevertheless, by the end of the 1990s income inequalities were still narrow, but the widening trend is alarming.

Whether other socioeconomic inequalities will also increase during the post-recession years in Finland, and whether this will be reflected as widening health inequalities by income, remains an open question. Health inequalities by income as well as other socioeconomic dimensions need continuous follow-up, and in addition to morbidity, other health indicators, including mortality, health behaviours and health services use, need to be examined. Finally, egalitarian health and welfare policies are needed to prevent widening health inequalities under the pressure of widening income inequalities.

The lessons to be learned from the Finnish case study are, first, that health inequalities by income remained unexpectedly stable although the country underwent a deep economic recession. The welfare state system is likely to have buffered against the economic pressures towards widening health inequalities. A piecemeal strategy of cutbacks and efforts to maintain the basic welfare structures contributed to this stability. Second, the welfare state may be less able to prevent the widening of inequalities during an economic boom. The strongest socioeconomic groups' share of the economic growth expands much faster than that of the weaker groups. Therefore, egalitarian health and welfare policies are needed not only during an economic recession but equally during a boom.

References

1. Atkinson A, Rainwater L, Smeeding T. *Income Distribution in OECD Countries*. OECD Social Policy Studies 18, 1995.
2. Cavelaars A, Kunst A, Geurts J, Helmert U, Lahelma E, Lundberg O *et al.* Differences in self-reported morbidity by income level in six European countries. In: Cavelaars A, ed. *Cross-national Comparisons of Socioeconomic Differences in Health Indicators*. Rotterdam: Thesis, Erasmus University, 1998: 49–66.
3. Mackenbach J, Kunst A, Cavelaars A, Groenhof F, Geurts J and the EU Working Group on Socioeconomic Inequalities in Health. Socioeconomic inequalities in morbidity and mortality in Western Europe. *Lancet* 1997: 349: 1655–9.
4. Kaplan GA, Pamuk E, Lynch JW, Cohen RD, Balfour JL. Income inequality and mortality in the United States: analysis of mortality and potential pathways. *Br Med J* 1996: 312: 999–1003.
5. Wilkinson RG. *Unhealthy Societies. The Afflictions of Inequality*. London: Routledge, 1996.
6. Stronks K, van de Mheen H, van den Bos J, Mackenbach J. The interrelationship between income, health and employment status. *Int J Epidemiol* 1997: 26: 592–600.
7. Kennedy B, Kawachi I, Glass R, Prothrow-Stith D. Income distribution, socioeconomic status and self-rated health in the United States: a multilevel analysis. *Br Med J* 1998: 317: 917–21.
8. Rahkonen O, Arber S, Lahelma E, Martikainen P, Silventoinen K. Understanding income inequalities in health among men and women in Britain and Finland. *Int J Health Serv* 2000: 30: 27–47.
9. Lundberg O, Lahelma E. Nordic health inequalities in the European context. In: Kautto M, Fritzell J, Hvinden B, Kvist J, Uusitalo H, eds. *Nordic Welfare States in the European Context*. London: Routledge, 2001: 42–65.
10. Prättälä R, Forssas E, Koskinen S, Sihto M. Lifestyle interventions in Finland – can they reduce inequalities in health? In: Mackenbach JP, Droomers M, eds. *Intervention and Policies to Reduce Socioeconomic Inequalities in Health*. Rotterdam: Department of Public Health, Erasmus University, 1999: 22–30.
11. *Health for All Policy in Finland 1991*. Copenhagen: WHO Regional Office for Europe, 1991.
12. Sihto M, Keskimäki I. Does a policy matter? Assessing the Finnish health policy in relation to its equity goals. *Critical Public Health* 2000: 10: 273–86.
13. Uusitalo H. *Social Policy in a Deep Economic Recession and After: The Case of Finland*. The Year 2000 International Research Conference on Social Security, International Social Security Association (ISSA), Helsinki, 25–27 September 2000.
14. Kosunen V. The recession and changes in social security in the 1990s. In: Heikkilä M, Uusitalo H, eds. *The Cost of Cuts. Studies on Cutbacks in Social Security and their Effects in Finland in the 1990s*. Helsinki: Stakes, 1997.
15. Rahkonen O, Lahelma E, Martikainen P, Silventoinen K. *Health Inequalities by Income in Finland from the 1980s to the 1990s*. J Epidemiol Community Health 2002 (in production).
16. Manderbacka K. Questions on survey questions on health. *Dissertation Series 30*. Stockholm: Stockholm University, Swedish Institute for Social Research, 1998.

17. Lahelma E, Arber S, Rahkonen O, Silventoinen K. Widening or narrowing inequalities on health? Comparing Britain and Finland from the 1980s to the 1990s. *Sociol Health Illness* 2000: 22: 110–36.

18. Lahelma E, Kivelä K, Roos E, Tuominen T, Dahl E, Diderichsen F *et al.* *Analysing Changes of Health Inequalities in the Nordic Welfare States.* 2001 Soc Sci Med 2002 (in production).

19. Kautto M. Two of a kind? Economic crisis, policy responses and well-being during the 1990s in Sweden and Finland. A balance sheet for welfare of the 1990s. *Government Official Reports* 2000: 83. Stockholm: Fritzes, 2000.

5   Municipal policies

The example of Barcelona

Carme Borrell, Joan R. Villalbí, Elia Díez,
M. Teresa Brugal and Joan Benach

Introduction

Barcelona, located in the northeast of the country, is the second largest city in Spain. Its population has decreased from 1,701,812 inhabitants in 1986 to 1,508,805 in 1996, and is increasingly ageing. After the restoration of democracy in the mid-1970s, the first democratic municipal elections were held in 1979, and a succession of coalitions led by the Socialist Party has governed the city. The city administration has had public health as part of its priorities for some time: a health information system was developed and new policies and interventions were set up. Barcelona was the first place in Spain to implement a Health Interview Survey (in 1983), and since 1984 an annual report on the health of the city has been presented to the city council by the Municipal Public Health Institute. This led to the identification of territorial inequalities in health, which in turn pointed to issues to be tackled by health policies or interventions. In this chapter we present four of the different interventions implemented in the city to reduce socioeconomic inequalities in health. These were selected because they have been subjected to formal evaluation and have produced research reports.

The extent of socioeconomic inequalities in health

Socioeconomic inequalities in health have been studied extensively in Barcelona during the past 15 years and show both geographic and individual inequalities. Several studies have shown that the poorer, historic inner-city district of Ciutat Vella, with 84,000 inhabitants, has health indicators well below city standards and below those of nine other districts of the city. Excess mortality has been reported in this district, which has higher premature mortality, higher infant mortality and lower life expectancy at birth (1–3). Other important negative health indicators include adolescent fertility, and the incidence of AIDS, drug overdose and tuberculosis (4, 5). Geographical inequalities in premature mortality increased between 1983 and 1994, from causes concentrated among the less privileged social classes (AIDS and drug overdose), as their increases were much higher in deprived neighbourhoods (6).

Inequalities in perceived health status were described with data from the 1986 health interview survey (2). Data from the 1992 Barcelona health survey showed persistent inequalities in perceived health status, health-related behaviours and health service utilization. The disadvantaged have worse perceived health and behaviours that tend to involve greater health risks (7, 8). Although the National Health Service facilitates access to services for all social classes free of charge, there are inequalities in other aspects related to healthcare, such as waiting times (9) or access to preventive health services (10).

Reduction of socioeconomic inequalities at the local level

Interventions on inequalities in health in Barcelona were prompted by three main factors: an overall thrust towards improving living conditions in working-class neighbourhoods; a drive to rehabilitate the old city, which was evolving into an inner-city area next to a gentrified historic quarter; and the input of annual health reports providing information on territorial inequalities in health and their main causes. The participation of Barcelona in the early phases of the Healthy Cities project (late 1980s) provided a global perspective on health at the city level, which was also instrumental in this process. Although many of the inequalities in health derive from factors beyond the capacity of action by local public health administrations, there are many options for intervention to improve health and access to healthcare.

Mother and child health programme

In order to reduce mother and child health inequalities in the district of Ciutat Vella, in 1987 an intervention was implemented in this low-income urban area aimed at increasing access to health and social services for pregnant women and their children based on early detection and nursing-home follow-up. Its impact was evaluated through a quasi-experimental design with a non-equivalent control group and multiple measurements. Infant mortality rates between Ciutat Vella and the rest of the city, both before 1983–6 and after the intervention have been compared (11).

The results show that the significant differences in mortality rates that existed before the intervention were reduced by the programme to a level that is no longer statistically significant. Infant mortality in Ciutat Vella, which was 17.8 per 1,000 births in 1983–6, fell to 7.1 in 1995–8; in the rest of the city, infant mortality was 8.2 per 1,000 births in 1983–6, and fell to 4.1 per 1,000 births (Figure 5.1). Although rates in the inner city are still higher, the gap has been greatly reduced. The evaluation shows that a comprehensive social and healthcare programme implemented in low-income areas may contribute to reduce inequalities in maternal and child health.

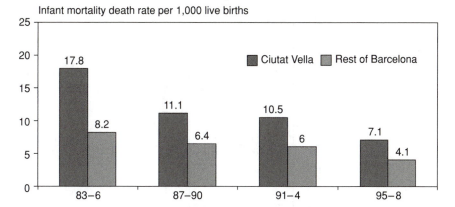

Infant mortality death rate per 1,000 live births

Figure 5.1 Cumulated infant mortality death rates (per 1,000 live births). District of Ciutat Vella and rest of Barcelona. Periods 1983–6, 1987–90, 1991–4, 1995–8

Tuberculosis control among the homeless and intravenous drug users

The homeless and other excluded groups are a priority in the global strategies of tuberculosis prevention and control in big cities, as a consequence of their poor compliance with treatment and of multiple concurrent social and health problems. In 1987 a social and health programme targeting homeless tuberculosis patients in the inner-city district of Ciutat Vella was developed. Relying on directly observed therapy programmes, it provided improved access to primary healthcare and social services, as well as housing accommodation if needed. The strategy included in this pilot programme was later expanded to cover other high-risk groups, specifically heroin users, through methadone maintenance programmes.

There was a significant decrease in the incidence of tuberculosis among the homeless in Ciutat Vella (from 32.4 per 100,000 inhabitants in 1987, to 19.8 per 100,000 in 1992, $p = 0.03$), compared to an unchanged rate elsewhere (1.6 per 100,000 inhabitants in 1987, and 1.7 per 100,000 in 1992, $p = 0.34$) (12).

The programme appears to be effective, as it has increased the proportion of high-risk patients who complete treatment successfully (13) (Table 5.1), including intravenous drug users (see next example of good practice). The pilot project was eventually broadened beyond the city by the Government of Catalonia to cover all non-compliant patients.

Drug abuse programmes

Heroin consumption appeared in Barcelona in the late 1970s and soon became concentrated in the poorer populations, located mostly in the inner-city districts. Simultaneously, an increased perception of crime by the media and

Table 5.1 Annual evaluation of adherence rate of tuberculosis therapy by tuberculous patients by criteria for high risk of not completing therapy. Barcelona, 1988–97

	1988	1989	1990	1991	1992	1993	1994	1995	1996	1997
HIV	74.6%	77.3%	66.1%	70.8%	75.3%	78.0%	84.4%	89.4%	91.5%	91.5%
Jail–prison	42.1%	53.5%	47.0%	56.5%	63.2%	81.7%	82.2%	90.4%	92.3%	91.5%
Homeless	42.4%	48.6%	54.5%	50.0%	61.3%	61.1%	83.3%	100%	91.7%	91.6%
Immigrants	60.6%	76.6%	73.5%	66.7%	53.2%	82.5%	84.5%	81.8%	90.2%	91.9%
City global	83.7%	87.6%	84.2%	81.1%	84.8%	89.4%	91.8%	93.8%	95.8%	95.1%

Notes:
Adherence rate of tuberculosis therapy is the percentage of tuberculous people who report to have taken the treatment and who have been cured.
HIV: Seropositive at human immunodeficiency virus.

Source: Adapted from Villalbí JR *et al.* 1999 (13)

the population pushed heroin addicts towards social exclusion. At first, social and health approaches were based on the promotion of abstinence and the criminalization of users, without visible results. This, and the emergence of AIDS, prompted a review of policies, which were directed towards a comprehensive and more pragmatic approach, grounded in public health. Thus four consecutive Drug Action Plans were implemented, involving different interventions in the city of Barcelona.

In 1987, the first City Drug Action Plan was approved by consensus among all political parties in the City Council, and was implemented. From the start, territorial analyses of the extent of the problem and its associated needs were carried out (14, 15). From 1990, with changes in legislation and following the model of other European cities, harm reduction programmes and a redesign of health and social services for drug users began. These aimed at providing help to drug users, both for health problems (for example, addiction, infectious disease and psychopathology) and for practical needs (for example, housing, food and work). These included diagnoses and treatment for organic problems, methadone maintenance programmes, syringe exchange programmes, outreach programmes, legal/labour assistance, and mobile harm reduction units (16, 17).

Table 5.2 shows the evolution of key indicators. The results suggest positive trends, thereby reinforcing a public health approach as a solid foundation for an action plan. However, future changes need to be monitored (cocaine addiction is a growing problem) and there is a need to ensure a continuing comprehensive response to new challenges.

The reform of primary healthcare

The reform of primary healthcare services in Spain began in 1984, modelled on the principles of the Alma Ata Conference. The new primary healthcare system is based on healthcare centres where professionals work in teams. The process of reform is cumulative, and currently covers over 70 per cent of the Spanish population. In Barcelona the reform covers only 50 per cent of the population, mainly because of technical problems (finding buildings, physicians who wish to change to the new system, etc.) but the process of reform has given higher priority to deprived areas and began in those with poor socioeconomic indicators (18). A recent study evaluated the impact of the reform of primary healthcare in 23 areas with lower socioeconomic status. The evolution of avoidable mortality rates over 1984–96 was compared in the areas already reformed and those where services were still unsatisfactory. At the end of the study period, mortality due to stroke and hypertension was lower in the areas that had benefited from an early reform of primary care services. Perinatal mortality showed a clear decline in all zones, and no relevant changes could be seen for tuberculosis and cervical cancer deaths, for which specific programmes covering all zones existed. Lung cancer mortality increased except in the early reformed areas, thereby

Table 5.2 Evolution of social and health indicators related to heroin over the four triennal Drug Action Plans. Barcelona 1986–97

	1986–8	1989–91	1992–4	1995–7	P
Health care and harm reduction					
Number of heroin treatments	853	1,365	2,116	2,042	NS
% MMP cover	Na	5.1%	14.9%	18.6%	<0.0001
Syringe exchanges for each drug user per year (average)	Na	0.6	4.9	23.7	0.001
Infectious diseases					
HIV incidence per 100 seronegative users	Na	5.53	4.02	2.73	<0.0001
HIV prevalence per 100	Na	Na	42%	31%	<0.0001
Anti HBc prevalence per 100	Na	Na	56%	36%	<0.0001
Adherence rate of tuberculosis therapy[a]	66.9%	68.2%	81.3%	92.0%	<0.0001
Tuberculosis in drug users. Number of cases	150	189	213	147	<0.05
Health care utilization: emergencies for drug consumption					
% Heroin emergencies[b]	Na	89.2%	63.8%	46.5%	<0.0001
% Heroin overdoses[c]	Na	24.3%	17.8%	15.9%	<0.0001
% Heroin craving[c]	Na	25.8%	17.2%	4.5%	<0.0001
Drug related death					
Annual rate of overdose (100,000 15–49 year old)	6.03 ± 1.7	15.14 ± 2.64	15.00 ± 2.1	14.27 ± 2.8	NS
Crimes related with drugs					
Violence index[d]	0.26	0.18	0.15	0.15	0.0001

Notes:
NS: Non statistically significative
Na: not available
MMP: Methadone Maintenance Programs
HIV: Human Immunodeficiency Virus.
a Adherence rate of tuberculosis therapy is the percentage of tuberculous people who report to have taken the treatment and who have been cured
b Percentage over all emergencies for drug consumption
c Percentage over all heroin emergencies
d Percentage of the general population that has declared being assaulted due to drugs in an Interview Survey done each year by the Local Council of Barcelona

Source: Adapted from Brugal MT *et al.* 1998 (16) and Manzanera R *et al.* 2000 (17)

eliminating the excess mortality that had existed in this zone at the beginning of the study. Death rates from cirrhosis and motor vehicle accident declined in all zones (19).

Conclusions

The study of socioeconomic inequalities in health has been a priority of the Municipal Public Health Institute since the 1980s, making Barcelona the place in Spain where this subject has been most analysed. Further, programmes have been implemented to tackle these inequalities, mainly in the inner-city area of Ciutat Vella. We have described four interventions carried out in the city, evaluations of which suggest that their implementation has been followed by reductions in health inequalities. As with other processes of change, it is hard to disentangle the specific contribution of each factor: these programmes, conducted in the late 1980s and early 1990s, have produced such results when the economic context in Spain was not favourable (high unemployment), but other social policies (in access to healthcare and education or in income support) were also addressing social inequalities in the country as a whole. Over the years, the expansion of AIDS has caused a clear increase in health inequalities in Spain, as in other European countries. Our experience also suggests that interventions confined to the healthcare sectors have serious limitations. It is necessary to involve other sectors of the administration and also the population to improve results.

The experience of Barcelona may be useful to other areas trying to reduce socioeconomic inequalities in health. In our view three aspects must be considered: the need for a strong and permanent political commitment to tackle these inequalities; an extensive information system focusing on socioeconomic inequalities in health; and the necessary instruments to intervene. In our experience, given these conditions it is possible to reduce avoidable mortality and morbidity as well as to improve equitable access to and utilization of healthcare services in relation to need.

References

1. Borrell C, Plasència A, Pañella H. Excés de mortalitat en un àrea urbana cèntrica: el cas de Ciutat Vella a Barcelona. (Excess mortality in an inner city area: the case of Ciutat Vella in Barcelona). *Gac Sanit* 1991: 5: 243–53.
2. Alonso J, Antó JM. Desigualdades de Salud en Barcelona (Health inequalities in Barcelona). *Gac Sanit* 1988: 2: 4–12.
3. Pasarín MI, Borrell C. ¿Dos patrones de desigualdades sociales en mortalidad en Barcelona? (Two patterns of social inequalities in mortality in Barcelona?). *Gac Sanit* 1999: 13: 431–40.
4. Nebot M, Borrell C, Villalbí JR. Adolescent motherhood and socioeconomic factors: an ecologic approach. *Eur J Public Health* 1997: 7: 144–8.
5. Pasarín MI, Borrell C, Brugal MT, Galdós-Tangüis H, García- Olalla P, Pañella

H. La salut a Ciutat Vella. (Health in Ciutat Vella). *Barcelona Societat* 1998: 9: 43–51.

6.   Borrell C, Pasarín MI, Plasència A, Ortún V. Widening inequalities in mortality: the case of a southern European city (Barcelona). *J Epidemiol Commun Health* 1997: 51: 659–67.

7.   Borrell C, Domínguez-Berjón F, Pasarín MI, Ferrando J, Rohlfs I, Nebot M. Social inequalities in health-related behaviours in Barcelona. *J Epidemiol Commun Health* 2000: 54: 24–30.

8.   Borrell C, Rué M, Pasarín MI, Rohlfs I, Ferrando J, Fernández E. Trends in social class inequalities in health status, health-related behaviors and health services utilization in a Southern European urban area (1983–94). *Prev Med* 2000: 31: 691–701.

9.   Borrell C, Fernandez E, Schiaffino A, Benach J, Rajmil L, Villalbí JR *et al.* Social class inequalities in the use of and access to health services in Catalonia (Spain): what is the influence of a supplemental private health insurance? *Int J Quality Health Care* 2001: 13(2): 117–25.

10. Rohlfs I, Borrell C, Pasarín MI, Plasència A. Social inequalities and realization of opportunistic screening mammographies in Barcelona (Spain). *J Epidemiol Commun Health* 1998: 52: 205–6.

11. Díez E, Villalbí JR, Benaque A, Nebot M. Desigualdades en salud materno-infantil: impacto de una intervención (Inequalities in mother and child health: the impact of an intervention). *Gac Sanit* 1995: 9: 224–31.

12. Díez E, Clavería J, Serra T, Caylà JA, Jansà I, Pedro R *et al.* Evaluation of a social health intervention among homeless tuberculosis patients. *Tubercle Lung Dis* 1996: 77: 420–4.

13. Villalbí JR, Galdos-Tanguis H, Cayla JA. El control de la tuberculosis basado en la evidencia: una aproximación de salud pública. (Evidence-based control of tuberculosis: a public health approach). *Med Clin (Barc)* 1999: 112 (Supl 1): 111–16.

14. Diaz A, Barruti M, Doncel C. *The Lines of Success. Laboratori de Sociologia ICESB. Area de Salut Pública.* Ajuntament de Barcelona, 1992.

15. Domingo-Salvany A, Hartnoll R, Antó JM. Opiate and cocaine consumers attending Barcelona emergency rooms: one year survey (1989). *Addiction* 1993: 88: 1247–56.

16. Brugal MT, Mestres M, Diaz de Quijano E, Caylà JA. Evolución temporal y factores asociados a la seroconversión por HIV en una cohorte de usuarios de drogas. (Time trends and associated factors to the HIV seroconversion in a cohort of drug users). *Rev Esp Salud Pública* 1998: 72 (Supl): 142–3.

17. Manzanera R, Torralba LL, Brugal MT, Armengol R, Solanes P, Villalbí JR. Afrontar los estragos de la heroína: evolución de diez años de un programmea integral en Barcelona. (Coping with heroin ravages: evolution of a 10 years comprehensive programme in Barcelona). *Gac Sanit* 2000: 14: 58–66.

18. Villalbí JR, Guarga A, Pasarín MI, Gil M, Borrell C. Corregir las desigualdades sociales en salud: la reforma de la atención primaria como estrategia. (Reducing social inequalities in health: the primary healthcare reform as a strategy). *Aten Primaria* 1998: 21: 47–54.

19. Villalbí JR, Guarga A, Pasarín MI, Gil M, Borrell C, Cirera E *et al.* Evaluación del impacto de la reforma de la atención primaria sobre la salud. (Evaluation of the primary healthcare reform impact). *Aten Primaria* 1999: 24: 468–74.

6 Work-related policies and interventions

Christer Hogstedt and Ingvar Lundberg

Introduction

Human production is the basis for both welfare and health. There is a clear correlation between gross national product (GNP), income level, living standards and average life expectancy when nations are compared, but also notable differences between different socioeconomic strata and occupational groups within nations. Most of the health improvements over time in most countries can be attributed to reduced poverty, improved education and improved living standards. Human productivity in different forms has been the basis for these improvements. One aspect of this is that the long-term unemployed or underemployed in all studies demonstrate poorer health status than the gainfully employed.

Differences in working conditions and work-related health status have been reported for centuries. The impetus for improvement has been the often appalling working conditions, especially for manual workers, who are often poorly educated and have low incomes. With the organization of trade unions, better knowledge, strengthened legislation and improved equipment many basic working conditions in industrialized countries have improved. This has generally improved health, although not necessarily diminishing demonstrable health inequalities, as the occupational groups with a better education have also benefited from welfare improvements and increased economic resources.

The main focuses for improvements in work-related health are awareness of health aspects in the planning of work and production, the eradication or control of known hazards and improvements in the work environment. But even when these 'classic' occupational hazards have been corrected, inequalities in health remain between higher and lower positions in the workforce, indicating the potential for further improvement. Interventions might thus lead to reduced disparity, as well as serving to clarify the complicated mechanisms behind such inequalities.

Occupation is the most important criterion of social stratification in advanced societies and is the basis of socioeconomic group categorizations. Esteem and social approval depend largely on one's type of job, professional training and level of occupational achievement. Furthermore, type and quality

Table 6.1 The distribution of selected working conditions in occupational groups according to the Second European Survey on Working Conditions

Working condition	Legislators and managers	Professionals	Technicians	Clerks	Service and sales workers	Agricultural workers	Craft and related trades workers	Plant and machine operators	Elementary occupations	Armed forces
Breathing in vapours	12	11	12	7	14	36	48	43	32	32
Moving heavy loads	23	12	17	11	35	70	55	47	49	28
Not able to choose or change methods of work	10	14	21	28	28	27	34	49	42	41
Job involving monotonous tasks	43	33	33	48	39	57	46	60	60	46
Job involving learning new things	82	95	87	77	73	61	74	57	47	79

of occupation, and especially the degree of self-direction at work, strongly influence personal attitudes and behavioural patterns in areas not directly related to work, such as leisure, family life, education and political activity.

Occupational exposures provide attractive explanations for social class differences in health, as their class distribution is often extremely skewed, with almost all exposed individuals being in the lower social strata. Table 6.1 shows the distribution of certain working conditions in occupational groups in European Union (EU) countries according to the Second European Survey on Working Conditions (1). The table is not based on socioeconomic groups, but different groups of blue- and white-collar workers are easily discernible. The figures vary by country (usually with more favourable conditions in northern countries and less favourable ones in Greece, Spain and Portugal), sex (usually with more favourable psychosocial conditions among men) and sector. However, in each country the distribution by occupational class mimics the overall European distribution.

In societies open to social mobility, selection processes operate that assign more fortunate individuals to more rewarding jobs and the less fortunate to less satisfactory jobs or none at all. It has been shown that, at least among men, such selection may be related to risk factors for later disease, such as smoking, alcohol consumption and symptoms of anxiety and depression (2). Such selection is particularly strong for the first job, and it is well known that class differences in health (in terms of relative risks) peak when the young enter a social class defined by their own occupation (3). Hence what work life and working conditions may do is to modify a process already begun. Work life will usually add more risk factors to social class for many, but may also occasionally undergo changes that benefit primarily these classes.

Contribution of working conditions to the explanation of socioeconomic inequalities in health

Cancer

Overall socioeconomic inequalities in cancer incidence are marginal in Finland and Sweden. However, stomach cancer and lung cancer show a higher incidence among blue- than among white-collar workers (4, 5).

Exposure to occupational carcinogens in relation to social class differences in cancer occurrence has been studied by Bofetta *et al.* (6). It has been estimated that occupational exposure is responsible for about 4 per cent of all human cancers in industrialized countries. These are concentrated among manual workers and the lower social classes. On the basis of the 1971 cancer mortality data from England and Wales, Bofetta *et al.* (6) estimated that occupational exposure is responsible for about a third of the total cancer difference between high (I, II and III-NM) and low (III-M, IV and V) social classes, and for about half of the difference for lung and bladder cancer.

The major cause of occupational cancer in recent decades has been asbestos, an exposure confined almost exclusively to working-class men in various occupations. In recent lung cancer studies in Sweden the population aetiological fraction of asbestos exposure was 4–10 per cent among men (7, 8), and it is likely that these fractions are similar in other countries. Asbestos was banned in Sweden in 1975 and in several other European countries during the 1970s and 1980s, which may have contributed to the decreasing incidence of lung cancer among men in these countries. Asbestos also causes mesothelioma, a pleural tumour with a poor prognosis which occurs long after the first exposure. It has no other known cause than exposure to asbestos and similar minerals, and the incidence without asbestos exposure is extremely low. Because of the exposure to asbestos the incidence of these tumours is expected to peak around 2010–2020 in Sweden, Denmark and England, and when the peak occurs more than 3,000 men in the United Kingdom (UK) alone are expected to die annually from this cause (9). The asbestos bans are one of the major achievements in non-infectious disease prevention so far.

Musculoskeletal disorders

Approximately 30–40 per cent of cases of musculoskeletal disorders are considered to be work-related in the Nordic countries (10). For occupations that are highly exposed to risk factors for musculoskeletal problems, the proportion may be as high as 50–90 per cent.

Data from the Second European Survey on Working Conditions (1) identified the industries (across the EU member states) where 40 per cent or more of the workers were exposed for at least 25 per cent of the working time to three or more of the risk factors: working in painful positions, moving heavy loads, short repetitive tasks, repetitive movements. These industries included agriculture, forestry and fisheries, mining and manufacturing, construction, wholesale, retail and repairs, hotels and restaurants.

The occupational groups with the greatest exposures were agriculture and fishery workers, craft and retail trade workers, plant and machine operators, and workers in unskilled occupations. The industries with the least exposure to these risk factors included transport and communication, financial and intermediation, real estate and business activity, and public administration. The occupational groups with the least exposure were legislators and managers, professionals, technicians and clerks. Although such classifications may be misleading because a job title may cover a wide range of tasks, these data are informative as to the social class distribution of risk factors for musculoskeletal disorders.

Not only are many workers in the EU highly exposed to such risk factors, but the magnitude of the exposure seems to be increasing (11).

Coronary heart disease

There is a growing recognition of the impact of stressful working conditions on health. Evidence of health-related harm is associated with lack of authority and the possibility of learning new skills, that is, low control, at work, as well as an imbalance between effort and reward (12). Again, such exposure is more common among lower socioeconomic groups.

Several studies from different countries have demonstrated two to four-fold differences in the incidence of coronary heart disease and mortality rates between different occupations and work characteristics. Decision latitude and job strain, that is, the demand control model, has shown a relationship between mainly low control (but also the combination of high psychological demands and low control) and an elevated risk of developing myocardial infarction. In the Whitehall study Marmot *et al.* (13) found that men and women in the lowest employment grade had a 50 per cent increased risk, compared to men in the highest grade, of developing symptoms or signs of coronary heart disease. In both genders low control at work explained most of this difference; conventional risk factors made smaller contributions.

It should also be noted that excessive tobacco consumption may be a way of coping with poor working conditions (14). This analysis is useful because it suggests practical ways to do something about the inequalities caused by such working conditions.

Mental health

In the Whitehall II investigation it was found that social support at work protected against psychological distress, whereas effort–reward imbalance, low decision latitude and high psychological demands increased the risk of impaired psychological function (15–17).

In a prospective cohort study from France with one year between the two investigations it was shown that high psychological demands, low decision latitude and poor social support predicted depressive symptoms. Work life events (transfers, reorganizations, etc.) were also associated with an increased risk of depressive symptoms (18).

A few publications have explicitly examined working life conditions as explanations for social class differences in mental health. The Whitehall investigation reported that work characteristics – mainly skill discretion and decision-making authority – explained most of the socioeconomic gradient in well-being and depression in male as well as female civil servants (19). A decline in mental functioning over time was more common among lower-grade than among higher-grade men. Differences in job decision latitude and material problems were major explanations. Among women there were no consistent socioeconomic differences in mental functioning (20).

There are large socioeconomic differences in alcoholism among men. In a study of Swedish men there was a fivefold difference in the risk of hospitaliza-tion as a result of alcoholism between intermediate and higher non-manual workers and unskilled manual workers. This difference was reduced to about twofold by taking account of risk indicators established in adolescence; also, after accounting for work control and demands in adulthood no excess risk remained (2, 21).

Overview of effective interventions and policies

Work environment interventions may affect health differences between social classes by diminishing exposure to the determinants of health problems in the lower socioeconomic groups and by diminishing the effects of ill-health on downward social mobility, particularly from working-class occupations to exclusion from the labour market. In general the same work environment measures will fulfil both these aims.

As shown earlier, working conditions often seem to explain a substantial part of the inequalities in coronary heart disease, as well as mental health and musculoskeletal disorders. This suggests that the work environment should be a major arena for preventive programmes intended to reduce social class differences, but very few, if any, such programmes have been instituted. However, in most countries there is a usually employer-dependent occupational health sector that works to increase productivity, quality and efficiency by improving health. Health inequalities are not a target of such organizations, but rather ill-health whatever its cause.

Moreover, in order to improve productivity, quality and efficiency work life is continuously and rapidly reshaped by market forces, and any intervention intended to improve health will occur against this background. Reviews of intervention projects repeatedly emphasize the difficulty of performing scientifically rigorous projects in this constantly changing environment (discussed later).

For work environment interventions to diminish social class differences in health they must meet two requirements. First, they should reduce ill-health. As will be shown, this is often very difficult to prove. Second, they should benefit the lower social classes. Most work environment interventions aimed at established risk factors will benefit the lower social strata because this is where they are more common. These requirements will be discussed in relation to physical as well as psychosocial hazards in the work environment.

Physical working conditions

Chemical hazards

Working conditions involving health hazards change with the progress of production. Chemical hazards were mainly linked to certain industrial processes, but with automation and increasing productivity there is no longer a need to expose large groups of blue-collar workers to high levels of chemical agents. In industry today much smaller groups are exposed to lower levels of chemical hazards than 30 or 50 years ago. National hygiene standards have reflected these developments and force employers to keep exposures below certain limits. In the case of asbestos (mentioned earlier) its mere use has been severely restricted. The effectiveness of reducing carbon disulphide exposures has been demonstrated by lower coronary heart disease rates (22).

Although effects on social class differences have not been shown, they may be inferred as chemical exposures have affected almost only blue-collar workers.

Muscular load

Work-related musculoskeletal disorders constitute a major problem in many industrialized countries, as shown earlier, and a large number of studies have been published describing interventions that aim to improve musculo-skeletal health by changing certain aspects of the work environment. These have been the subject of recent reviews which unanimously point to the difficulty of evaluating their effects (23–25). The studies suffer from limita-tions concerning the documentation of interventions, lack of control groups, lack of adequate observation periods, generalizability to other settings and too-small study groups. In general, the sustainability of intervention effects seems unproven because of short follow-up periods and, more importantly, the constantly changing environment. Hence, there is no evaluated inter-vention programme that can be applied in other settings with any firm expectation of success. A reasonable conclusion, however, is that interven-tions that attempt to involve the entire organization (including both work-ers and management) in a continuous effort to improve health by reducing identified risk factors, are more often successful (24). More attempts need to be encouraged in this potentially promising field. Probably a focus more on process than on effectiveness could prove as beneficial in musculoskeletal as in stress interventions (discussed later). Most risk factors related to muscular load are distributed so that improvements will benefit lower socioeconomic groups.

Psychosocial conditions and stress

As the technology and organization of production have changed, other fea-tures of the work environment have come to be seen as health hazards, for example, lack of control, or effort–reward imbalance. Such conditions have always affected lower socioeconomic groups more than the higher. The lower the occupational class, for example, the more likely are people to experience low decision latitude and the less reward they are likely to get. There has been growing concern that certain production processes introduced in the post-war period in Europe and America have caused a deterioration in working conditions by introducing alienating and dehumanizing conditions.

Reviews of case studies

A number of articles have reviewed workplace interventions to reduce stress (26–32) (Table 6.2). It is noted that although the literature on the adverse health effects of certain psychosocial conditions is abundant, intervention

Table 6.2 Review of workplace interventions

Objective of the review	Target population	Inclusion criteria	Review type	Conclusion	Reference
To review risk factors for the onset of low back pain and associated disability and to critically summarize intervention studies attempting to achieve prevention	Workers in workplaces without (occupational) low back pain complaints ((O)LBP)	The authors do not specify how they selected the articles to be included	The authors have not conducted their own review. Instead they refer to several reviews of (O)LBP epidemiology	Primary prevention measures focus on reducing the incidence of new episodes of (O)LBP. To achieve their goal, primary prevention interventions typically follow two paths: They aim to: 1. change the workers (job training, behaviour modification, increasing trunk strength). This is the most reported type of intervention, however mixed results are reported. 2. change the work (ergonomic interventions). Very few interventions have produced a clear reduction in (O)LBP incidence. Several reasons: – high cost of interventions – lack of underlying commitment of staff and employees – difficulty in identifying what needs to be changed – uncertainty concerning how best to monitor effect – relatively weak study designs	25

To identify effective ergonomic interventions for improved musculoskeletal health in the workplace and to make recommendations for quality criteria in ergonomic interventions research	Workers in workplaces	Relevant literature was identified by inclusion criteria. Quality criteria were applied to identify studies describing effective interventions	No formal review	Organizational culture interventions with multiple interventions and high stakeholder commitment to reduce identified risk factors were particularly effective. Modifier interventions focusing on workers at risk and using measures which actively involved the individual were also effective	24
To understand why there is conflicting information on whether workplace interventions are effective in preventing low-back disorders	Workers in workplaces without (occupational) low back pain complaints ((O)LBP) although some workers who participated may have had back pain or filed a previous claim	Six studies selected where 1. the intent was to demonstrate primary prevention of low-back disorders 2. An occurrence rate of recordable back injuries or episodes of lost time from work was among the outcomes 3. The studies reported outcomes of interventions that occurred specifically at the workplace 4. The outcomes of the studies were successful. However, the studies were based on different principles: change in organization, introduction of ergonomic devices, back-belt use and back strengthening exercises	Studies were not selected on the basis of methodological quality but rather because, with one exception, they appeared in peer reviewed journals. Four of the six studies did not include a contemporaneous control group and five of the six did not randomize study subjects	The quality of the study design often inversely related to the reported effectiveness of the intervention. Enough pragmatically oriented studies have been conducted to suggest that workplace interventions may have an effect on low-back disorders. More conclusive explanatory studies should be conducted	23

Table 6.2 (Cont'd)

Objective of the review	Target population	Inclusion criteria	Review type	Conclusion	Reference
To establish criteria for success in work-site stress prevention programmes (selected stress prevention programmes aim at modifying the work situation rather than by attending to stress symptoms after the fact)	The majority of studies involve high strain job categories with low decision latitude and high psychological demands (for example, clerical and service workers, auto machinists and operatives, steelworkers and electrical assemblers)	Nineteen case studies commissioned by the International Labour Organization (ILO) of stress prevention programmes in the worksite from nine industrialized and developing countries (Sweden, US, Italy, Mexico, Germany, Japan, UK, Canada and India)	No formal review	Self-sustaining, successful, programmes were characterized by: – employee feelings of self-worth enhanced by understanding stress reactions as normal and legitimate – workers' participation in designing intervention – top management support Failing programmes were characterized by: – programmes treating symptoms only – entirely technical solutions imposed from the top – management retains constant control of the dialogue	27
To analyse and compare various selected projects orientated towards primary stress prevention rather than individual approaches directed towards accommodating stress	Ten Dutch projects from several branches of industry (ministry, prison, cigarette factory, oil company, scaffolding company, bricklaying,	Projects were selected if: – they included a primary preventive work-orientated intervention (for example, job enrichment or increasing workers' autonomy in decision-making)	Six projects were selected since (one of the) authors of this article had been involved as a consultant or (action) researcher.	Successful projects are characterized by: – a stepwise and systematic approach – adequate diagnosis and risk analysis – a combination of measures (work and worker orientated)	30

(continued)	hospital, homes for the elderly, telecommunications and home-care institute) aimed at reducing work stress, physical work load, and sickness absenteeism	– they utilized an adequate stress audit (problem analysis) – they used a minimum methodological standard (evidence obtained without a control group or randomization but with an evaluation) – evaluative data on 'soft' (health complaints) and 'hard' (sickness absenteeism, productivity) outcome variables was available	Four other projects were tracked down through a network approach	– workers involvement (involvement and commitment of both employees and middle management) – top management support
To review current challenges in the conceptualization, design and evaluation of organizational interventions to improve occupational health	Workers in workplaces	No specific inclusion criteria mentioned	No formal review	Less emphasis should be put on identifying causal associations and more on describing the intervention process. Interventions should be examined for conceptualization, design and implementation and mediating mechanisms involved. These processes are likely to be more generalizable than the eventual effect of the programme. Qualitative methods need to be used more

Table 6.2 (Cont'd)

Objective of the review	Target population	Inclusion criteria	Review type	Conclusion	Reference
To contribute to reduce the gap between stress research and practice. To obtain knowledge on evidence-based work stress prevention in Europe	Nine case studies from nine EU countries and different branches of industry (forest industry, hospital, pharmaceutical company, public sector, bus company, mail sorting, airport management company and school of nursing)	Selection criteria were: 1. A prevention and intervention programme had to be carried out 2. Cases should meet a minimum methodological standard (evidence without a control group or randomization, but with an evaluation)	Network approach. Through a network approach national experts were identified in 14 European countries. Each of the national experts was asked to identify and present a national case study in stress prevention	Success factors the same as in (30). Preventive measures based on these factors may simultaneously benefit health and increase productivity.	29
Cardiovascular disease prevention through workplace interventions	Workers in workplaces (for example, viscose rayon workers, policemen, tax accountants, nursing homes, technical services, pharmaceutical company, bus drivers, bank employees)	Ten studies were selected which were considered to be informative in relation to the objective of the review (interventions concerning physical and chemical factors, interventions related to work schedules and interventions on psychosocial job characteristics)	No formal review	Intervention studies need integration to be successful, integration between interventions at different levels; between primary, secondary and tertiary prevention; between mass, high-risk, and environmental approaches; between different disciplines. Intervention research give insights in aetiology as well as feasibility that can not be gained in any other way.	31

| To select, compare, and analyse interventions and preventive actions that international bus companies have taken to decrease occupational stress and sickness absenteeism among bus drivers | Bus drivers from four EU countries (Germany, the Netherlands, Sweden and Denmark) | Selection criteria were:
1. Projects had to be directed at bus drivers in city and rural transport
2. A prevention and intervention programme had to be carried out
3. Cases should meet a minimum methodological standard (evidence without a control group or randomization, but with an evaluation) | Cases were selected through (a) networking among international researchers and through the study of the scientific and 'grey' literature and (b) national and international organizations of employers and employees | Stress prevention that combines adequate interventions and proper implementation may benefit health and increase productivity | 28 |

studies to improve them are few. There are several reasons for this: companies are inclined towards individual-orientated interventions (such as stress management); there is a lack of strong designs in evaluation research; many interventions are not evaluated; and study designs often show serious methodological flaws. Regardless of their main aim, success factors in work environment interventions seem to include an adequate analysis of risk factors and risk groups, interventive measures fit to this analysis, and sustained commitment from top management as well as lower management and workers.

To date, initiatives have been confined to separate workplaces and the scale of the operations has been insufficient to measure the influence of changes in health indicators across occupational groups. There also needs to be political commitment at the highest levels to encourage larger-scale changes. Sweden has made some progress on this front. The Swedish Working Life Fund (the equivalent of 1,300 million Euros), raised by a levy on business, offered financial grants as incentives for companies to make improvements in the worst conditions in line with the 1991–5 legislation. Unfortunately, such large-scale intervention was never systematically evaluated, as no evaluation was planned from the beginning and *a posteriori* evaluations of the interventions in particular sectors did not produce coherent results.

Participatory ergonomic teams for hospital orderlies

High rates of work-related injuries are seen among healthcare workers involved in lifting and transferring patients. A prospective trial examined work injuries and other outcomes among hospital orderlies before and after an intervention, using other hospital employees as controls (33).

A participatory ergonomics team was formed with three orderlies, one supervisor, and technical advisers. This team designed and implemented changes in training and work practices. All 100–110 orderlies in the 1,200-bed urban hospital were studied using passively collected data, and around 70 per cent of them responded to questionnaires.

The ergonomics team members received an initial eight-hour training session, which included exercises for team-building, the provision of basic technical information on hazard identification and control, and supervised exercises in observation and measurement. The team met weekly to identify job factors that contributed to injuries among orderlies, and to seek solutions to perceived job hazards. The team had limited authority to make changes in work processes. The three authors provided technical assistance by meeting regularly with the team to address questions and provide information as needed. Team members were responsible for identifying and prioritizing safety problems and for evaluating and implementing possible solutions.

Several factors contributing to injury were identified, the two major ones being the lack of standard procedures for lifting and moving patients, and inconsistent training procedures for employees. There were also concerns about specific types of lifts, the underuse of mechanical lifting equipment, and the occurrence of injuries when moving hospital equipment such as beds and scales.

The intervention began by implementing standardized lifting techniques and training all orderlies in their use. The team members established standard techniques for twelve common types of lift and transfer, including those requiring mechanical aids. Manual lifts and transfers were all performed by two persons; the procedures emphasized such precautions as using a draw sheet, positioning beds at convenient heights, and the avoidance of a bent-waist posture while lifting. Special procedures were developed for very heavy patients.

A lifting manual was written by the team members, and training included both practical experience working with a senior orderly and a written examination that had to be completed satisfactorily before the trainee could work independently. New employees were required to complete training successfully before being allowed to work independently.

By the end of the 2-year intervention period the risks of injury, per 100 workers, were reduced by around 60 per cent and were close to levels among other hopital employees. Lost work time due to injury, per 100 workers, was reduced by 75 per cent and had fallen to about the same level as among other hospital employees. Annual workers' compensation costs declined markedly. The proportion of workers with musculoskeletal symptoms declined and there were statistically significant improvements in job satisfaction, perceived psychosocial stressors, and social support among the orderlies.

Preventing stress among bus drivers

The origin of this programme was the wish of the Stockholm bus company to improve the operating efficiency of a major downtown bus route. The intervention emphasized physical design changes and technological innovation to reduce traffic congestion and lessen passenger demands on the drivers (34, 35). Measures included:

- an increase in the number and length of separated bus lanes, mainly in the middle lane of the road;
- a reduced number of bus stops;
- active signal priority, with green lights to oncoming buses;
- automated passenger information on all approaching bus stops and adjoining transfer routes. Computerized information on the arrival of the next bus was displayed at the bus stops.

As this intervention might also improve drivers' health, the researchers suggested to the bus company a work environment and health assessment of the intervention and this proposal was accepted. The participants were full-time bus drivers who were already working on the intervention route or control routes. Data were collected before and after the intervention through questionnaires, observation of job hassles en route, and certain psycho-physiological measurements. The final analysis was based on only a few drivers (8–13 in the intervention group and 10–31 controls). It was found that perceived stress and the number of hassles on the route decreased significantly among the intervention drivers. Heart rate also decreased significantly in this group, and systolic blood pressure was significantly decreased among both intervention and control drivers.

This project obviously has many advantages when it comes to promoting health as well as reducing social class differences in health by changing the work environment: It is aimed at a high-risk group of blue-collar workers for whom work stress is suspected as a major cause of their increased incidence of myocardial infarction. The preventive efforts were aimed at diminishing the causes of this stress, rather than supporting individual handling of it. These causes were largely the same as those identified by the bus company as reducing efficiency among the drivers. Hence the efficiency requirements were well matched to what would be likely to promote health.

The programme involved drivers on a route with particular stress problems as well as drivers on a control route with less stress exposure, where no measures were taken, thereby facilitating an evaluation of the effectiveness of the programme.

The programme could be evaluated in terms of subjective and objective signs of stress, and showed a reduction of subjective stress as well as signs of stress in the intervention group. It could be shown that a reduction in job hassles greatly contributed to this stress reduction, that is, a mechanism for the beneficial effect of the programme was found.

Through the common interest of the drivers, the bus company and a large political majority in the Stockholm City Council, the measures taken have been largely sustainable and to some extent even extended, and should thus, all things being equal, have improved health among bus drivers and diminished social class differences in health.

Conclusions

Work and production are the basis for all means of welfare, including health. Large differences in health outcomes between different occupational groups are found even in the most advanced countries, where the most obvious health hazards have been eliminated, regulated and controlled. Research from the past two decades has demonstrated the importance of workers' influence on the pace and content of work and its effects on coronary heart disease, mental health and musculoskeletal disorders, but many workplaces still have unacceptable safety risks and exposures. The most obvious intervention to improve the health situation is therefore to correct these hazards.

Interventions are continuously carried out by companies to improve efficiency; sometimes they involve changes in working conditions which are risk factors for disease and illness, but very seldom is health itself evaluated. A very small fraction of such interventions are ever published and contribute to general knowledge. Assessment of interventions and programmes to protect or promote health, as well as the publication of such efforts, needs to be encouraged. Analysis of health consequences for the workers of major restructuring processes is a reasonable demand in terms of company efficiency as well as workers' health.

As shown in this chapter, working conditions often seem to explain a substantial part of social class differences in coronary heart disease, as well as mental health and musculoskeletal disorders. This suggests that the working environment should be a major arena for preventive programmes intended to reduce social class differences. A systematic exploration of the role of working conditions in explaining social class differences in general health and specific disorders is thus warranted, but such an effort must take account of the continuous selection processes that give those with good health and few risk factors the best jobs and those with bad health and many risk factors worse jobs or none at all.

References

1. Paoli P. *Second European Survey on Working Conditions*. European Foundation for the Improvement of Living and Working Conditions. Dublin, 1997.
2. Hemmingsson T, Lundberg I, Diderichsen F, Allebeck P. Explanations of social class differences in alcoholism among young men. *Alcoholism: Clinical and Experimental Research* 1998: 4: 662–8.
3. West P, Macintyre S, Annandale E, Hunt K. Social class and health in youth: findings from the West of Scotland twenty-07 study. *Social Science and Medicine* 1990: 30: 665–73.
4. Pukkala E. Cancer risk by social class and occupation: a survey of 109,000 cancer cases among Finns of working age. In: *Contributions to Epidemiology and Biostatistics* 7. Karger. Basel 1995.
5. Vågerö D, Persson G. Occurrence of cancer in socioeconomic groups in Sweden. An analysis based on the Swedish Cancer Environment Registry. *Scand J Soc Med* 1986: 14: 151–60.
6. Boffetta P, Kogevinas M, Westerholm P, Saracci R. Exposure to occupational carcinogens and social class differences in cancer occurrence. *IARC Scientific Publications* 138: 331–41. Lyon, 1997.
7. Jarvholm B, Larsson S, Hagberg S *et al*. Quantitative importance of asbestos as a cause of lung cancer in a Swedish industrial city. *Eur Respir J* 1993: 6: 1271–5.
8. Gustavsson P, Jakobsson R, Nyberg F, Pershagen G, Järup L, Scheele P. Occupational exposure and lung cancer risk: a population-based case-referent study in Sweden. *Am J Epidemiol* 2000: 152: 32–40.
9. Peto J, Hodgson J, Matthews F, Jones J. Continuing increase in mesothelioma mortality in Britain. *Lancet* 1995: 345: 535–9.

10. Hagberg M, Wegman DH. Prevalence rates and odds ratios of shoulder-neck diseases in different occupational groups. *British Journal of Industrial Medicine* 1987: 44: 602–10.

11. Dhondt S, Houtman I. *Indicators of Working Conditions in the European Union.* Loughlinstown, Co. Dublin: European Foundation for the Improvement of Living and Working Conditions; Luxembourg: Office for Official Publications of the European Communities, Lantham, Md.: Bernan Associates (distributor), 1997.

12. Steenland K, Fine L, Belkic K, Landsbergis P, Schnall P, Baker D, Theorell T, Siegrist J, Peter R, Karasek R, Marmot M, Brisson C, Tuchsen F. Research findings linking workplace factors to CVD outcomes. *Occupational Medicine* 2000: 15: 7–68.

13. Marmot M, Bosma H, Hemingway H, Brunner E, Stansfeld S. Contribution of job control and other risk factors to social variations in coronary heart disease incidence. *Lancet* 1997: 350: 235–9.

14. Marmot M, Theorell T. Social class and cardiovascualr disease: the contribution of work. *Int J Health Services* 1988: 18: 659–74.

15. Stansfeld SA, Fuhrer R, Head J, Ferrie J, Shipley M. Work and psychiatric disorder in the Whitehall II study. *J Psychosom Res* 1997: 43: 73–81.

16. Stansfeld SA, Bosma H, Hemingway H, Marmot MG. Psychosocial work characteristics and social support as predictors of SF-36 health functioning. *Psychosom Med* 1998: 60: 247–55.

17. Stansfeld SA, Fuhrer R, Shipley MJ, Marmot MG. Work characteristics predict psychiatric disorder: prospective results from the Whitehall II study. *Occup Environ Med* 1999: 56: 302–7.

18. Niedhammer I, Goldberg M, Leclerc A, Bugel I, David S. Psychosocial factors at work and subsequent depressive symptoms in the Gazel cohort. *Scand J Work Environ Health* 1998: 24: 197–205.

19. Stansfeld S, Head J, Marmot M. Explaining social class differences in depression and well-being. *Social Psychiatry & Psychiatric Epidemiology* 1998: 33: 1–9.

20. Martikainen P, Stansfeld S, Hemingway H, Marmot M. Determinants of socio-economic differences in change in physical and mental functioning. *Soc Sci Med* 1999: 49: 499–507.

21. Hemmingsson T. *Explanations of Differences in Alcoholism Between Social Classes and Occupations among Swedish Men – a register based follow up study.* Karolinska institutet, Stockholm, 1999.

22. Nurminen M, Hernberg S. Effects of intervention on the cardiovascular mortality of workers exposed to carbon disulphide: A 15-year follow up. *Br J Ind Med* 1985: 42: 32–5.

23. Volinn E. Do workplace interventions prevent low-back disorders? If so, why?: a methodological commentary. *Ergonomics* 1999: 42: 258–72.

24. Westgaard RH, Winkel J. Ergonomic intervention research for improved musculoskeletal health: A critical review. *International Journal of Industrial Ergonomics* 1997: 20: 463–500.

25. Frank J, Kerr M, Brooker AS, DeMaio S, Maetzel A, Shannon H, Sullivan T, Norman R, Wells R. Disability resulting from occupational low back pain. Part I: What do we know about primary prevention? A review of the scientific evidence on prevention before disability begins. *Spine* 1996: 21: 2908–17.

26. Karasek R, Theorell T. Healthy Work. *Stress, Productivity and the Reconstruction of Working Life*. New York: Basic Books, 1990.

27. Karasek R. Stress prevention through work reorganisation: A summary of 19 international case studies. In: *International Labour Organisation, Conditions of Work Digest*, volume 11, number 2, Geneva: ILO, 1992: 23–41.

28. Kompier M, Aust B, van den Berg AM, Siegrist J. Stress prevention in bus drivers: Evaluation of 13 natural experiments. *J Occup Health Psychol* 2000: 5: 11–31.

29. Kompier M, Cooper C, Geurts S. A multiple case study approach to work stress prevention in Europe. *Europ J Work Organization Psychol* 2000: 9: 371–400.

30. Kompier M, Geurts S, Gründemann R, Vink P, Smulders P. Cases in stress prevention: The success of a participative and stepwise approach. *Stress Medicine* 1998: 14: 155–68.

31. Kristensen T. Workplace intervention studies. *Occupational Medicine: State of the Art Reviews* 15, 2000: 293–305.

32. Griffiths A. Organisational interventions: Facing the limits of the natural science paradigm. *Scand J Work Environ Health* 2000: 6: 589–96.

33. Evanoff BA, Bohr PC, Wolf LD. Effects of a participatory ergonomics team among hospital orderlies. *Am J of Industrial Medicine* 1999: 35: 358–65.

34. Rydstedt L, Johansson G, Evans G. The human side of the road: Improving the working conditions of urban bus drivers. *J Occup Health Psychol* 1998: 3: 161–71.

35. Evans G, Johansson G, Rydstedt L. Hassles on the job: a study of a job intervention with urban bus drivers. *J Organiz Behav* 1999: 20: 198–208.

7 Food and nutrition policies and interventions

Ritva Prättälä, Gun Roos, Karin Hulshof and Marita Sihto

Introduction

In this chapter we explore socioeconomic inequalities in diet, with a particular focus on European food and nutrition policies. To find out whether there are empirical studies on the impact of universalist versus selectivist food and nutrition policies and interventions, literature searches based on Medline and Social Science Citation Index were performed. Two cases, Finland and The Netherlands, are described in terms of policies and interventions that affect socioeconomic inequalities in diet.

Contribution of food and nutrition to the explanation of socioeconomic inequalities in health

A review in 15 European countries showed that high educational level is associated with a more healthy diet (1, 2). Those with a higher education, with the exception of southern European countries, tend to consume more vegetables, fruits and cheese and less fats and oils. Differences in the intakes of energy-yielding nutrients are less evident, but those with a high level of education tend to have a smaller intake of fat (1). The diets of the less advantaged are not in all respects less healthy than the diets of the advantaged. For example, in Finland the lower social groups consume more rye bread and potatoes (3, 4).

Obesity also varies with socioeconomic status. According to a study based on 26 mostly European populations, lower education was associated with higher body mass index (BMI) in about half of male and almost all of the female population. Over the past ten years there has been a small shift towards a stronger inverse association (5).

Different energy needs and cultural and social factors have been suggested as causes of nutritional inequalities (4–8). Social groups have different priorities regarding food consumption and different ideas about what constitutes healthy eating (9). A higher educational level tends to be associated with a wider knowledge about healthy diet (10). Poverty and low income may restrict the ability to buy food on the basis of health and limit access to healthy foods (11, 12).

Dowler *et al.* (11) summarize European findings on the effects of poverty and low income. Foods preferred by the poor vary according to cultural practice, region and place of residence. Poor people tend to consume less fresh fruit and vegetables and more cheap, high-fat, high-sugar foods than those who are better off. For people on a low income the choice of food depends critically on access, how much money they can allocate to food and how much it costs. In order to avoid being hungry, poor people choose familiar, filling foods and are less concerned about the nutrient content – even though they know they should eat more fruits and vegetables and avoid excess fat.

Nutrient deficiencies may be observed in connection with serious social or health problems, but there is not much evidence of lack of energy and macronutrients among the European poor. For example, according to German surveys income has no major influence on nutrient intake (13). In cases where differences do exist, the less advantaged have lower levels of intakes of certain minerals and vitamins, such as iron and vitamin C (14).

When socioeconomic differences in food and nutrition are observed, they are generally in line with health inequalities. The poor in affluent societies do not suffer from dramatic energy and nutrient deficiencies: in fact, overnutrition seems to be more common than undernutrition.

The contribution of behavioural factors, including food behaviour, to socioeconomic inequalities in health is not well understood (6). On the other hand, health behaviours such as food consumption and obesity explain a large proportion of the overall mortality and morbidity in Europe (15–18). Where socioeconomic inequalities in behaviours are in line with those in mortality and morbidity, they can be assumed to contribute to the overall inequalities.

Overview of interventions and policies

Policies and interventions to reduce nutritional inequalities can be universalistic or selectivist. Universal measures are directed to the population as a whole, with the idea that all citizens should have equal access to healthy foods. This approach does not always aim explicitly to diminish inequalities. Selective measures aim at improving the condition of the least advantaged.

Food-related inequality and the balance between the universalist and selectivist principles have been central themes in European food and nutrition policies. Since the nineteenth century, food and nutrition policies have gone through four phases characterized by different emphases on universalism and selectivism (19). In the introductory phase in the middle of the nineteenth century food policies were philanthropic in origin and their impact was highly selective. This approach changed when poverty became politicized and governments became concerned with both industrial and military manpower. Also, the second phase was related to the selective identification of groups at risk and meeting their needs. The third phase was generated after the Second World War, when food policies became associated with welfare state programmes and acquired the principle of universality. The fourth phase emerged by the 1970s, when social welfare provisions were considered to take too high a share of the gross national product. Governments began to limit the high-cost universal policies and to choose more selectivist approaches. The universalist and selectivist phases can be identified even if there is considerable variation in timing in the different European regions. In the following, recent interventions and policies are discussed from the point of view of universalism and selectivism.

Food and nutrition interventions

The search identified 32 interventions (Table 7.1). Specific information about the way this review was conducted is included in the Appendix.

Most interventions followed the selective approach: they were targeted at the less advantaged groups, such as low-income mothers, ethnic groups in deprived areas, or homeless young people. The search also located two reviews, one of North American programmes (20) and another one of programmes in Atlantic Canada (21).

Devaney *et al.* (20) reviewed four selectivist North American food and nutrition programmes, the Food Stamp Program (FSP), the Special Supplemental Food Program for Women, Infants and Children (WIC), the National School Lunch Program (NSLP) and the School Breakfast Program (SBP), which were intended to mitigate the effects of poverty on low-income children. The authors based their judgements on the effectiveness of these programmes on the accumulated evidence produced by repeated studies. They considered them to be successful in providing food assistance to low-income children and in benefiting children proportionately more than other population groups. However, there was little scientific information on their long-term effects.

Selective interventions have been criticized for not diminishing the differences between higher and lower socioeconomic groups. McIntyre *et al.* (21) studied nine selective children's feeding programmes in Atlantic Canada, analysing school meal programmes through observation and interviews with recipients and operators. Even if the programmes were aimed at feeding children who did not get enough food at home, it was recognized that the majority of those who attended were not poor: their reasons for attending were convenience and socializing. In addition, the programmes tended to contribute to stigmatization: 'everyone knew who the kids were who really needed to be there'. The authors concluded that these programmes reproduced, rather than reduced, inequalities.

Typically, evaluations concluded that the intervention had at least some of the expected outcomes (Table 7.1). For example, effective interventions have included not only a well planned and structured programme, but also a monitoring and reinforcement system designed for the needs of the target

Table 7.1 Interventions to reduce nutritional inequalities

Objective	Target population	Intervention	Effect of intervention	Evidence	Reference
Intervention aimed at low SES-groups, reported to be effective					
Cardiovascular disease prevention	Low-income adults at risk for CVD (USA)	1. Validated risk assessment 2. Structured diet treatment programme 3. Monitoring and reinforcement system	Patients report more behaviourally focused counselling from their physician, greater understanding of recommended dietary change and more confidence in ability to make dietary changes	Quasi-experimental design	61
Improvement of nutritional status (fruits and vegetables)	Low-income elders (USA)	Farmers' market coupons redeemable for fresh produce at farmers' markets	Fruits and vegetables are most frequently purchased with the coupons (very weak study)	Cross-sectional survey (no control group)	62
Nutritional risk (anaemia, inadequate weight gain etc.)	Pregnant and postpartum women, infants and young children who qualify for benefits (USA)	Federal nutrition program ($35 monthly vouchers for the purchase of high-nutrient foods)	The programme helps poor mothers and poor children by producing healthier pregnancy outcomes, higher birthweights and fewer fetal deaths	Observational study	63
Improve dietary behaviour	Low-income women (USA)	Computer-based intervention: a. tailored soap opera b. interactive 'info-mercials'	Reduction in fat consumption not different between study groups. But the intervention group reports improvement in knowledge, stage of change and eating behaviours	RCT	64
Cardiovascular disease prevention	Recent adult immigrants (primarily Latinos) (USA)	Five 3-hour classes which incorporate heart health/nutrition education, designed specifically for multicultural adults with limited English proficiency	Effects of the intervention on nutrition knowledge and fat avoidance, only short-term effects on total cholesterol : total HDL and systolic blood pressure	Two-group repeated-measures design	65

Table 7.1 (Cont'd)

Objective	Target population	Intervention	Effect of intervention	Evidence	Reference
Improve dietary behaviour	Low-income Hispanic-American families (USA)	12-week culture-specific cancer prevention curriculum encouraging adoption of a low-fat, high-fibre diet	Parental support is related to changes in diet, nutrition knowledge. Dietary changes were seen only in the experimental group	RCT	66
Improvement of nutritional status	Adults holding Healthcare Cards (low income earners) (Australia)	a. Recommended spending model b. Resources addressing barriers to healthy eating c. Group activities to enhance knowledge and skills	Positive changes in participants' self-reported dietary, cooking and shopping behaviours	Observational study with pre/post tests. No control group	67
Cardiovascular risk reduction	Primary school children in low SES neighbourhoods (Australia)	3 groups: 1. School-based CVD risk-reduction programme (BOM) 2. BOM + programme for teachers and school canteens 3. Control	Group 2 reports reduction in blood pressure, total cholesterol and triglyceride concentration and increase in nutrition and health knowledge	Quasi-experimental design	68
Reduction of fat intake	Low-income adults (USA)	Low-fat nutrition education curriculum and additional materials	24-hour dietary interviews suggest a positive effect on low-fat eating (no statistical significance)	Quasi-experimental design	69
Fruit and vegetable consumption	Low-income women (USA)	a. Nutrition sessions by peer educators b. Printed materials and visual reminders c. Direct mail	Daily consumption increases. Intervention participants show greater changes in stages of change, knowledge, attitudes and self-efficacy	Randomized crossover design	70–73

Aim	Population	Intervention	Result	Study type	Ref.
Lower food costs to promote better nutrition	Isolated low-income communities in Northern Canada (Canada)	Food mail (selective transportation subsidy)	Costs of nutritious perishable food have been reduced, and consumption of these foods doubled within 3 years	Observational study	74
Iron deficiency	Low-income children (UK)	Dietary education screening for iron deficiency, sickle cell disease and thalassaemia	Screening children was acceptable and successful	Observational study	75
Reduction of fat intake	Low-literacy, low income adults (USA)	6-week classroom-based intervention followed by 12-week maintenance intervention (by telephone or mail)	Improvement in nutrition knowledge, attitudes and self-efficacy. Greater reduction in % of calories from total fat and saturated fat	RCT	76
Nutritional status	Low-income children (USA)	Housing subsidies	Receiving housing subsidy is associated with increased growth	Observational study	77
Fruit and vegetable consumption	Community health centres (low-income residents) (USA)	a. Minimal intervention b. Worksite intervention c. Worksite + family intervention	Controlled for baseline variables such as worksite, education and occupation; total fruit and vegetable intake increased by 19 per cent in the worksite + family group, 7 per cent in the worksite group and 0 per cent in the minimal intervention group	RCT	78–80
Fat intake	Adults with low literacy skills (USA)	Classroom-based dietary fat intake reduction curriculum	23 per cent of intervention group with moderate baseline dietary fat intake met intervention goal (<30 per cent of calories from total fat). Participants with high baseline intake were much less successful	RCT	81

Table 7.1 (Cont'd)

Objective	Target population	Intervention	Effect of intervention	Evidence	Reference
Intervention aimed at low SES-groups, reported to be non-effective					
Iron deficiency anaemia	Children (inner city, deprived population) (UK)	Health education information at key ages by face to face contact (+materials)	No difference in iron intake between the two groups	RCT	82
Nutrition education	LSES women (UK)	Groups: a. Video and booklet (motivational material) b. Video and booklet	No differences in nutritional knowledge scores between groups	Quasi-experimental design	83
Energy status	Poor elderly persons (USA)	Food Stamp Program (FSP)	The FSP was not consistently associated with differences in energy status	Observational study	84
Iron deficiency	Poor elderly persons (USA)	Food Stamp Program (FSP)	The FSP was not consistently associated with better iron nutrition	Observational study	85
Improvement of nutritional status	Children from lower socioeconomic background (Canada)	Children's feeding programmes	Children's feeding programmes result in stigmatization of participants and families. They reproduce, rather than reduce, inequalities	Observational study	21
Nutrition	Low-income primary school children (UK)	Increase in Family Credit (to compensate for right to free school meals)	This policy change has led to a significant drop in uptake of school meals	Observational study	86
Fruit and vegetable consumption	Low-income families with young children (USA)	a. Advertising campaign b. Cooking events	Self-reported fruit and vegetable intake did not change	Quasi-experimental design	87

Intervention aimed at general population, reported to be at least as effective in low as in high SES-groups

Cardiovascular disease prevention	Adults (Sweden)	Small-scale, action-orientated and community-based programme with a multiple risk factor approach.	Relative risk of hypercholesterolaemia dropped substantially and significantly. No clear changes in perceived good health	Repeated cross-sectional surveys in study area (random sample Sweden Monica study, reference population)	88
Fat consumption	Adults (The Netherlands)	Computer-tailored written nutrition education	No difference in impact between educational groups. Respondents with low education more positive about tailored letters	RCT	89
Fruit and vegetable consumption	Elementary school children (4th and 5th grades) (USA)	6-week, 18-session curriculum	Although some small increases were observed, substantially increasing fruit and vegetable intake seems to be a problem that resists school-based nutrition education	Quasi-experimental design	90
Cardiovascular disease prevention	Middle-aged men with high-risk for coronary heart disease (Norway)	Diet advice	Analysis of social class reveals that the favourable results in the intervention group were present in all social strata, despite the unexpected finding that lower-class men experienced a lower CHD incidence than men of higher socioeconomic status	RCT	23
Preventing weight gain	Adults (USA)	Three conditions: a. Education through monthly newsletters b. Education + incentives c. Control	Positive changes in frequency of weighing and healthy dieting practices. No differences in weight. No differences between SES groups on outcomes	Quasi-experimental design	91

Table 7.1 (Cont'd)

Objective	Target population	Intervention	Effect of intervention	Evidence	Reference
Pellagra (nutritional deficiency disease)	General population (USA)	Niacin and other B vitamins fortification of cereal-grain products (federal regulations, state laws and other national activities)	Results provide support for the belief that food fortification played a significant role in the elimination of pellagra in the USA	Chronological comparison of recorded annual cases, deaths and death rates from pellagra for selected critical years	92
Fruit and vegetable consumption	Elementary school children (4th grade) (USA)	Behavioural curricula, parental involvement/ education, school food service changes, and industry involvement and support	Increase in lunchtime fruit and combined fruit/vegetable consumption and daily fruit consumption as well as total daily calories attributable to fruits and vegetables	RCT	93

Intervention aimed at general population, reported to be less effective in low than in high SES-groups

Objective	Target population	Intervention	Effect of intervention	Evidence	Reference
Growth	Children (England, Scotland)	1. School meals 2. Lunches prepared at home	No relation between rate of growth and school meals in UK. In Scotland, indication that children with school meals have smaller rate of growth	Observational study	94
Height	Primary school children (England, Scotland)	School meals and school milk policies	No consistent association between provision of school meals or school milk and the rate of growth when stratified according to poverty status and ethnic background	Observational study	95

group. Interventions that, in addition to information and personal assistance (for example, food coupons), take into account the cultural, economic and social conditions of the group are the most effective. Evaluation studies of selective interventions do not, however, answer questions about the distribution of inequalities in a society. For example, an intervention directed at homeless men may improve their diet, but little can be concluded on differences between the homeless and other men.

Den Hartog's (22) historical study of the Dutch school feeding programmes summarizes well the problems of using selective approaches in food-related interventions:

> School feeding is an example . . . which did not take fully into account . . . the social meaning of food. It was based on wrong principles by linking school feeding with poverty. A food policy measure associated by the beneficiaries with a social stigma will have no lasting effect.
>
> (Den Hartog 1994 (22))

Universalist interventions dealing with dietary or other behavioural changes have been criticized for benefiting more the privileged groups. The Oslo study (23), a universalist intervention, showed a similar impact on middle-aged men in all socioeconomic groups. Also in the North Karelia project, a community intervention in Eastern Finland aimed at changing, for example, dietary behaviour in the community, the beneficial effects were observed in all socioeconomic groups (24). These and a few other interventions aimed at the general population suggest that universalist lifestyle interventions do not automatically widen the gap between socioeconomic groups: in fact, there is very little evidence of widening (Table 7.1).

Food and nutrition policies

Literature searches through the Social Science Citation Index yielded 20 references dealing with food and nutrition policies and socioeconomic inequalities, only three of which had a special focus on Europe. Studies analysing food and nutrition policies in relation to health inequalities were very rare. The search did not identify any comparative descriptions of food and nutrition policies in European countries, nor did it yield references to studies analysing long-term trends in nutritional inequalities and relating these to parallel policies and social change within a country.

Most reports were prescriptive (normative) (25): they discussed what types of policies ought to be adopted to improve the nutritional situation of the less privileged without investigating the impacts of policies empirically.

In producing normative food and nutrition policy documents the WHO European office has had a central role. The First Action Plan for Food and Nutrition Policy European region (26) states that reducing inequalities is one of its main aims. The emphasis is universalist. The document recommends attempts to encourage the consumption of vegetables and fruit through financial mechanisms. Partnerships with food retailers, mass catering agencies and local food producers should also be strengthened. The specified goal related to nutritional inequalities is: 'By the year 2005, all countries should have implemented policies to increase access to vegetables and fruit, especially for low-income groups, older people and the most vulnerable'.

The WHO European office has also collected information on current food and nutrition policies in the member states. A survey on food and nutrition policies (27) mailed to the 57 member countries included 'caring for the deprived and vulnerable' as a policy topic. This was mentioned in the majority of the 36 country reports. The respondents listed some selective interventions and policy actions: food and consumer knowledge as a part of introductory programmes for refugees; local projects in schools and women's groups; and developing food products for children. Parts of the described programmes were broader structural measures of a universalist nature, such as school feeding programmes, food norms for catering services, and strengthening of basic health services. In addition, the member states mentioned general policy actions improving the health and welfare of the deprived (27).

To exemplify measures to reduce nutritional inequalities two cases will be presented, Finland and The Netherlands, because:

- In both countries the intake of saturated fat has been considered an important public health problem and several programmes have been set up to deal with it.
- The long research traditions of social and public health nutrition and health inequalities in the two countries have resulted in relevant dietary studies and other documents.
- The Finnish health and nutrition policies have a strong universalist emphasis, whereas in The Netherlands selective measures can also be identified.

The cases trace chronological changes in food and nutrition policies, in food-related inequalities, and in general socioeconomic developments that could have affected these inequalities.

Example: Finland

The Finnish nutrition policies have followed the Nordic welfare ideology where universalism has been the general principle (28, 29). With regard to nutrition this means promoting equal access to recommended foods for everyone, with no particular emphasis on the underprivileged.

Universalism is apparent in the development of catering services. Meals eaten outside the home are common in Finland (30) and special dietary guidelines have been developed for school, hospital and workplace kitchens and so on. All Finnish children have received a free meal at elementary school since 1948. The same benefit has gradually also included primary and secondary school pupils. University students have received subsidized meals since 1979 (31).

Finland has a long tradition of nutrition committees and dietary recommendations (1, 25). Since the early 1980s these recommendations have systematically emphasized the need to reduce the intake of saturated fats. Finns have been advised to reduce their consumption of butter, cream, high-fat cheeses and other high-fat milk products, and to replace them sparingly with margarine, vegetable oils, skimmed milk and other low-fat milk products. Food-related inequalities have not been high on the political agenda: they were recognized in the documents of the early 1980s, but programmes to tackle them have not been suggested (32).

Since the 1970s several campaigns have supported the implementation of these dietary recommendations. The North Karelia project (33), originally directed at one Finnish province with exceptionally high cardiovascular morbidity and mortality, is probably the most famous. A healthy diet and reduced intake of saturated fats was a central goal of the project, and similar favourable changes were observed in all socioeconomic groups. In general, dietary recommendations have been well accepted (34), even in less advantaged groups such as working-class men (35, 36).

The Finnish agricultural policy has not been nutrition orientated. However, political changes over the past 20 years have been favourable for nutrition. Measures to reduce dairy production have been designed and, since 1990, milk subsidies have been paid on the basis of protein rather than fat content (37). Furthermore, a new type of rape plant high in monounsaturated fat was bred. Lately also, the food industry has been actively involved in developing products containing less fat and a larger proportion of vegetable oil.

The Finnish food price, subsidy and tax policy measures have traditionally favoured dairy fats rather than fats/oils of plant origin (37). However, since 1995 membership of the European Union (EU) has improved the competitiveness of plant oils and margarines: the price of margarine has dropped from 70 per cent to 60 per cent of that of butter (38).

The Finnish trends in fat consumption have been favourable for health. For example, during the past twenty years the overall consumption of vegetable oils and margarines has increased, whereas consumption of butter has decreased (30, 39).

In the early 1980s male farmers and blue-collar workers consumed more saturated fats than did white-collar workers (40), but since the 1990s hardly any socioeconomic differences in the intake of fats have been observed (4, 41). Educational differences in the use of butter on bread and in drinking high-fat milk diminished between 1978 and 1998, along with a clear decrease in the use of these foods. The use of low-fat milk and margarine followed an opposite pattern: their consumption increased without a significant change in educational differences (42, 43).

Many structural changes in Finnish society have promoted healthy nutrition since the late 1970s. Standards of living and the general educational level have risen. Urbanization has continued – and indeed has increased since Finland joined the EU. These changes have created circumstances whereby the public's interest in healthy nutrition has increased, and everyone is better able to choose the recommended foods.

The Finnish case shows that socioeconomic differences in the use of butter and high-fat milk decreased at the same time as their total consumption decreased. In evaluating the factors that contributed to these changes, two issues need to be considered. First, this decrease started before nutritional inequalities were even on the agenda. Second, no selective interventions have been directed at reducing fat intake in the lower socioeconomic groups. These favourable changes took place because:

- The foods to be avoided – butter and high-fat milk – had healthier alternatives, such as margarine and skimmed milk.
- Choosing the healthier alternatives did not increase costs – the price of margarine relative to that of butter declined.
- The healthier alternatives were served by mass catering – margarine and low-fat milk were served in schools, hospitals, workplace canteens, etc.
- People were aware of the dietary recommendations and accepted them.

Example: The Netherlands

In The Netherlands, food and nutrition policies and interventions have followed the universalist principles as well, but since the early 1990s programmes targeted at the underprivileged have been emphasized (44, 45). Lifestyle-related risk factors, such as smoking, excessive alcohol use, lower consumption of vegetables and fruit, and less physical activity, have been mentioned as reasons for socioeconomic inequalities (46).

An example of a universalist measure is the school milk programme, which since 1937 has offered the opportunity for pupils in primary and secondary schools to obtain subsidized milk (47); in contrast to Finland, however, no school meal system is available in The Netherlands. From 1958 to 1977 all university students had the opportunity to have a hot meal at a relatively low price. However, owing to students' improved social position, good kitchen facilities in their lodgings and the increase in lunch opportunities within the universities, the participation rates became very low, and at the end of 1977 the programme ceased (48).

In 1984 a comprehensive nutrition report was adopted by parliament as a policy document. In 1986 dietary guidelines for a healthy diet, including nutrient goals, were issued (49), and in 1991 these were revised (50). The need to reduce the population's fat intake, especially the consumption of saturated fats, was underlined. The documents also recommended the surveillance of dietary patterns to obtain an insight into the consumption of food and the ensuing intake of energy and nutrients, so as to enable the identification of risk groups.

Although low education and low socioeconomic status are associated with a higher fat consumption and a less healthy diet (7, 51, 52), most national interventions have been offered to the general population and are only analysed by socioeconomic status afterwards. However, out of the four nationwide dietary interventions implemented between 1993 and 1998, three were selective to the less advantaged (53).

Reduction of fat intake was in the early 1990s the special focus of national intervention programmes and campaigns, for example, the 'Fat Watch'. This recognized socioeconomic differences in fat intake but, because all socioeconomic groups still had an intake higher than the guideline, universalist measures were implemented, because it was thought that a selective strategy would increase costs (54). As part of the campaign, nationwide nutrition education tours were set up in the supermarkets by local health services. This type of intervention might contribute to the reduction of socioeconomic differences, as a pilot study showed that more than half of the participants had a low level of education; the tours were attended especially by women aged at least 40 (55).

Underestimation of personal fat intake has been identified as an important barrier to the reduction of fat consumption (56). In 1997, a campaign aiming to make people aware of their fat consumption, to stimulate the consumption of fruits and vegetables and to decrease the intake of saturated fat, was started. The target group was women aged 22–50 years, housekeepers who have a family with children 7–12 years old and who belong to a low or very low social class (57). In 1998, the minister concluded that programmes that target deprived groups need to be tailored to local situations. Nowadays several programmes for deprived or lower socioeconomic groups, implemented by local health services, also focus on dietary patterns.

The Dutch food industry has been involved in the development of products with lower fat content. Over the past decade a number of new products have been launched, and this might have affected fat intake (58). Moreover, in the mid-1990s the food industry reduced the *trans* fatty acid content of margarines. This might especially benefit the poor, because they are major consumers of cheaper margarines (59).

Originally, farm prices for milk were based on the fat content, but since 1990 they have been based on both fat and protein content. Together with the increased supply of low-fat milk products, this has influenced the shift from whole milk and milk products to semi-skimmed and skimmed varieties.

Although the average fat intake of the Dutch population declined by 10 per cent in the period 1987/8–1997/8 (60), socioeconomic inequalities still exist. There is no empirical evidence on diminishing socioeconomic inequalities in food habits. Some universalist interventions, such as shopping tours with dieticians and the reduction in the *trans* fatty acid content of margarines, have, however, been shown to reach particularly the lower socioeconomic groups. The effects of the recent selective interventions cannot yet be evaluated.

In the case of The Netherlands it is too early to draw conclusions about the effects of the recent selective interventions. The universalist interventions seem to have benefited particularly the less advantaged. The decision of the food industry to modify the composition of margarines favoured by the lower socioeconomic groups did not require any behavioural changes and caused no additional costs or changes in the taste of the margarine.

Conclusions

There is very little information on the long-term effects of interventions aiming to reduce socioeconomic inequalities in nutrition. An intervention targeted at a specific disadvantaged group does not tell us about the distribution of inequalities within a whole society. Therefore, comparative analyses on the impacts of food and nutrition policies on nutritional inequalities are needed.

Despite the lack of such studies, the following can be recommended:

1. Carefully tailored selective measures, which are sensitive to the cultural and social conditions of the target group, may improve the diet of the underprivileged. In the long term, however, they may also reproduce inequalities.
2. Universalist measures may reduce nutritional inequalities if they increase the chance of healthier food choices among large population groups.

References

1. Roos G, Prättälä R, *FAIR-97-3096 Disparities Group (tasks 4 and 5). Disparities in Food Habits: Review of Research in 15 European Countries.* (Publications of the National Public Health Institute B24/1999.) Helsinki: National Public Health Institute, 1999.
2. Irala-Estevez JD, Groth M, Johansson L, Oltersdorf U, Prättälä R, Martinez-Gonzalez MA. A systematic review of socioeconomic differences in food habits in Europe: consumption of fruit and vegetables. *Eur J Clin Nutr* 2000: 54(9): 706–14.
3. Prättälä R, Helasoja V, Mykkänen H. The consumption of rye bread and white bread as dimensions of health lifestyles in Finland. *Public Health Nutr* 2001: 4(3): 813–19.
4. Roos E, Prättälä R, Lahelma E, Kleemola P, Pietinen P. Modern and healthy?: socioeconomic differences in the quality of diet. *Eur J Clin Nutr* 1996: 50(11): 753–60.
5. Molarius A. *Determinants of Relative Weight and Body Fat Distribution in an International Perspective (Dissertation).* Rotterdam: Erasmus University, 1999.
6. Smith GD, Brunner E. Socioeconomic differentials in health: the role of nutrition. *Proc Nutr Soc* 1997: 56(1A): 75–90.

7. Hulshof KF, Lowik MR, Kok FJ, Wedel M, Brants HA, Hermus RJ *et al.* Diet and other life-style factors in high and low socioeconomic groups (Dutch Nutrition Surveillance System). *Eur J Clin Nutr* 1991: 45(9): 441–50.

8. Karisto A, Prättälä R, Berg M-A. The good, the bad and the ugly: differences in changes in health related lifestyles. In: Kjaernes U, Holm L, Ekström M, Fuerst E, Prättälä R, eds. *Regulating Markets – Regulating People: On Food and Nutrition Policy.* Oslo: Novum Press, 1993.

9. Lang T. Access to healthy foods: part II. Food poverty and shopping deserts: what are the implications for health promotion policy and practice. *Health Educ J* 1998: 57: 202–11.

10. Margetts BM, Martinez JA, Saba A, Holm L, Kearney M, Moles A. Definitions of 'healthy' eating: a pan-EU survey of consumer attitudes to food, nutrition and health. *Eur J Clin Nutr* 1997: 51 Suppl 2: S23–9.

11. Dowler E, Barlösius E, Feichtinger E, Köhler B. Poverty, food and nutrition. In: Köhler B, Feichtinger E, Barlösius E, Dowler E, eds. *Poverty and Food in Welfare Societies.* Berlin: WZB, Edition Sigma, 1997.

12. James WPT, Nelson M, Ralph A, Leather S. The contribution of nutrition to inequalities in health. *Br Med J* 1997: 314: 1545–9.

13. Karg G, Gedrich K, Weyrauch S. Nutrition in the Federal Republic of Germany: Exploring the socioeconomic situation of households. In: Köhler B, Feichtinger E, Barlösius E, Dowler E, eds. *Poverty and Food in Welfare Societies.* Berlin: WZB, Edition Sigma, 1997.

14. Evans N. Nutrition of single homeless and marginalised people in London. In: Köhler B, Feichtinger E, Barlösius E, Dowler E, eds. *Poverty and Food in Welfare Societies.* Berlin: WZB, Edition Sigma, 1997.

15. McGinnis JM, Foege WH. Actual causes of death in the United States. *JAMA* 1993: 270(18): 2207–12.

16. Vartiainen E, Puska P, Pekkanen J, Tuomilehto J, Jousilahti P. Changes in risk factors explain changes in mortality from ischaemic heart disease in Finland. *Br Med J* 1994: 309: 23–7.

17. Stronks K, Mheen van de H, Looman C, Mackenbach JP. Behavioural and structural factors in the explanation of socioeconomic inequalities in health: an empirical analysis. *Sociol Health Illness* 1996: 18: 653–74.

18. Puska P. Nutrition and mortality: the Finnish experience. *Acta Cardiol* 2000: 55(4): 213–20.

19. Burnett J, Oddy DJ, eds. *The Origins and Development of Food Policies in Europe.* London: Leicester University Press, 1994.

20. Devaney BL, Ellwood MR, Love JM. Programs that mitigate the effects of poverty on children. *Future Child* 1997: 7(2): 88–112.

21. McIntyre L, Travers K, Dayle JB. Children's feeding programs in Atlantic Canada: reducing or reproducing inequities? *Can J Public Health* 1999: 90(3): 196–200.

22. den Hartog A. Feeding schoolchildren in The Netherlands: conflict between state and family responsibilities. In: Burnett J, Oddy D, eds. *The Origins and Development of Food Policies in Europe.* London: Leicester University Press, 1994: 70–89.

23. Holme I, Hjermann I, Helgeland A, Leren P. The Oslo Study: diet and anti-smoking advice. Additional results from a 5-year primary preventive trial in middle-aged men. *Prev Med* 1985: 14(3): 279–9.

120   *Ritva Prättälä* et al.

24. Pekkanen J, Vartiainen E, Tuomilehto J, Puska P. Differences between educational groups in risk factor trends. In: Puska P, Tuomilehto J, Nissinen A, Vartiainen E, eds. *The North Karelia Project. 20 year Results and Experiences.* Helsinki: National Public Health Institute, 1995.

25. Murcott A, Prättälä R. Comparing food and nutrition policies. A very small start. In: Kjaernes U, Holm L, Ekström M, Fürst E, Prättälä R, eds. *Regulating Markets – Regulating People.* On food and nutrition policy. Oslo: Novus Press, 1993.

26. WHO Regional Office for Europe. *The First Action Plan for Food and Nutrition Policy. European Region of WHO 2000–2005.* Copenhagen: WHO Regional Office for Europe, 2000.

27. WHO Regional Office for Europe. *Comparative Analysis of Nutrition Policies in WHO European Member States.* Copenhagen: WHO Regional Office for Europe, 1998.

28. Kautto M, Heikkilä M, Hvinden B, Marklund S, Ploug N. Introduction: Nordic welfare states in the 1990s. In: Kautto M, Heikkilä M, Hvinden B, Marklund S, Ploug N, eds. *Nordic Social Policy. Changing Welfare States.* London: Routledge, 1999.

29. Sihto M, Keskimäki I. Does a policy matter? Assessing the Finnish health policy in relation to its equity goals. *Critical Public Health* 2000: 10(2): 273–86.

30. Lahti-Koski M, ed. *Nutrition in Finland.* Helsinki: National Public Health Insitute, 1999.

31. Prättälä R. North European meals: Observations from Denmark, Finland, Norway and Sweden. In: Meiselman H, ed. *Dimensions of the Meal. The Science, Culture, Business and Art of Eating.* Maryland: Aspen, 2000.

32. Milio N. Food and nutrition policy. In: *Health for All Policy in Finland.* Copenhagen: WHO Regional Office for Europe, 1991.

33. Puska P, Tuomilehto J, Nissinen A, Vartiainen E, eds. *The North Karelia Project. 20 year Results and Experiences.* Helsinki: National Public Health Institute, 1995.

34. Urho U-M, Luova T, Packalén L, Hasunen K. Ruoka ja terveys – mitä suomalaiset ajattelevat? Kysely väestölle sekä ravitsemuksen ja terveydenhuollon asiantuntijoille, 1993 (Food and health – what do Finns think? A questionnaire to the population and nutrition and health experts, 1993). (Sosiaali- ja terveysministeriön selvityksiä 1994: 2.) Helsinki: Sosiaali- ja terveysministeriö, 1994.

35. Prättälä R. Puun ja kuoren välissä. Metsurit ja kirvesmiehet puhuvat terveellisistä elintavoista (Between a rock and a hard place. Loggers and carpenters talking about healthy lifestyles). (LEL *Työeläkekassan Julkaisuja* 32: 1997.) Helsinki: LEL Työeläkekassa, 1998.

36. Uusitalo H, Prättälä R, Uutela A. Työn luonne, sosiaalisuus ja työaikainen ateriointi (Type of work, social orientation and meals at work). *Sosiaalilääketieteellinen Aikakauslehti* 1996: 33: 25–31.

37. National Nutrition Council. *Nutrition Policy in Finland. Country Paper Prepared for the FAO/WHO International Conference on Nutrition in Rome 1992.* Helsinki: 1992.

38. Voutilainen E. Margariinitiedotus (Finnish margarine information centre). Personal communication. 18.4.2000.

39. Roos Gun, Lean Michael, Anderson Annie. Dietary Interventions in Finland, Norway and Sweden – lessons for Scotland Part I. Trends in food consumption and diet-related diseases. *Health Bull* 1997: 55(6): 432–43.

40. Uusitalo U, Pietinen P, Leino U. *Food and Nutrient Intake among Adults in East and Southwest Finland – a Dietary Survey of the FINMONICA Project in 1982* (Publications of the National Public Health Institute B1/1987). Helsinki: National Public Health Institute, 1987.

41. *The 1997 Dietary Survey of Finnish Adults* (Publications of the National Public Health Insitute B8/1998). Helsinki, National Public Health Institute, 1998.

42. Helakorpi S, Uutela A, Prättälä R, Puska P. *Health Behaviour and Health among the Finnish Adult Population, Spring 1999* (Publications of the National Public Health Institute B19/1999). Helsinki: National Public Health Institute, 1999.

43. Prättälä R, Berg M-A, Puska P. Diminishing or increasing contrasts? Social class variation in Finnish food consumption patterns 1979–1990. *Eur J Clin Nutr* 1992: 42 (Suppl): 16–20.

44. Mackenbach JP. Socioeconomic health differences in The Netherlands: a review of recent empirical findings. *Soc Sci Med* 1992: 34(3): 213–26.

45. Mackenbach JP. Socioeconomic inequalities in health in The Netherlands: impact of a five year research programme. *Br Med J* 1994: 309: 1487–91.

46. Mackenbach JP, Verkley H, eds. *Volksgezondheid Toekomst Verkennningen 1997. II Gezondheidsverschillen* (Public Health Status and Forecasts 1997. II, Health inequalities). Maarssen: Elsevier/De Tijdstroom, 1997.

47. Hartog den C. 40 jaar schoolmelkvoorziening (40 years' school milk supply). *Voeding* 1978: 39(6): 162–70.

48. Bakker PJA (1978). Twintig jaar studentenvoeding – 1958–77 (Twenty years' students' nutrition – 1958–77). *Voeding* 1978: 39(10): 296–99.

49. *Guidelines for a Healthy Diet. Recommendations Drawn up by the Committee on Guidelines for a Healthy Diet.* The Hague: Netherlands Nutrition Council, 1986.

50. *Reassessment of the advice on fat consumption contained in 'Guidelines for a Healthy Diet'.* The Hague: Netherlands Nutrition Council, 1991.

51. Brants HAM, Aarnink EJM, Hulshof KFAM *et al. Vetconsumptie in Nederland. Vol. 1. Doelgroepsegmentatie* (Fat intake in The Netherlands. Vol. 1. Target group segmentation). (National Food Consumption Survey 1987/1988). Zeist: TNO Nutrition and Food Research, 1989. TNO-report V89.436.

52. Hulshof KFAM, Löwik MRH. Socioeconomic differences in dietary quality. Experience from two national surveys in The Netherlands. In: Köhler BM, Feichtinger E, Dowler E, Winkler G, eds. *Public Health and Nutrition. The Challenge.* Berlin: Sigma, 1999: 127–37.

53. Droomers M, Mackenbach JP. *Interventions and Policies on Socioeconomic Differences in Health-related Behaviour in The Netherlands 1993–8.* Rotterdam: Erasmus University, Department of Public Health, 1999.

54. Löwik MRH, Hulshof KFAM, Riedstra M, Brants HAM, van Wechem SN. High fat intake: policy implications for The Netherlands. In: Wheelock V, ed. *Implementing Dietary Guidelines for Healthy Eating.* London: Blackie, 1997: 302–15.

55. van Assema P, Cremers S, van Dis I. Nutrition education tours in the super-market: the results of a pilot project in The Netherlands. In: Worsley A, ed. *Multidisciplinary Approaches to Food Choice.* Adelaide: 1996.

56. van Wechem SN, Brug J, van Assema P, Kistemaker C, Riedstra M, Lowik MR. Fat Watch: a nationwide campaign in The Netherlands to reduce fat intake – effect evaluation. *Nutr Health* 1998: 12(2): 119–30.

57. Netherlands Nutrition Centre. www.voedingscentrum.nl/menu.asp?ST_ID=64.

58. Hulshof KFAM, Beemster CJM, Westenbrink S, Löwik MRH. Reduction in fat intake in The Netherlands: the influence of food composition data. *Food Chem* 1996: 57: 67–70.

59. Katan MB. Exit *trans* fatty acids. *Lancet* 1995: 346: 1245–6.

60. *The Way the Dutch Eat, 1998. Results of the National Food Consumption Survey 1997–8.* The Hague: Netherlands Nutrition Centre, 1998.

61. Ammerman AS, DeVellis BM, Haines PS, Keyserling TC, Carey TS, DeVellis RF *et al.* Nutrition education for cardiovascular disease prevention among low income populations – description and pilot evaluation of a physician-based model. *Patient Educ Couns* 1992: 19(1): 5–18.

62. Balsam A, Webber D, Oehlke B. The farmers' market coupon program for low-income elders. *J Nutr Elder* 1994: 13(4): 35–42.

63. Brown JL, Gershoff SN, Cook JT. The politics of hunger: when science and ideology clash. *Int J Health Serv* 1992: 22(2): 221–37.

64. Campbell MK, Honess-Morreale L, Farrell D, Carbone E, Brasure M. A tailored multimedia nutrition education pilot program for low-income women receiving food assistance. *Health Educ Res* 1999: 14(2): 257–67.

65. Elder JP, Candelaria JI, Woodruff SI, Criqui MH, Talavera GA, Rupp JW. Results of language for health: cardiovascular disease nutrition education for Latino English-as-a-second-language students. *Health Educ Behav* 2000: 27(1): 50–63.

66. Fitzgibbon ML, Stolley MR, Avellone ME, Sugerman S, Chavez N. Involving parents in cancer risk reduction: a program for Hispanic American families. *Health Psychol* 1996: 15(6): 413–22.

67. Foley RM, Pollard CM. Food Cent$ – implementing and evaluating a nutrition education project focusing on value for money. *Aust NZ J Public Health* 1998: 22(4): 494–501.

68. Gore CJ, Owen N, Pederson D, Clarke A. Educational and environmental interventions for cardiovascular health promotion in socially disadvantaged primary schools. *Aust NZ J Public Health* 1996: 20(2): 188–94.

69. Hartman TJ, McCarthy PR, Park RJ, Schuster E, Kushi LH. Results of a community-based low-literacy nutrition education program. *J Commun Health* 1997: 22(5): 325–41.

70. Havas S, Anliker J, Damron D, Langenberg P, Ballesteros M, Feldman R. Final results of the Maryland WIC 5-a-day promotion program. *Am J Public Health* 1998: 88(8): 1161–7.

71. Havas S, Anliker J, Damron D, Feldman R, Langenberg P. Uses of process evaluation in the Maryland WIC 5-a-day promotion program. *Health Educ Behav* 2000: 27(2): 254–63.

72. Anliker J, Damron D, Ballesteros M, Havas S. Using the stages of change model in a 5 a day guidebook for WIC. *J Nutr Educ* 1999: 31: 175.

73. Anliker J, Damron D, Ballesteros M, Feldman R, Langenberg P, Havas S. Using peer educators in nutrition education research: Lessons learned from the Maryland WIC 5-a-day promotion program. *J Nutr Educ* 1999: 31: 347–54.

74. Hill F. Food mail: the Canadian alternative to food stamps. *Int J Circumpolar Health* 1998: 57 (Suppl 1): 177–81.

75. James J, Lawson P, Male P, Oakhill A. Preventing iron deficiency in preschool children by implementing an educational and screening programme in an inner city practice. *Br Med J* 1989: 299: 838–40.

76. Howard-Pitney B, Winkleby MA, Albright CL, Bruce B, Fortmann SP. The Stanford Nutrition Action Program: a dietary fat intervention for low-literacy adults. *Am J Public Health* 1997: 87(12): 1971–6.

77. Meyers A, Frank DA, Roos N, Peterson KE, Casey VA, Cupples LA *et al.* Housing subsidies and pediatric undernutrition. *Arch Pediatr Adolesc Med* 1995: 149(10): 1079–84.

78. Sorensen G, Hunt MK, Cohen N, Stoddard A, Stein E, Phillips J *et al.* Worksite and family education for dietary change: the Treatwell 5-a-day program. *Health Educ Res* 1998: 13(4): 577–91.

79. Sorensen G, Stoddard A, Macario E. Social support and readiness to make dietary changes. *Health Educ Behav* 1998: 25(5): 586–98.

80. Sorensen G, Stoddard A, Peterson K, Cohen N, Hunt MK, Stein E *et al.* Increasing fruit and vegetable consumption through worksites and families in the Treatwell 5-a-day study. *Am J Public Health* 1999: 89(1): 54–60.

81. Winkleby MA, Howard-Pitney B, Albright CA, Bruce B, Kraemer HC, Fortmann SP. Predicting achievement of a low-fat diet: a nutrition intervention for adults with low literacy skills. *Prev Med* 1997: 26(6): 874–82.

82. Childs F, Aukett A, Darbyshire P, Ilett S, Livera LN. Dietary education and iron deficiency anaemia in the inner city. *Arch Dis Child* 1997: 76(2): 144–7.

83. Fine GA, Conning DM, Firmin C, De Looy AE, Losowsky MS, Richards ID *et al.* Nutrition education of young women. *Br J Nutr* 1994: 71(5): 789–98.

84. Lopez LM, Habicht JP. Food stamps and the energy status of the U.S. elderly poor. *J Am Diet Assoc* 1987: 87(8): 1020–4.

85. Lopez LM, Habicht JP. Food stamps and the iron status of the U.S. elderly poor. *J Am Diet Assoc* 1987: 87(5): 598–603.

86. Somerville SM, Rona RJ, Chinn S, Qureshi S. Family Credit and uptake of school meals in primary school. *J Public Health Med* 1996: 18(1): 98–106.

87. Weaver M, Poehlitz M, Hutchison S. 5 a day for low-income families: evaluation of an advertising campaign and cooking events. *J Nutr Educ* 1999: 31: 161–9.

88. Brännström I, Weinehall L, Persson LA, Wester PO, Wall S. Changing social patterns of risk factors for cardiovascular disease in a Swedish community intervention programme. *Int J Epidemiol* 1993: 22(6): 1026–37.

89. Brug J, van Assema P. Differences in use and impact of computer-tailored dietary fat-feedback according to stage of change and education. *Appetite* 2000: 34(3): 285–93.

90. Domel S, Baranowski T, Davis H *et al.* Development and evaluation of a school intervention to increase fruit and vegetable consumption among 4th and 5th grade students. *J Nutr Educ* 1993: 25: 345–9.

91. Jeffery RW, French SA. Preventing weight gain in adults: the pound of prevention study. *Am J Public Health* 1999: 89(5): 747–51.

92. Park YK, Sempos CT, Barton CN, Vanderveen JE, Yetley EA. Effectiveness of food fortification in the United States: the case of pellagra. *Am J Public Health* 2000: 90(5): 727–38.

93. Perry CL, Bishop DB, Taylor G, Murray DM, Mays RW, Dudovitz BS *et al.* Changing fruit and vegetable consumption among children: the 5-a-Day Power Plus program in St. Paul, Minnesota. *Am J Public Health* 1998: 88(4): 603–9.
94. Rona RJ, Chinn S, Smith AM. School meals and the rate of growth of primary school children. *J Epidemiol Community Health* 1983: 37(1): 8–15.
95. Rona RJ, Chinn S. School meals, school milk and height of primary school children in England and Scotland in the eighties. *J Epidemiol Commun Health* 1989: 43(1): 66–71.

8 Smoking policies

Stephen Platt, Amanda Amos, Wendy Gnich and Odette Parry

Introduction

In common with most other health-related behaviours, cigarette smoking varies markedly by sociodemographic characteristics, in particular socio-economic status. However, the pattern of socioeconomic inequalities in smoking is itself variable, according to the stage of the smoking epidemic in a particular country.

In the earlier decades of the smoking epidemic in high-income countries, smokers were more likely to be affluent than poor. In the past four decades, however, the pattern in these countries has been reversed, reflecting a combination of relatively lower uptake rates and higher cessation rates in more affluent groups. Drawing on a widely used four-stage model of the global smoking epidemic (1), some countries in southern Europe can be located currently at stage 2 (for example, Portugal), when smoking rates peak at between 50 per cent and 80 per cent among men while the trend among women is rising, or at stage 3 (for example, Spain, Italy, France), when prevalence rates among men decrease and women's smoking rates peak at 35–45 per cent.

Northern European countries with the longest history of smoking, on the other hand, are located at stage 4, when smoking prevalence declines among both men and women (2, 3). The most recent international comparison of variation in cigarette smoking by educational level (a proxy indicator of socioeconomic status) shows that in mature smoking economies a higher prevalence is associated with lower educational attainment. Smoking is now statistically abnormal and normatively deviant in higher socio-economic status groups and communities. It is overwhelmingly associated with social and material disadvantage, and concentrated in areas of low income and multiple deprivation. Based on an analysis of data from the British Household Panel Survey, Graham (4) shows that, among women smokers, over 60 per cent experience one or more of four forms of disadvantage (low-skilled worker, tenant, social security claimant or lone mother), whereas among non-smokers over 60 per cent experience none of these disadvantages.

Contribution of smoking to the explanation of socioeconomic inequalities in health

About 1.2 million deaths (14 per cent of all deaths) in Europe (World Health Organization (WHO) European region) each year can be attributed to tobacco products (primarily cigarettes). It is estimated that, unless more effective measures are implemented to help the current 200 million European adult smokers to stop, or at least to reduce their consumption, tobacco products will be responsible for 2 million deaths a year (20 per cent of all deaths) by 2020.

The impact of the differential smoking rates across socioeconomic groups is profound. An analysis of data from four countries where the smoking epidemic is mature (Canada, Poland, the United Kingdom and the United States) indicates that tobacco is responsible for more than half the difference in adult male mortality between those in the highest and the lowest socioeconomic groups (5). The widening survival gap between more advantaged and more disadvantaged men in the UK between 1970–2 and 1990–2 (6) can be attributed in large measure to cigarette smoking.

Overview of effective interventions and policies

Two broad types of policy initiative intended to tackle the smoking epidemic can be differentiated: those relating to the supply of tobacco products and those relating to the demand for them. Initiatives undertaken at European level should also be distinguished from those taken at country level.

Demand-side interventions and policies

Raising tobacco taxes

Despite the addictive components of tobacco, there is research evidence that smokers' demand for tobacco is strongly affected by price. Higher taxes reduce cigarette consumption (7, 8) and postpone the initiation of smoking (9). For example, tax increases in Canada between 1982 and 1993 led to a steep increase in the real price of cigarettes and consumption fell considerably. When tax was reduced in an attempt to counter smuggling, consumption rose sharply again until a subsequent tax increase in 1995, when consumption levelled off (5). Increases in the price of tobacco appear to have a greater impact in low- and middle-income countries than in high-income countries.

In high-income countries increases in taxation do appear to reduce consumption disproportionately among the lower socioeconomic groups (8). Paradoxically, however, increases in the price of cigarettes appear to have very little impact on smoking prevalence (10). Thus, despite their overall positive effects, policies to increase tobacco taxation can be seen as regressive, penalizing continuing smokers within the very poorest group of society, which is least able to find a way out of addiction. A reduction in the scale of health inequality requires that interventions and public policies relevant to smoking should take account of the needs of the poorest. For example, a proportion of tobacco tax revenues could be hypothecated to address both the dimensions of disadvantage that bind people to smoking as well as providing specifically targeted smoking interventions (4, 11–13).

Health education and information

There is a considerable amount of indirect evidence to support the claim that overall levels of cigarette smoking are responsive to health education messages. At earlier stages in the tobacco epidemic (when general awareness of the health risks of smoking is low), information 'shocks' (such as the influential Report of the US Surgeon General in 1964) can have a dramatic effect on smoking prevalence. An analysis of trends between the 1930s and the 1970s in the United States suggests that the combined effect of three such information shocks was to reduce consumption by about 30 per cent. In a wide range of European countries, for example, Finland, Greece, Switzerland, Turkey and the United Kingdom, a broadly similar impact has been demonstrated. The introduction of warning labels on cigarette packets has been linked to an 8 per cent fall in consumption over 6 years. On the other hand, school-based anti-smoking programmes have been shown to have only a weak (temporary) effect, at best. However, there is some evidence that comprehensive programmes dealing with a range of substance use or health issues may be more effective (14), although such programmes rarely assess their impact in relation to young people's socioeconomic status.

Bans on advertising and promotion

Studies of partial cigarette advertising bans have found little or no effect on smoking, an unsurprising finding given the ability of the tobacco industry to make use of alternative media outlets. The conclusion of an analysis of smoking bans in 22 high-income countries over the period 1970–92 was that a comprehensive approach can reduce smoking. On the basis of the findings of this study, it has been estimated that the European Union Directive which will ban all tobacco advertising and promotion by 2006 could reduce cigarette consumption within the European Union by nearly 7 per cent. Another study of 100 countries showed that the downward trend in consumption was steeper over time (1980/2–1990/2) in countries with relatively complete bans on advertising and promotion than in those without such bans (5).

The pursuit of financial compensation for tobacco-related health damage from the major tobacco companies, particularly in the United States, is intended also to lead to a reduction in aggressive marketing of tobacco products in Europe and the rest of the developed world, and can therefore be considered a potentially powerful demand-side measure. It remains to be seen whether or not the level of compensation will be sufficient to have the desired effect. Additionally, it should be recognized that one possible, albeit unintended, consequence may be an exacerbation of the existing trend towards the promotion of tobacco products in the developing world, boosting demand and accelerating progression from stage 2 to stage 4 smoking status. Although there is at present little evidence to support the view that this is inevitable (15), it is clearly essential that rapid progress be made towards the global implementation of a comprehensive ban on all tobacco promotion to ensure that increased protection for (especially poorer) smokers in Europe and North America is not offset by greater vulnerability among (especially poorer) smokers in the burgeoning tobacco markets of Africa and Asia.

Smoking restrictions

Restrictions on smoking in public places, for example, restaurants and transport facilities, are becoming increasingly common in high-income countries, including those in Europe. A systematic review of interventions for preventing smoking in public places concludes, on the basis of 11 studies using relatively weak experimental designs, that carefully planned and resourced, multicomponent strategies effectively reduce smoking in public places, whereas less comprehensive strategies are less effective (16). With respect to the impact of workplace smoking cessation programmes and smoking policies, a recent review concludes that group programmes are more effective than minimal treatment programmes, and that policy interventions reduce both cigarette consumption at work and workplace environmental tobacco smoke exposure (17). However, Parry and Platt (18) draw attention to the danger that the implementation of workplace no-smoking policies may widen differences between smokers and non-smokers at work, thereby also (because of the socioeconomic patterning of smoking behaviour) exacerbating class/occupational differences within the workplace.

Nicotine replacement therapy and other cessation interventions

A recent systematic review concludes that all of the commercially available forms of nicotine replacement therapy are effective as part of a strategy to promote smoking cessation, increasing quit rates approximately 1.5–2-fold (19). It is estimated that brief advice by a clinician increases the percentage of smokers abstaining for at least 6 months by about 2.5 per cent, compared to no advice (20). Adding nicotine replacement therapy (patches, gums, sprays, inhalers) to brief advice results in an increase of 6 per cent of smokers abstaining for at least 6 months, compared to brief advice alone or with placebo. Intensive support (for example, smokers' clinic) plus nicotine replacement therapy results in an increase of 8 per cent compared to intensive support alone or with placebo (21). Results of a systematic review of nursing interventions for smoking cessation indicate the potential benefits of advice and counselling given by nurses to patients, with reasonable evidence that such interventions can be effective (22). Numerous other interventions for smoking cessation have been evaluated, with evidence of effectiveness established for individual behavioural counselling, group behaviour therapy programmes, medication and self-help.

Free telephone helplines offering advice and support to smokers who want to stop, often combined with mass media campaigns, have also become popular in view of their accessibility to all sections of the population, and have been found to increase cessation rates (23–25).

Evidence of the impact of cessation interventions is compelling with regard to reducing *overall* smoking prevalence. However, in this context it is important to assess the extent to which such interventions might reduce *socioeconomic inequalities* in smoking. Table 8.1 summarizes information on 25 relevant studies published over the past 15 years. Specific information about how the studies were selected is incorporated in the Appendix. Of the 16 studies targeted at low socioeconomic groups, half have demonstrated effectiveness and half have not. There are also nine studies which, although not targeted at low socioeconomic groups, have produced findings about differential impact according to socioeconomic status. In five studies the intervention was at least as effective in low as in high socioeconomic groups, whereas in four studies the intervention was shown to be less effective in low than in high socioeconomic groups.

Likely impact of demand-side interventions and policies on smoking-related health inequalities

On the whole there is little direct evidence that permits any definitive judgement to be made about the possible or actual effects of country-level demand-side measures on reducing smoking-related inequalities. It is possible that the rate of smoking in the lowest socioeconomic groups would have been even higher, and the gap between the highest and lowest groups even greater, in the absence of these policy initiatives and practical actions. However, that would be a rather weak and defensive claim, lacking conviction. Where there are relevant data, for example, derived from studies of the effectiveness of cessation interventions, it is difficult to escape the conclusion that there is a long way to go before programmes are devised that are likely to benefit low socioeconomic groups or reduce smoking-related health inequalities.

At the policy level, the United Kingdom (UK) is the only country to have targeted disadvantaged groups (and, by implication, reduce smoking-related inequalities) as part of a comprehensive national tobacco control strategy. In addition, the UK government has recently announced that nicotine

Table 8.1 Interventions designed to promote smoking cessation: evidence of effectiveness in low socioeconomic groups

Target population	Intervention	Effect of intervention	Evidence	Reference
Interventions aimed at low socioeconomic groups, reported to be effective				
Residents (predominantly African-American) aged 18+ years of urban communities characterized by low income and high socioeconomic deprivation (USA)	Community organization approach (smoking cessation classes, billboards, door-to-door campaigns, a 'gospelfest') and mass media	Prevalence of smoking declined significantly more in the intervention communities (from 34 per cent to 27 per cent) than in the control communities (34 per cent to 33 per cent). A difference favouring the intervention was found for those with annual incomes over $20,000, but not for those with incomes below this level	Quasi-experimental design, incorporating repeat cross-sectional study	38
Female smokers attending low-income planned parenthood clinics (15–35 years) (USA)	9-minute video, 12–15 minutes of behavioural counselling, clinician advice to quit and follow-up telephone calls	Six weeks post intervention (10.2 per cent quit rate vs. 6.9 per cent) Six months post intervention (6.4 per cent vs. 3.8 per cent, not significant)	Randomized controlled trial	39
Low-income women (Canada)	Smoking cessation course	Programme produced quit rates comparable to those reported for cessation programme directed at the general population	Before–after study design/no control group	40
Adults (16–60 years) in disadvantaged low-income communities, mostly of Hispanic origin (USA/Mexico)	Health education intervention which made extensive use of mass media. Activities also undertaken in schools. A more intensive contact programme, including individual counselling and telephone support, was received by some of the intervention group	For moderate smokers (>10 cigarettes a day) smoking cessation was significantly greater in the experimental group than in the control group	Quasi-experimental design, incorporating cohort study	41

Population/Setting	Intervention	Outcome	Study design	
Adults (aged 18+ years) living in urban, predominantly African-American neighbourhoods, half classed as 'low income', half as 'moderate income' (USA)	'Passive' intervention communities received mass media intervention to raise general awareness of smoking cessation. 'Active' intervention communities received in addition a multicomponent intervention (including health advocacy, distribution of educational materials, telephone quit line)	All main outcome measures (point prevalence of non-smoking, period prevalence of quit attempts, smoke-free days and daily cigarette consumption) were significantly improved in 'active' communities compared to 'passive' communities. Moderate-income areas tended to show a smaller change than lower-income areas	Quasi-experimental design, incorporating cohort study	42
African-American adults aged 18+ years living in an economically deprived inner-city urban area with a high unemployment rate (USA)	Church parishes randomized to intensive intervention received pastoral sermons on smoking, testimonies from those trying to quit, training of lay cessation counsellors, individual and group support, and screening at church health fairs. Minimal self-help intervention churches received screening and distribution of a self-help booklet only	There was a significant net effect of both intensive and minimal intervention over a community reference group (spontaneous quit rate)	Randomized controlled trial, incorporating cohort study	43
Whole adult population (especially middle-aged men) resident in mainly rural small towns with very high rates of cardiovascular disease, low socioeconomic status, low educational levels and high unemployment (Finland)	Broad-based community intervention with extensive use of mass media. Anti-smoking programme focused on four main areas: general public information, organization for preventative services, training of personnel, and promotion of a smoke-free environment.	Reduction in smoking prevalence and tobacco consumption in the intervention area was significant only for men. Effects did not differ for males and females from different socioeconomic groups. Net increases in tobacco consumption among men were larger for those with lower levels of educational attainment	Quasi-experimental design, incorporating repeat cross-sectional study	44

Table 8.1 (Cont'd)

Target population	Intervention	Effect of intervention	Evidence	Reference
Interventions aimed at low socioeconomic groups, reported to be non-effective				
Adults (18–65 years) living in a low-income inner-city neighbourhood (Canada)	Community-based heart disease prevention programme (smoking cessation workshops, smoking cessation contest)	No substantial decline in the prevalence of smoking. Proportion of heavy smokers (>25 cigarettes a day) declined	Quasi-experimental design, 3-year repeat independent sample survey and 5-year longitudinal cohort sample	45
Low-income women (Canada)	Smoking cessation guide	None of the subjects stopped smoking, but a majority reduced the number of cigarettes smoked	Before–after study design/no control group	46
Adults (18–65 years) living in a community with low socioeconomic status (Australia)	1. Single group counselling session 2. Specially prepared pamphlet	There were no major differences in changes in smoking behaviour (number of cigarettes smoked per day, quitters, attempting to quit) between the two groups	Randomized parallel-group trial	47
Adults (18–64 years) living in low-income areas with low educational attainment and high unemployment (USA)	Small group risk factor screening, educational events, smoking cessation contests, a quit line, cessation groups and distribution of self-help quit kits. School programmes also undertaken. Focus on cardiovascular disease reduction	Although trends in smoking moved in a favourable direction there was no significant difference between experimental and control communities. Less educated males showed smaller decreases in smoking in the experimental community compared to the control community	Quasi-experimental design, incorporating repeat cross-sectional and cohort studies	48

Population	Intervention	Results	Study design	Reference
Population aged 18+ years living in rural, low-income communities (USA)	Health education through mass media and, more directly, through presentations and community events. Other activities included screening at local fairs, a quit and win contest, and distribution of self-help kits. Focus on cardiovascular disease reduction	There was no significant overall effect of the intervention on smoking prevalence. Downward trend in smoking over the course of the study was minimal	Quasi-experimental design, incorporating cohort study	49
Adults living in rural, predominantly African-American, communities, medically underserved, with high unemployment, low education levels and high poverty rates (USA)	Cardiovascular disease education programmes. Health messages disseminated through mass media and community events	Although there were reductions in smoking prevalence in both experimental and control communities, there was no significant net effect. Further analysis of data from the intervention areas (not available for the control areas) shows that reduction in smoking prevalence was greater among those with post high-school education	Quasi-experimental design, incorporating repeat cross-sectional study	50
Adult population (particularly women) living in low income, socioeconomically deprived communities with low educational attainment (Canada)	Activities aimed at developing personal skills, creating supportive environments and building healthy public policy, in support of cardiovascular disease reduction. Also screening for cardiovascular disease risk factors, smoking cessation contests, workshops and support groups, community events, and distribution of educational materials	There was no significant net effect. Trends in smoking prevalence were equally favourable in both intervention and control communities	Quasi-experimental design, incorporating cohort and repeat cross-sectional studies	51
Whole adult population, but special efforts were made to reach unemployed and low-income groups (Ireland)	Training for health, education and catering personnel, health assessment programme, school-based health education, distribution of educational material, special community events and media coverage. Policy-level intervention proved difficult	There was no significant net effect. Trends in smoking prevalence were equally favourable in both intervention and control communities	Quasi-experimental design, incorporating repeat cross-sectional study	52, 53

Table 8.1 (Cont'd)

Target population	Intervention	Effect of intervention	Evidence	Reference
Interventions aimed at general population, reported to be at least as effective in low as in high socioeconomic groups				
Whole adult population, although emphasis was given to heavy smokers (>25 per day) (USA/ Canada)	Multifaceted programme delivered through four main channels: public education (through mass media), healthcare providers, workplaces and cessation resources	No significant net intervention effect for the total sample. However, a significant net intervention effect was found for the light-to-moderate smokers in the cohort study. This was largely attributable to behavioural change among the less educated (those with high-school education only)	Randomized controlled trial, incorporating repeat cross-sectional and cohort studies	54, 55
Males with high risk for coronary heart disease (35–57 years) (USA)	Smoking cessation counselling programme	The intervention found a similar effect on both black and white participants of varying educational and socioeconomic backgrounds	Randomized controlled tria	56
Middle-aged men with high-risk for coronary heart disease (Norway)	Smoking cessation counselling	Anti-smoking advice was especially effective in lower class intervention group men (reduction in number of cigarettes a day)	Randomized controlled trial	57
Adult smoking patients of six GP practices (UK)	Study groups: 1. Verbal and written advice from GP 2. Advice + demonstration of exhaled CO 3. Advice + further help from health visitor	Giving advice and demonstration of exhaled CO is the most effective intervention in the lower social classes (approximately 14.5 per cent quitters after 1 year)	Randomized controlled trial	58
Adult smokers (25–59 years) (Australia)	Mass media-led anti-smoking campaign	The relative decrease in smoking of the least educated is not significantly different from that of the most educated group	Quasi-experimental design	59
Employees (USA)	No-smoking policy (education programmes, company-sponsored quit courses)	The programme induced positive behavioural and attitudinal changes to smoking	Observational study	60

Interventions aimed at general population, reported to be less effective in low than high socioeconomic groups

Population	Intervention	Results	Study design	Reference
General population (New Zealand)	Smoking cessation course	Unemployed, self-employed and students had low success rates compared to professional and technical workers	Cross-sectional survey	61
Adults (25–69 years) (Germany)	Community-based primary prevention programmes for cardiovascular disease (interventions are aimed at smoking, nutrition, physical activity and hypertension)	Decrease in smoking among higher social classes and increase in smoking among lower classes	Three independent cross-sectional surveys	62
Population aged 12+ years (USA)	Multifactorial health education campaign, emphasizing use of mass media, aimed at reducing cardiovascular disease	Significantly greater reduction in smoking prevalence in the experimental cities (compared to control cities). However, differences in smoking trends between experimental and control cities were not found for those with less than a high-school education.	Quasi-experimental design, incorporating repeat cross-sectional and cohort studies	63
Whole adult population in a small rural town with a high cardiovascular disease risk (Sweden)	General health education using mass media and direct education. Other activities included screening and counselling, political debate and community events	There was no significant net intervention effect. Trends were not in a favourable direction in the intervention community and remained unchanged in the control area. Subgroup analysis showed that the probability of being a smoker was reduced only among the highly educated groups	Quasi-experimental design, incorporating repeat cross-sectional and cohort studies	64, 65

replacement therapies will be made available on National Health Service prescription (free to those in receipt of social security benefits). There has been little attempt in other stage 4 countries to target this type of treatment towards the poorest sections of society, where cessation needs are greatest and where levels of motivation to stop may be low (26).

Supply-side interventions and policies

Restrictions on youth access to tobacco

Although interventions with retailers can lead to large decreases in the number of outlets selling tobacco to young people, the effectiveness of attempts to establish sustainable comprehensive restrictions on the sale of cigarettes to underage children has not been demonstrated. This may explain why there is little evidence for an effect of such interventions on smoking prevalence among young people (27, 28). These restrictions are difficult to enforce and can be circumvented in a number of ways, including false identification documents, proxy purchasing (for example, asking an older relative or friend to purchase on one's behalf), and collusion by shopkeepers.

Crop substitution and diversification

This measure is relevant to only a few European Union (EU) countries – specifically Belgium, Germany, Greece, Italy, France, Spain, Portugal and Austria – where tobacco is grown. There have been several experimental schemes to substitute other crops for tobacco, but there is no evidence relating to any European country that these have successfully contributed to a reduction in tobacco consumption. The two main problems are the high profitability of tobacco and the ready availability of other suppliers to replace those farmers who attempt crop substitution.

Price supports and subsidies on tobacco production

The EU spends hundreds of millions of pounds – £584 million (approximately 930 million euros) in 1998 (29) – on subsidies for tobacco production in the eight member states where tobacco is grown. It is unlikely that the removal of government price supports and subsidies would affect consumption in the EU, as most of this tobacco is exported to developing countries, and the impact on production is unclear.

Restrictions on international trade

Attempts to control the international trade in tobacco and tobacco products must take account of the global trend towards increased free trade. Although there is evidence that trade liberalization has contributed to an increase in consumption in low- and middle-income countries, international free trade rules discourage trade restrictions, which in any case are likely to prompt retaliatory action that could reduce national income and economic growth. Countries have a right to adopt and enforce measures to protect public health, provided that such measures are applied equally to both domestic and imported products.

Action to combat smuggling

With nearly a third of internationally exported cigarettes lost to smuggling, it can be seen that this constitutes a major challenge to, and opportunity for, supply-side management of tobacco consumption. This is particularly true in Europe, where levels of cigarette smuggling have increased dramatically, losing European governments over $6 billion (approximately 6.7 billion euros) a year in tax revenues (30). According to the World Bank (5), 'economic theory suggests that the tobacco industry itself will benefit from the existence of smuggling'. A recent report from the UK House of Commons Select Committee on Health (31) alleged that some tobacco companies were 'complicit' in organized tobacco smuggling by being prepared to supply large quantities of cigarettes to sources in continental Europe used by organized bootlegging operations. The Committee urged consideration of criminal proceedings against British American Tobacco (BAT), Britain's largest tobacco company, which has been accused of orchestrating, managing and controlling cigarette smuggling (claims the company strenuously denies). Noting that there is currently very little research on the effectiveness of anti-smuggling measures, the World Bank (5) lists a number of options that policy-makers might wish to consider. Given the apparently easy access to cheaper smuggled cigarettes among lower-income smokers in the UK, action to combat smuggling in that country could have a significant impact on overall smoking prevalence.

Likely impact of supply-side interventions and policies on smoking-related health inequalities

The potential contribution of supply-side policy interventions in reducing the global availability of tobacco products is unknown, but is unlikely to be large (32). It is difficult to envisage how any of the measures considered earlier will play a significant role in reducing smoking-related health inequalities.

European-level interventions

Concerted action to reduce smoking prevalence and smoking-related diseases across Europe has been pledged by both the World Health Organization and the European Union/Commission.

World Health Organization interventions and policies

Described as 'a major landmark in the World Health Organization's 50-year history' (33), Resolution WHA52.18 (May 1999) calls for the development of a Framework Convention on Tobacco Control (FCTC) and related protocols. These might address issues such as taxation, smuggling, tax-free tobacco products, advertising/sponsorship, cigarette content and testing methods, package design/labelling, information sharing, agricultural diversification, and the regulation of tobacco.

The FCTC is intended to build on the extensive investment in the prevention of smoking and reduction of smoking-related harm already committed by WHO. At the European level, the WHO Third Action Plan for a Tobacco-Free Europe (1997–2001) proposes five key strategies for reducing tobacco-related harm: regulation of the market; litigation and product liability; smoke-free environments; support for smoking cessation; and education, public information and mobilization of public opinion. The Action Plan identifies a reduction in tobacco use as the single most important public policy action to improve population health, and addresses tobacco products as the key to achieving this goal. Consequently, the WHO established a European Partnership Project on Tobacco Dependence, which targets the reduction of tobacco-related morbidity and mortality among dependent smokers. Although certain initiatives will be Europe-wide, the initial focus is on four target countries: France, Germany, Poland and the United Kingdom.

Despite the emphasis of the WHO policy framework on reducing the 'health gap' between socioeconomic groups within countries (target 2 of the new HEALTH 21 policy for the European Region (34)), there is a surprising lack of reference to issues of equity and inequality in the WHO policy statements on tobacco control.

European Commission/Union interventions and policies

Smoking prevention has been identified as one of the public health priorities at the European Community level since the establishment of the Europe Against Cancer programme in 1986. Ten years later the Commission published a White Paper on smoking prevention in which action at both state and Union levels was identified. Included among the latter were the development of improved data collection on and monitoring of smoking, and the updating and extension of legislation. The EU has already laid down directives to harmonize the labelling of tobacco products, regulate the maximum tar yield of cigarettes, and ban all forms of advertising and sponsorship for tobacco products. Proposals under examination include the introduction of further reductions or new ceilings on the noxious ingredients of cigarettes, and changes to the warning messages on tobacco packaging.

The FCTC is likely to increase joint strategic planning and action on tobacco between WHO and the EU. In October 1999 the EU Council of

Ministers authorized the Commission to participate in negotiations leading to the creation of an FCTC.

The Women, Low Income and Smoking Initiative

Established in 1996, this 3-year project was based on Action on Smoking and Health (ASH) Scotland, and funded by the Health Education Board for Scotland (11). The project adopted a community development, 'bottom -up' approach based on the findings of a widespread consultation with community workers and health promoters. This emphasized the need to reframe the issues around smoking in ways that were more sensitive to women's needs and their day-to-day lives (35). The project provided grants of £500–£3000 (approximately €800–4,800) and evaluation support to 19 community-based initiatives that focused on women and smoking. The projects used a variety of different approaches, including drama, fitness, stress reduction, cessation, diversionary activities, poetry and social support.

Several key lessons for policy and practice have been learned from this initiative. First, the reduction of smoking among women on low income must be addressed within the wider context of strategies to tackle poverty, disadvantage and health. Second, women on low income who want to stop smoking need support from family, friends and community services. There is a dearth of community services that could help women address their smoking. Third, although small grants can stimulate and support innovative work on this issue, longer-term funding is required to develop and sustain any major impact on smoking prevalence. Fourth, there is a need for indirect, as well as direct, approaches to promoting smoking cessation among low-income women. Indirect approaches provided women with opportunities to develop new skills and increase their confidence and self-esteem. Few of the available smoking education materials were appropriate for women on low income. Fifth, knowledge and competence to undertake and evaluate tobacco-related work varied enormously among community-based support staff. More training and partnership working with health services is needed. Sixth, evaluation can be challenging for community projects. The use of a diverse range of methods to collect process and outcome data is essential. These need to reflect the philosophy and diversity of the work, the aims and objectives, the resources available, and the participants and organizations involved. Finally, more research is needed to inform the development of effective community approaches to tackling smoking among low-income women.

Conclusions

The potential for tackling health inequalities through concerted policy and practice interventions on smoking is extremely high, particularly in northern and central Europe. At present there is a conspicuous failure to seize this opportunity, with both continental- and country-level approaches tending to concentrate on the target of reducing overall tobacco consumption, rather than addressing the persistently large gap between smoking rates in higher and lower socioeconomic groups. The typical supply-side policy interventions (discussed earlier), although likely to reduce overall tobacco consumption, are as likely (if not more so) to enhance existing smoking-related inequalities as to reduce them. The first priority of national government health departments and European health organizations must be to reorientate their approach to the problem by focusing primarily on the reduction of smoking rates in the poorest and least powerful sections of society. The regressive impact of the price weapon (through raising taxes) on the poorest smokers who are unable to stop must be counteracted by active promotion of the availability of free nicotine replacement therapy (as in the UK) and other cessation services which are sensitive to poorer smokers' needs and circumstances. At the same time, the underlying economic and psychosocial processes that enhance the risk of smoking, smoking dependence and unsuccessful cessation attempts among the poor (4, 10, 12, 36) also need to be addressed through the introduction (or maintenance) of policies that reduce income inequalities and improve the living standards of individuals, households and communities reliant upon social security benefits (37).

References

1. Lopez AD, Collishaw NE, Piha T. A descriptive model of the cigarette epidemic in developed countries. *Tobacco Control* 1994: 3: 242–7.
2. Cavelaars A, Kunst A, Geurts J, Crialesi R, Grotvedt L, Helmert U *et al.* Educational differences in smoking: international comparison. *Br Med J* 2000: 320: 1102–7.
3. Graham H. Smoking prevalence among women in the European Community 1950–90. *Soc Sci Med* 1996: 43: 243–54.
4. Graham H. Promoting health against inequality: using research to identify targets for intervention – a case study of women and smoking. *Health Educ J* 1998: 57: 292–302.
5. World Bank. *Curbing the Epidemic. Governments and the Economics of Tobacco Control*. Washington, DC: World Bank, 1999.
6. Drever F, Whitehead M. *Health Inequalities: Decennial Supplement*. London: The Stationery Office, 1997.
7. US Department of Health and Human Services (USDHHS). Responses to increases in cigarette prices by race/ethnicity, income and age groups – United States, 1976–93. *MMWR* 1998: 47(29): 605–9.
8. Townsend J, Roderick P, Cooper J. Cigarette smoking by socioeconomic group, sex and age: effects of price, income and health publicity. *Br Med J* 1994: 309: 923–7.
9. Lewit EM, Hyland A, Kerrebrock N, Cummings KM. Price, public policy, and smoking in young people. *Tobacco Control* 1997: 6 (Suppl 2): S17–24.
10. Marsh A, McKay S. *Poor Smokers*. London: Policy Studies Institute, 1994.
11. Gaunt-Richardson P, Amos A, Howie G, McKie L, Moore M. *Women, Low Income and Smoking – Breaking down the Barriers*. Edinburgh: ASH Scotland/ Health Education Board for Scotland, 1999.

12. INWAT Europe (2000) *Report of the INWAT Europe Seminar on Women and Tobacco, June 1999*. http://www.inwat.org/eseminarreport.PDF.

13. Marsh A. Tax and spend: a policy to help poor smokers. *Tobacco Control* 1997: 6: 5–6.

14. Reid DJ, McNeill AD, Glynn TJ. Reducing the prevalence of smoking in youth in Western countries: an international review. *Tobacco Control* 1995: 4: 266–77.

15. Warner K. The economics of tobacco: myths and realities. *Tobacco Control* 2000: 9: 78–89.

16. Serra C, Cabezas C, Bonfill X, Pladevall-Vila M. Interventions for preventing tobacco smoking in public places. In: *The Cochrane Library, Issue 3*. Oxford: Update Software, 2000.

17. Eriksen MP, Gottlieb NH. A review of the health impact of smoking control at the workplace. *Am J Health Promotion* 1998: 13: 83–104.

18. Parry O, Platt S. Smokers at risk: implications of an institutionally bordered risk-reduced environment. *Health and Place* 2000: 6: 117–23.

19. Silagy C, Mant D, Fowler G, Lancaster T. Nicotine replacement therapy for smoking cessation. In: *The Cochrane Library, Issue 3*. Oxford: Update Software, 2000.

20. Silagy C. Physician advice for smoking cessation. In: *The Cochrane Library, Issue 3*. Oxford: Update Software, 2000.

21. Raw M, McNeill A, West R. Smoking cessation: evidence based recommendations for the healthcare system. *Br Med J* 1999: 318: 182–5.

22. Rice VH, Stead LF. Nursing interventions for smoking cessation. In: *The Cochrane Library, Issue 3*. Oxford: Update Software, 2000.

23. Wakefield M, Borland R. Saved by the bell: the role of telephone helpline services in the context of mass-media anti-smoking campaigns. *Tobacco Control* 2000: 9: 117–19.

24. Owen L. Impact of a telephone helpline for smokers who called during a mass media campaign. *Tobacco Control* 2000: 9: 148–54.

25. Platt S, Tannahill A, Watson J, Fraser E. Effectiveness of antismoking telephone helpline: follow up survey. *Br Med J* 1997: 314: 1371–5.

26. Batten L, Graham H, High S, Ruggiero L, Rossi J. Stage of change, low income and benefit status: a profile of women's smoking in early pregnancy. *Health Education J* 1999: 58: 378–88.

27. DiFranza JR. Youth access: the baby and the bath water. *Tobacco Control* 2000: 9: 120–1.

28. Stead LF, Lancaster T. A systematic review of interventions for preventing tobacco sales to minors. *Tobacco Control* 2000: 9: 169–76.

29. House of Lords (2000) Col79L *Hansard*, 28th June.

30. Joossens L, Raw M. Cigarette smuggling in Europe: who really benefits? *Tobacco Control* 1998: 7: 66–71.

31. House of Commons Select Committee on Health (2000) *Second Report: the Tobacco Industry and the Health Risks of Smoking*. http://www.publications.parliament.uk/pa/cm199900/cmselect/cmhealth/27/2702.htm

32. Jha P, Chaloupka FJ. The economics of global tobacco control. *Br Med J* 2000: 321: 358–61.

33. Puska P, Bettcher D, Yach D. Framework convention on tobacco control. Possible European linkages. *Eur J Pub Health* 2000: 10: 5–6.

34. World Health Organization (WHO). HEALTH 21. *The Health for All Policy Framework for the WHO European Region*. Copenhagen: WHO, 1999.

35. Crossan E, Amos A. *Under a Cloud – Women, Low Income and Smoking.* Edinburgh: Health Education Board for Scotland, 1994.

36. Graham H. *When Life's a Drag: Women, Smoking and Disadvantage.* London: HMSO, 1993.

37. *Independent Inquiry into Inequalities in Health. Report.* London: The Stationery Office, 1998.

38. Fisher EB, Auslander WF, Munro JF, Arfken CL, Brownson RC, Owens NW. Neighbors for a smoke free north side: evaluation of a community organization approach to promoting smoking cessation among African Americans. *Am J Pub Health* 1998: 88: 1658–63.

39. Glasgow RE, Whitlock EP, Eakin EG, Lichtenstein E. A brief smoking cessation intervention for women in low-income planned parenthood clinics. *Am J Pub Health* 2000: 90: 786–9.

40. O'Loughlin J, Paradis G, Renaud L, Meshefedjian G, Barnett T. The 'Yes, I Quit' smoking cessation course: does it help women in a low income community quit? *J Commun Health* 1997: 22: 451–68.

41. McAlister AL, Ramirez AG, Amezcua, C, Pulley L, Stern MP, Mercado S *et al.* Smoking cessation in Texas–Mexico border communities: a quasi-experimental panel study. *Am J Health Promotion* 1992: 6: 274–9.

42. Darity WA, Chen TTL, Tuthill RW, Buchanan DR, Winder AG, Stanek E *et al.* A multi-city community based smoking research intervention project in the African-American population. *Int Q Commun Health Educ* 1998: 17: 117–30.

43. Voorhees CC, Stillman FA, Swank RT, Heagerty PJ, Levine DM, Becker DM. Heart, body and soul: impact of church-based smoking cessation interventions on readiness to quit. *Prev Med* 1996: 25: 277–85.

44. Puska P, Nissinen A, Tuomilehto J. The community-based strategy to prevent coronary heart disease: conclusions from the ten years of the North Karelia Project. *Ann Rev Pub Health* 1995: 6: 117–93.

45. O'Loughlin JL, Paradis G, Gray-Donald K, Renaud L. The impact of a community-based heart disease prevention program in a low-income, inner-city neighborhood. *Am J Pub Health* 1985: 6: 147–93.

46. O'Loughlin JL, Lampron GP, Sacks-Silver GE. Evaluation of a smoking cessation guide for low income, functionally illiterate women: a pilot study. *Can J Pub Health* 1990: 81: 471–2.

47. Reid C, McNeil JJ, Williams F, Powles J. Cardiovascular risk reduction: a randomized trial of two health promotion strategies for lowering risk in a community with low socioeconomic status. *J Cardiovasc Risk* 1995: 2: 155–63.

48. Carleton RA, Lasater TM, Assaf AR, Feldman HA, McKinlay S. The Pawtucket Heart Health Program Writing Group. The Pawtucket Heart Health Program: Community changes in cardiovascular risk factors and projected disease risk. *Am J Pub Health* 1995: 85: 777–85.

49. Goodman RM, Wheeler FC, Lee PR. Evaluation of the heart to heart project: lessons from a community-based chronic disease prevention project. *Am J Health Promotion* 1995: 9: 443–55.

50. Brownson RC, Smith CA, Pratt M, Mack NE, Jackson-Thompson J, Dean CG *et al.* Preventing cardiovascular disease through community-based risk reduction: the Bootheel heart health project. *Am J Pub Health* 1996: 86: 206–13.

51. O'Loughlin JL, Paradis MD, Gray-Donald K, Renaud L. The impact of a community-based heart disease prevention program in a low income, inner-city neighborhood. *Am J Pub Health* 1999: 89: 1819–26.

52. Shelley E, Daly L, Collins C, Christie M, Conroy R, Gibney M *et al.* Cardio-vascular risk factor changes in the Kilkenny health project: a community health promotion program. *Eur Heart J* 1995: 16: 752–60.

53. Shelley E, Collins C, Daly L. Trends in smoking prevalence: the Kilkenny health project population surveys 1985–91. *Irish Med J* 1995: 89: 182–5.

54. The Commit Research Group. Community Intervention Trial for Smoking Cessation (COMMIT). I. Cohort results from a four-year community interven-tion. *Am J Pub Health* 1995: 85: 183–92.

55. The Commit Research Group. Community Intervention Trial for Smoking Cessation (COMMIT). II. Changes in adult cigarette smoking prevalence. *Am J Pub Health* 1995: 85: 193–200.

56. Connett JE, Stamler J. Responses of black and white males to the special intervention program of the Multiple Risk Factor Intervention Trial. *Am Heart J* 1984: 108: 839–48.

57. Holme I, Hjermann I, Helgeland A, Leren P. The Oslo Study: diet and antismoking advice. Additional results from a 5-year primary preventive trial in middle-aged men. *Prev Med* 1985: 14: 279–92.

58. Jamrozik K, Vessey M, Fowler G, Wald N, Parker G, Van Vunakis H. Con-trolled trial of three different antismoking interventions in general practice. *Br Med J* 1984: 288: 1499–503.

59. Macaskill P, Pierce JP, Simpson JM, Lyle DM. Mass media-led antismoking campaign can remove the education gap in quitting behavior. *Am J Pub Health* 1992: 82: 96–8.

60. Shirres G. Successful implementation of a no-smoking policy. *Collegian* 1996: 3: 30–8.

61. Brown J, Parr W, Bates M. Evaluation of a smoking cessation programme that uses behaviour modification. *NZ Med J* 1999: 112: 399–402.

62. Helmert U. Social class and risk factor changes at the midpoint of the German Cardiovascular Prevention Study. In: Abel T, Geyer S, Gerhardt U, eds. *Medical Sociology: Research on Chronic Illness.* Bonn/Berlin: 1993.

63. Fortmann SP, Taylor CB, Flora JA, Jatulis DE. Changes in adult cigarette smoking prevalence after 5 years of community health education: The Stanford 5-city project. *Am J Epidem* 1993: 137: 82–96.

64. Weinehall L, Westman G, Hellsten G, Boman K, Hallmans G, Pearson TA *et al.* Shifting the distribution of risk: results of a community intervention in a Swedish program for the prevention of cardiovascular disease. *J Epidemiol Commun Health* 1999: 53: 243–50.

65. Brannstrom I, Weinehall L, Persson LA, Wester PO, Wall S. Changing social patterns of risk factors for cardiovascular disease in a Swedish community intervention program. *Int J Epidemiol* 1993: 22: 1026–37.

9 Children, an important target group for the reduction of socioeconomic inequalities in health

Andreas Mielck, Hilary Graham and Sven Bremberg

Introduction

Children are an important group for interventions aimed at reducing health inequalities. First, there are large socioeconomic inequalities – and thus also health inequalities – among children. Child poverty, as measured by the proportion of children living in households with incomes less than half the average, ranges from less than 4 per cent in Sweden and Norway to about 20 per cent in the United Kingdom (UK) and Italy (1). In some countries, such as Germany, childhood poverty has increased dramatically in recent years (2). Second, childhood is a key life stage, with exposure to disadvantage in childhood having lasting effects on socioeconomic status and on health in adult life. Third, there is strong evidence that childhood health inequalities can be reduced. Finally, and underlining these three arguments, European countries are giving greater recognition to the right of all children to the best possible start in life, a right endorsed in the United Nations Convention on the Rights of the Child (www.unicef.org/crc).

In this chapter, 'children' refers to those aged up to 18 years. The chapter mainly deals with inequalities by family income, parental education or parental occupation.

Socioeconomic inequalities in health among children

Description

Child health has improved dramatically in Europe over the past 100 years, but there are still pronounced inequalities. These include intrauterine growth and growth in childhood (3, 4). Because these dimensions, together with weight gain, are associated with adult disease, risk factors influencing health and development in early life are also seen to hold an important key to reducing health inequalities in adulthood (5).

Table 9.1 Health inequalities among children in Germany

	Prevalence (in per cent, controlling for age and sex) Social class of the parents[a]					
	1 (lower)	2	3	4	5 (upper)	Total
Distribution in the study	5.3	38.1	24.2	26.2	6.2	100.0
Poor general health[b]	16	7	8	5	1	7
Headache[b]	22	11	13	11	9	12
Backache[b]	16	10	9	7	7	9
Poor sleep[b]	26	17	18	15	16	17
Helplessness[c]	14	7	6	5	3	6
Loneliness[d]	19	14	9	8	9	11

Notes:
a Index of education and occupation of the parents and of the financial situation of the family
b Daily or more than once per week; c very often; d often
b,c,d different categories used in the questionnaire for different questions)
Study population: 3,328 boys and girls aged 11–15 years (survey conducted 1994)

Source: Kloche & Hurrelmann (8)

There are also marked socioeconomic gradients in negative dimensions of child health, including infant mortality and childhood morbidity. Data from the 1990s for England and Wales, for example, show that infant mortality rates in the lower social classes are 1.71 times higher than in the upper classes; the corresponding mortality difference for children aged 0–14 years is 3.30 times (6). Health inequalities among children are also evident from data on morbidity (2). A survey conducted in 1994 in Germany, for example, shows that in the lower social classes the prevalence of physical and psychological morbidity is up to 16 times higher than in the upper classes (Table 9.1). Similar results are found for other measures of morbidity, such as limiting long-standing illness and dental health (6). As Spencer (7) puts it: 'There is a consistent positive correlation between low socioeconomic status and adverse late pregnancy and child health outcomes in developed countries which holds for mortality at all ages and for measures of medically defined morbidity and parent-reported morbidity.'

Although socioeconomic inequalities in child health are evident across Europe, their scale varies. For example, as Figure 9.1 indicates, the socioeconomic gradient in infant mortality is more pronounced in Greater London (England) than in Stockholm (Sweden).

Potential causes and consequences of health inequalities among children

Explanations of health inequalities track the socioeconomic patterning of child and adult health back through a series of intermediate factors to

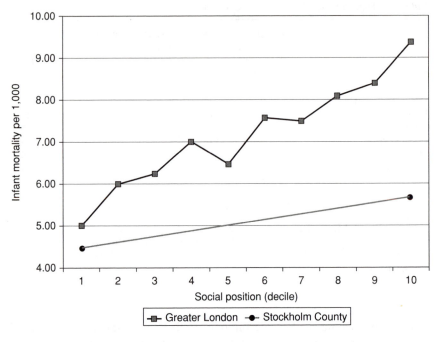

Figure 9.1 Infant mortality in Greater London 1990–5 and Stockholm county
1987–95 by social position of residential area

Source: The information was provided by the Health of Londoners Project – Directorate of
Public Health (Martin Bardsley) and by the Stockholm County Register. Comparable data
were collected from London and from Stockholm county, yet the size of the Stockholm
county population was only one-fifth of that of London. Therefore, the information from
Stockholm county is presented as a regression line, and not as specific points as for London,
in order to increase the readability of the graph.

individual socioeconomic status. Health inequalities are seen as the outcome
of differences in exposure to intermediate risk factors (see Chapter 1). These
are typically grouped into:

*   Material/environmental, for example, housing, environmental pollution
*   Service related, for example, access to and utilization of healthcare
    services
*   Psychosocial, for example, social support, parental interest, stress at
    school
*   Behavioural, for example, nutrition, active and passive smoking.

Poor socioeconomic circumstances tend to be associated with an adverse
profile of adolescent health behaviours. Concerning smoking, in northern
European countries in particular it is young people on disadvantaged educational trajectories – that is, heading towards leaving school early and without
qualifications – who are more likely to become regular and persistent smokers

in adult life. There is increasing evidence that early exposure to advantage and disadvantage has lifelong effects, making childhood a particularly critical period for interventions designed to reduce health inequalities. First, we know that children growing up in lower socioeconomic groups are more likely to follow educational pathways that expose them to greater risks of unemployment and reliance on social security benefits in adulthood (3). Secondly, there is evidence that children born into poorer circumstances accumulate more material risks (for example, overcrowded homes and poverty), more psychological risks (for example, loss of a parent) and more behavioural risks (for example, poorer diet, greater exposure to passive smoking) as they move through childhood. Thirdly, exposure to poor material conditions in infancy and childhood has been identified as having a long-term effect on adult health, independent of adult socioeconomic status (9–11). Other research has studied the effects of exposures in utero and found evidence that under-nutrition in pregnancy programmes an individual's susceptibility to disease in adulthood (12). However, there is evidence to suggest that the contribution of childhood factors to disease risk in later life differs for different diseases. For example, deprivation in childhood may play a particularly important role in the aetiology of certain diseases, such as stroke and stomach cancer; for other diseases socioeconomic conditions at other life-course stages may be just as or more important (13).

Overview of effective interventions and policies

Three basic strategies to reduce childhood health inequalities can be identified: (a) reduction of socioeconomic inequalities by 'levelling up' living standards for children in lower socioeconomic groups; (b) interventions aimed at improving the health status of all children, without a special focus on children in lower socioeconomic groups; (c) interventions aimed specifically at improving the health status of children in lower socioeconomic groups. The first strategy may be the most difficult, but it is likely to be crucial for the effectiveness of the others. However, the second and third types of intervention are more likely to be evaluated through methods regarded as scientifically rigorous; this section therefore focuses on examples of these interventions.

The following limitations of the evidence on these interventions should be noted:

- Evaluated interventions are the exception. As a result, a vast range of innovative interventions remain unmentioned here.
- Assessing outcomes requires research designs that are both longitudinal and scientifically rigorous. Otherwise, important effects – anticipated and unanticipated – can go undetected. The Head Start programme in the United States (USA), for example, one of the best known and successful childhood intervention programmes, was initially regarded as

a failure; it was only with later follow-up, measuring longer-term and broader outcomes, that it was re-evaluated as a success (14, 15).

• How children and their parents measure effectiveness and evaluate interventions is important, but user perceptions are rarely incorporated into designs of evaluated interventions (16). Interventions perceived as stigmatizing may reduce participation among the groups most in need of support (15).

Major risk factors

The health problems that lead to the greatest number of disability adjusted life years (DALY) in Europe have been identified in recent reports (17–19). For European children aged 0–14 years, the eight most important causes of ill-health are neonatal disorders, congenital defects, sudden infant death syndrome (SIDS), accidental injuries, mental health problems, infections, malignant tumours and asthma. There are socioeconomic gradients in morbidity and/or mortality for all these conditions, except for malignant tumours (7, 20, 21), thus, measures intending to reduce health inequalities in children should also address the socioeconomic conditions that increase their prevalence and severity. To be more specific: the interventions should focus on well established risk factors that are more common in socially disadvantaged groups, and which have an important influence on these seven conditions.

For physical health problems only a limited number of risk factors fulfil these requirements. The main ones are environmental hazards (childhood accidents, respiratory problems), economic stress (multiple health problems), parental tobacco smoking (low birthweight, SIDS, infections, asthma), lack of breastfeeding (SIDS, infections, asthma), sleeping prone (SIDS), lack of routine immunizations (infections) and multiple risk factors for accidental injuries. Additional but less well established risk factors are family stress, weak family social support, inadequate nutrition and access to healthcare. The main risk factors for mental health problems are family stress, weak family social support, insecure infant–carer attachment, low caregiver sensitivity to an infant, maternal depression, lack of quality preschool cognitive and emotional training, lack of quality school education (including risk factors such as schools with more than 500 students, lacking pedagogic leadership, etc.).

Universalist versus selectivist approaches

To reduce inequalities in health it might be appropriate to address either the most disadvantaged children, all children, or any fraction in between. The relationship between social position and health outcomes is usually continuous, however. The information from Greater London, upon which Figure 9.1 is based, indicates that the cumulated fraction of mortality, which can be attributed to low social position, is 44 per cent. The most disadvantaged decile (that is, the lowest 10 per cent of the population) contributes only 9 per cent. Accordingly, the most disadvantaged decile contributes only a fifth of the total risk attributed to low social position. Therefore, in order to reduce socioeconomic health inequalities it is not sufficient to restrict the interventions to children living in poverty.

List of interventions

In Tables 9.2 and 9.3 studies have been included if they address a risk factor that is relevant according to the discussion earlier; if they target socially disadvantaged children or families either as the only group studied or as part of a more general population; and if they have been evaluated. As the major purpose of this chapter is to present and discuss examples that can serve as role models, it is essential that the effect of the intervention has been evaluated and that the evaluation has been published.

The search for reports to be included in the tables was based on several sources. There are two major reviews of interventions aimed at reducing health inequalities, which include studies published in any language. One was conducted by the University of York and focuses on interventions that have been evaluated in an experimental or quasi-experimental design; it includes 94 studies published between 1984 and 1994 (22), most of them ($n = 68$) from the USA. The other review was conducted at the University of Amsterdam (23, 24) and includes studies published until 1993. The search for 'grey literature' (reports not officially published) focused on publications from The Netherlands and the United Kingdom. The review covers 129 publications on interventions, 31 of them being 'grey literature', and again most come from the USA. The criteria for including a study were similar in both cases but not identical. The second review did not exclude studies without an experimental or quasi-experimental design, for example. Additional and more up to date information was obtained from our own network and from an additional literature search. For example, we searched Medline for studies published between 1966 and August 2000, and we searched in the Documentation Centre Socioeconomic Inequalities in Health (Department of Public Health, Erasmus University, Rotterdam). Specific information about this last review is incorporated in the Appendix.

All studies presented in the tables were conducted in Western Europe. Interventions were included only if they had been evaluated by one of the following research designs: (a) randomized controlled trial (RCT), (b) controlled experiment (that is, experiment with control group), (c) observational study with control group, or (d) experiment or time series without a control group.

It is also important to distinguish interventions according to the specific age group, and there are good arguments for some gender-specific interventions. In the tables and figures presented, however, no distinction is made between boys and girls, as this information is largely unavailable and there

Table 9.2 Interventions aimed primarily at children and adolescents

Objective	Target population	Intervention	Effect of intervention	Evidence	Reference
Intervention aimed at low socioeconomic status groups, reported to be effective					
Nutrition	Low-income school children (7–8-year-old) (UK)	Provision of free school milk	Modest height gain (2.9 mm in experimental group) and weight gain	RCT	39
Iron deficiency	Low-income children (UK)	Dietary education Screening for iron deficiency, sickle cell disease and thalassaemia	Screening children was acceptable and successful	Observational study	40
Dental health (caries)	Low-income mothers with young children (UK)	5 groups: 1. Dental health education (DHE) focused on diet 2. DHE focused on oral hygiene instruction 3. Combination 4. Combination (only once a year) 5. Control	Groups 1, 2 and 3 with regular home visits (first 2 years every 3 months, last year twice) are effective in preventing the occurrence of nursing caries	RCT	41
General health	Low-income children (UK)	Reorganization of child health clinic (intensified medical care, including more personal attention and a problem-orientated child record	Increased number of clinical visits and increased detection and treatment of defects	Time series	42
Accidental injuries	Deprived areas, general population (UK, Sweden)	Community interventions; feedback of local data to authorities in charge of local environmental injury risks	Reduction of accidental injuries	Controlled experiments	43, 44

Health problem	Population	Intervention	Outcome	Study type	Ref.
Mental health problems	Low socioeconomic status district (UK)	Structured schooling; clear and realistic targets for the students, feedback from teachers to students, headmaster leadership, etc.	Less behavioural problems, improved social adjustment	Observational study	45
Mental health problems	Low socioeconomic status groups (UK)	Schools with less than 500 students	Less behavioural problems, improved social competence	Observational Study	46
Accidental injuries	Families in deprived areas (UK)	Separation of residential areas from motor traffic	Reduction of fatal injuries	Observational study	47
Intervention aimed at low socioeconomic status groups, reported to be non-effective					
Iron deficiency anaemia	Children (inner-city, deprived population) (UK)	Health education information at key ages by face to face contact (+materials)	No difference in iron content of diets between the two groups	RCT	48
Nutrition	Low-income primary school children (UK)	Increase in Family Credit (to compensate for right to free school meals)	This policy change has led to a significant drop in uptake of school meals	Observational study	49
Intervention aimed at general population, reported to be at least as effective in low as in high socioeconomic status groups					
Mental health problems	Low socioeconomic status adolescents (15/16 y.) and general population[a] (see paragraph 3.3: 'It Is Your Decision') (Sweden)	Training in active problem solving	Increased self-initiated health-enhancing activities, best effect in low socioeconomic status children	Controlled experiment	34, 35
Mental health problems	General population, including low socioeconomic status families (Sweden and other countries)	Child-centred quality daycare	Reduction of behavioural and social problems, effect size increases by age of child	Observational studies[b]	50–52

Table 9.2 (Cont'd)

Objective	Target population	Intervention	Effect of intervention	Evidence	Reference
Dental health (caries)	5-year-old children (UK)	Fluoridation of the drinking water in different communities	Fluoridation reduces but does not eliminate social inequalities	Observational study	53
Mental health problems	General population, including low socioeconomic status groups (several countries)	Less than 20 students in each class	Metastudy of 109 interventions: improved academic achievement and social adjustment[c]	Controlled experiments	54
Tobacco smoking	General population, including low socioeconomic status groups (Finland)	Increased tobacco tax	Reduced smoking in low-income group[d]	Time series	55
Dental health	Children (UK)	Fluoridation of water	A reduction of over one-third in caries experience between 1976 and 1981. Between 1981 and 1987 no further reduction	Quasi-experimental design	56
Amblyopia	Children (UK)	Vision screening service	The relationship between social deprivation and the age at presentation of asymptomatic amblyopia seems to have disappeared	Observational study	57
Dental health (caries)	Children with signs of dental caries and with no recent treatment (UK)	Letter to the parents saying that the child would benefit from a detailed dental examination	Increased visits to dentists, greatest effect in the low socioeconomic status group	RCT	58

Intervention aimed at general population, reported to be less effective in low than in high socioeconomic status groups

Topic	Population	Intervention	Results	Study design	Ref.
Growth	Children (England, Scotland)	1. School meals 2. Lunches prepared at home	No relation between rate of growth and school meals in UK. In Scotland indication that children with school meals have smaller rate of growth	Observational study	59
Height	Primary school children (England, Scotland)	School meals and school milk policies	No consistent association between provision of school meals or school milk and the rate of growth when stratified according to poverty status and ethnic background	Observational study	60
Dental health	5-year-old school children (UK)	Dental health education (toothbrushes, take-home materials)	Improvement in plaque scores took place only in non-deprived schools	Pre-/post-test design. No control group	61
Dental health	Preschool children (UK)	Low-fluoride toothpaste	No difference between low and high fluoride toothpaste. However, caries and plaque more common among low-income children	RCT	62

Intervention aimed at general population, objective of the intervention relevant to low socioeconomic status groups

Topic	Population	Intervention	Results	Study design	Ref.
Tobacco smoking	General population, including low socioeconomic status groups (Norway)	Provocative media campaign in Norway	Reduced smoking	Controlled experiments	63
Accidental injuries	General population, including low socioeconomic status groups (UK)	Child resistant containers for drugs	Reduction of accidental injuries	Time series	64

Table 9.2 (Cont'd)

Objective	Target population	Intervention	Effect of intervention	Evidence	Reference
Accidental injuries	General population, including low socioeconomic status groups (UK)	Wearing of bicycle helmet	70 per cent reduction of head injuries	Observational study	65
Mental health problems	General population, including low socioeconomic status groups (Norway)	Multilevel school programmes targeting students, teachers and parents	50 per cent reduction of bullying	Controlled experiment	66
Accidental injuries	General population, including low socioeconomic status groups (UK)	Building of separate bicycle lanes	20 per cent reduction of accidental injuries	Observational study	67
Tobacco smoking	General population, including low socioeconomic status groups (UK)	School education combined with community interventions	2 UK and 1 Finnish study: reduced smoking	Controlled experiments	68
Road traffic accidents (pedestrian and cyclist)	Children, including low socioeconomic status groups (UK)	Introduction of 20 mph zones in residential areas	Pedestrian and cyclist accidents fell by 70 per cent and 48 per cent respectively (overall reduction: 67 per cent); no 'accident migration' to neighbouring areas	Controlled before/after study	69

Notes:
a Target group 'general population', but effect specifically reported for low socioeconomic status subpopulation as well
b Effects demonstrated with similar methods in 11 US studies, including RCTs (94, 95)
c Mainly studies from the USA
d Also demonstrated in a US study (96)

Table 9.3 Interventions aimed primarily at families

Objective	Target population	Intervention	Effect of intervention	Evidence	Reference
Intervention aimed at low socioeconomic status groups, reported to be effective					
Mental health problems	Low socioeconomic status mothers with a firstborn 6-month-old infant (The Netherlands)	Participation in a training programme aiming at the enhancement of maternal sensitive responsiveness	Increased maternal sensitivity and increased incidence of secure mother–infant attachment at 3.5-year follow-up	Controlled experiment	70, 71
Child safety	Low-income families with children below age 5 (UK)	General practitioner advice about child safety, provision of low-cost safety equipment, use of equipment and safe practices at home	Increased use of socket covers, locks on cupboards for storing cleaning materials, door slam devices; safer practice in storage of medicine	RCT	72
Accidental injuries	Families with children living in deprived areas (UK)	Home visits to prevent childhood accidents, information about the TV series 'Play it Safe' aimed at preventing childhood accidents	Families who were visited at home were more likely to make at least one change to improve safety	Controlled experiment	73
Perinatal disorders	Families living in deprived areas (UK)	Home visiting, local parentcraft classes, community centres	47 per cent in experimental group gave up smoking cf. 25 per cent in control group	Controlled experiment	74
Childhood development	Travelling community mothers (Ireland)	Community mothers' programme with lay volunteers	Encouraging results, especially regarding dietary habits, maternal well-being and developmental stimulation of the children; still low uptake of vaccinations	RCT	75

Table 9.3 (Cont'd)

Objective	Target population	Intervention	Effect of intervention	Evidence	Reference
Mental health problems	Mothers of children below age 5 living in deprived areas (UK)	Group discussions with mothers on topics such as child behaviour and childhood illnesses	Improvement of the psychological well-being of the mothers	RCT	76
Nutritional disorders	Mothers of children aged 1–4 living in deprived areas (UK)	Food diary of the children's diet filled out by the mother, home visits to discuss the child's diet	Improved diet	Time series	77
Childhood development	Mothers having their first child and living in deprived areas (Ireland)	Home visits by volunteer mothers from the community who had been specially trained for this programme	Improvement of a number of health indicators (psychological well-being, diet, immunization, etc.)	Controlled experiment	78
Nutritional disorders	Families with children aged 1–6 months living in deprived areas (Ireland)	Home visits by public health nurses offering advice on nutrition	Improved diet	RCT	79
Multiple	Families living in deprived areas (UK)	Letter from the family clinic informing about preventive services, home visits to promote the use of preventive services	Increased use of preventive services	Time series	80
Mental health problems	Low socioeconomic status families (UK)	Home visiting by midwifes	7 years follow-up, child health and development slightly improved	RCT	81

Mental health problems	Low socioeconomic status families (UK)	Mellow Parenting (group session supporting parenting skills), video feedback used	Reduced negative parent–child interaction[b]	Experiment, no control group	82
Multiple	Pregnant women living in deprived areas	Promotion of prenatal care by a better integration of community-based services	Improved prenatal care participation	Observational study	83

Intervention aimed at general population, reported to be at least as effective in low as in high socioeconomic status groups

SIDS, infections, asthma	General population, including low socioeconomic status groups (Sweden)	Counselling at child health centres	Decreased smoking, larger effect in low socioeconomic status group	Observational study	84
Breastfeeding	General population, including low socioeconomic status women[c] (UK)	Provision of lactation nurse	Increased breastfeeding	RCT	85
Perinatal disorders	General population, including low socioeconomic status families (France)[c]	Additional social support	Some studies demonstrate decreased incidence of low birthweight	Controlled experiments	86, 87
Infections	Families with poor immunization uptake	Information of non-immunized children to GPs and health visitors, clear advice on immunization, immunization referral service	Improved uptake of immunizations in all socioeconomic status groups, inequality did not diminished until 95 per cent overall uptake	Time series	88
Multiple	General population, including low socioeconomic status groups (several countries)	Social security benefits	High family benefits are associated with low infant mortality	Observational study	89

Table 9.3 (Cont'd)

Objective	Target population	Intervention	Effect of intervention	Evidence	Reference
Intervention aimed at general population, objective of the intervention relevant to low socioeconomic status groups					
Mental health problems	General population, including low socioeconomic status families (UK)	Metastudy: three studies of child health nurses' non-directive counselling	Reduced depression, expected to decrease incidence of insecure attachment	Controlled experiments	90
SIDS	General population (UK)	Advice on supine sleeping	Metastudy: decrease of SIDS	Observational study	91
Mental health problems	General population, including low socioeconomic status families (The Netherlands and other countries)	Metastudy: 12 studies of training programmes[c]	Increased maternal sensitivity and increased incidence of secure mother–infant attachment	Controlled experiments	92
Accidental injuries	General population, including low socioeconomic status groups (Norway)	Information to authorities and parents about passive and active burn injury preventive measures	50 per cent reduction in burn injuries	Controlled experiment	93

Notes:
a Effects demonstrated with similar methods in RCT studies in USA (97) and Canada (98)
b Target group 'general population', but effect specifically reported for low socioeconomic status subpopulation as well
c Some studies from the USA are included

are hardly any such gender-specific interventions. In the future, more effort should be directed towards developing specially designed interventions for subgroups defined by age, gender, ethnic background and so on.

Tables 9.2 and 9.3 focus on interventions in Western Europe, but most interventions aimed at reducing childhood health inequalities have been conducted in the USA. Our own search revealed more than 50 publications from the USA dealing with such interventions. Because space is limited these studies cannot be reviewed here, and as there are major differences between the USA and Western Europe in terms of the welfare and healthcare systems, it is not always clear to what extent US findings can be transferred to Western Europe (24). Some principles of 'what works' are surely transferable, however. Kehrer and Wolin (25) in a randomized community-based trial demonstrated, for example, that in poor households the provision of income subsidies can effectively reduce the risk of low birthweight, and that this effect is most pronounced in the highest risk groups (for example, mothers under 18 who smoke). It is important to assess the potential contribution of US analyses to interventions in Western Europe.

The studies presented in Tables 9.2 and 9.3 clearly show that there are many effective interventions, about the same number being aimed primarily at children and adolescents on the one hand, and at families on the other. The health problems most often targeted are mental health and accidents. Looking at the childhood life course, effective interventions have been conducted for all age groups and it cannot be concluded that an intervention is more effective in one age group than in another, each age group seeming to have its specific potential for interventions aimed at reducing health inequalities. Many interventions are delivered by professional staff working in the major settings in which children live – the home and the school – and highlight the contribution that both can play in tackling health inequalities in childhood. Eight of the 47 studies are based on a randomized controlled trial, and 11 other studies are based on a controlled experiment. It can therefore be concluded that it is often possible to evaluate the effect of an intervention using a rigorous method. It is also important to note that most interventions presented here have been conducted in the United Kingdom, and that from a number of countries (such as Germany) there are no interventions at all.

In order to demonstrate how interventions aimed at reducing childhood health inequalities could be carried out, two examples of good practice are described below in more detail. We were looking for examples from two different countries, using two different approaches but both including an evaluation. The first, 'Sure Start', comes from the UK, and the second, 'It is your decision', from Sweden.

'Sure Start'

Sure Start is a new early-childhood programme designed to promote the development of children aged 0–3 in disadvantaged areas (26). Its broad aim is to enable children in need to reach a stage of physical, intellectual and social development to enable them to 'thrive when they reach school', by providing a one-stop gateway to a range of services 'within pram-pushing distance' and backed up by outreach services and domiciliary support. The services include childcare, primary healthcare, early education and income support for families. Services are open to all children in the age range in the catchment area and, on a means-tested basis, are free to low-income families. Sure Start projects are developed with parents and typically build on existing local schemes/networks. Variation is therefore a feature of the initiative, with the result that there is no uniform service input against which expected process and outcome measures can be evaluated. From a health inequalities perspective it is an intervention targeted at a key life stage – the first 3 years of life – and a key life transition, entry to school, with the potential to improve the home environment and the socioeconomic and health trajectories of children.

The development of Sure Start is distinctive in that it has drawn on social science evidence on the effectiveness of early interventions (27). In line with this evidence, its combined focus on parents, on children and on the provision of services sensitive to the needs of disadvantaged communities maximizes the chance of its having a positive effect on child health and development. Projects have an obligation to monitor outputs and outcomes. A wider, independent evaluation is planned, with the new UK millennium birth cohort study providing a baseline against which the progress of Sure Start children can be compared.

There are potential effects on the health of children – for example on their psychosocial well-being and nutritional status – which the evidence suggests may also carry forward into improved health in adulthood (4, 5, 7, 14, 15, 27). Longer-term effects could include the outcomes identified in other early intervention initiatives (for example, higher employment and skill levels in mothers, improved school performance, improved employment prospects).

These potential benefits for Sure Start children will be mediated (and blunted) by other influences on childhood disadvantage and their life-course effects on socioeconomic status and health. For example, it does not directly address the material circumstances of poor children: the one in four children living on state benefits (income support) are still in households well below the poverty line (28). The population impact of Sure Start is limited by its targeted approach: it aims to reach a third of children aged 0–3 years in poverty by 2004. It is targeted at disadvantaged areas (local authorities), but not necessarily at the most disadvantaged neighbourhoods within them or at the most disadvantaged children. It is also cost limited. The resources per child (1999–2002) are currently less than a quarter of those devoted to each student in higher education (29). Finally, being targeted at disadvantaged groups, its potential impact does not extend up the socioeconomic gradient.

'It is your decision': A student-centred health education model at school for adolescents

Socioeconomic health inequalities increase during development from adolescence to young adulthood (30). These changes might be explained by increasing disparity in life environments during this period of life. Certain psychological predispositions and vulnerabilities might also contribute. Individuals react differently to problems and opportunities: good mental health is consistently associated with active coping, for example, a focus on active problem solving (31, 32), instead of denial, aggression, depression and so on. The evidence suggests that active coping is less common in socially disadvantaged groups (33). Thus, some health inequalities might be counteracted by training adolescents in active coping. A school-based method for that purpose was developed in Sweden in 1985, and its effects have been confirmed in a Swedish (34, 35) and a Danish controlled study (36). The manual is also used in a German version (37).

The students participate in six 1-hour sessions, three in groups of five students, alternating with three individual sessions over a period of approximately 2 months. The students clarify what makes them feel good or bad by means of discussions and worksheets. In this way, the method intends to bring the students face to face with their own life situations. Out of this, the students are invited to draw up a health-enhancing goal of their own. During the subsequent sessions their progress with respect to this goal is discussed. Hence, the method forms a strategy for health enhancement which starts by identifying personally relevant health issues and continues with self-initiated activities promoting a personally relevant goal.

A first quasi-experimental pre/post control group study was carried out with 105 students, 15–16 years of age, in four schools in disadvantaged districts. Statistically significant differences in favour of the experimental group were found for self-reported problem-orientated activities concerning the school, activities aiming at improving well-being and self-esteem, and a tendency in the same direction for locus of control. The differences were more apparent in students of working-class origin than in middle-class students. This effect may be due to the concrete and perspicuous way of working, where drawing on worksheets was as important as verbal communication.

Almost all students selected a specific individual goal which they worked on during the sessions and in the period in between. These goals related mainly to psychological and social health, for example, to improve grades in a school subject, or to get along better with a specific friend. In the post-test interviews, 4 months after the last session, the students were asked to report on health-enhancing activities that they themselves had initiated after the last session, mainly concerning physical health. Most of these activities had not been treated as goals during the sessions. Thus, the students had improved their ability to carry out self-initiated health-promoting activities, a competence which is closely related to active coping.

Conclusions

A great number of interventions are shown to be effective in reducing childhood health inequalities, but it is obvious that much more could and should
be done to address this fundamental problem. Although interventions need
to address local needs and contexts, some general principles have been identified for success (for example, (22)). Interventions should:

- be vigorous, intensive, multifaceted and interdisciplinary;
- include face-to-face interventions with individuals and small groups in
  indigenous settings (home, school, workplace etc.);
- include an initial needs assessment, to help ensure that cultural values
  are respected;
- include agents from the target populations in the design and delivery
  phases;
- provide access to skills, services and material support, as well as advice
  and information.

No intervention can meet all these criteria perfectly. It is hoped, though,
that this list might be helpful in the planning phase of an intervention, when
different options are being developed and evaluated. 'Downstream' interventions should be mixed with 'upstream' ones. Downstream interventions
(such as vaccination for children in poor households) are probably less
expensive, but upstream interventions (such as improving the quality of
preschooling in deprived areas) are probably more effective. It is misleading
to discredit upstream interventions as too costly, as they might well be more
cost-effective than downstream interventions. There can be no doubt, however, that the most cost-effective way is to combine the two. Also, policies
addressing the total population (universalist policies) should be mixed with
those that specifically address low socioeconomic status groups (targeted
policies). Both have their pros and cons: universalist policies carry the risk
of missing those most in need, for example, and targeted policies carry the
risk of discrimination. We would argue that many universalist policies –
such as equal access to education and healthcare for all – are crucial for
reducing childhood health inequalities, but that targeted policies – such as
regular home visits to low-income mothers with young children (see Table
9.2, (41)) – are very important as well.

Our review suggests that many different interventions are carried out by
community and professional organizations, but there is no routine reporting
system for describing them. Most are not well known, and very few have
been systematically evaluated. It is therefore difficult to learn from their
experiences. This is why we strongly recommend that every intervention
involve some kind of evaluation, with a Europe-wide reporting system. One
of the most important contributions that public health researchers can make
is to participate in the development and evaluation of such interventions

(38). It is a challenging task to convince governments and agencies that interventions should be evaluated, and to find a compromise between a perfect scientific evaluation on the one hand and the constraints of the specific intervention on the other. Without this effort, it will not be possible to establish a set of effective interventions aimed at reducing childhood health inequalities.

References

1. UNICEF. *Child Poverty in Rich Nations, Innocenti Report Card No 1*. Florence: 2000 (www.unicef-icdc.org/publications/pdf/repcardle.pdf)
2. Mielck A. Armut und Gesundheit bei Kindern und Jugendlichen: Ergebnisse der sozial-epidemiologischen Forschung in Deutschland (Poverty and health in childhood and adolescence: results of social-epidemiology research in Germany). In: Klocke A, Hurrelmann K (Hrsg). *Kinder und Jugendliche in Armut. 2., vollständig überarbeitete Auflage*. Opladen: Westdeutscher Verlag, 2001; 230–53.
3. Power C, Matthews S. Origins of health inequalities in a national population sample. *Lancet* 1997: 350: 1584–5.
4. Gunnell DJ, Davey-Smith G Frankel G *et al.* Childhood leg length and adult mortality: follow-up of the Carnegie (Boyd Orr) Survey of Diet and Health in Prewar Britain. *J Epidemiol Commun Health* 1998: 52: 142–52.
5. *Acheson Report: Independent Inquiry into Inequalities in Health* (Chairman Sir Donald Acheson). London: The Stationery Office, 1999.
6. Drever F, Whitehead M, eds. *Health Inequalities*. London: Office for National Statistics, 1997.
7. Spencer N. *Poverty and Child Health*. Oxford: Radcliffe Medical Press, 1996.
8. Klocke A, Hurrelmann K. Armut und Gesundheit. Inwieweit sind Kinder und Jugendliche betroffen? (Poverty and health. How are children and adolescents affected?). *Zeitschr Gesundheitswiss* 1995 (2. Beiheft): 138–51.
9. Lundberg O. The impact of childhood living conditions on illness and mortality in adulthood. *Soc Sci Med* 1991: 36(8): 1047–52.
10. Power C. Social and economic background and class inequalities in health among adults. *Soc Sci Med* 1991: 32(4): 411–17.
11. Mheen D van de: *Inequalities in Health: To Be Continued? A Lifecourse Perspective on Socioeconomic Inequalities in Health*. Rotterdam: Erasmus University, 1998.
12. Barker D. *Mothers, Babies and Health in Later Life*. London: Churchill Livingstone, 1998.
13. Davey Smith G, Gunnell D, Ben-Shlomo Y. Lifecourse approaches to socio-economic differentials in cause-specific adult mortality. In: Leon D, Watt G, eds. *Poverty, Inequality and Health*. Oxford: Oxford University Press, 2000; 88–124.
14. McKey H, Condelli L *et al. The Impact of Head Start on Children, Families and Communities. Final Report of the Head Start Evaluation, Synthesis and Utilization Project*. Washington: US Department of Health and Human Services, 1985.
15. Oliver C, Smith M. *The Effectiveness of Early Interventions*. Perspectives on Education Policy Series. London: Institute of Education, 2000.

16.   Alderson P. How much do children care about effectiveness? In: Alderson P, Brill S *et al.*, eds. *What Works? Effective Social Interventions and Child Welfare*. London: Barnardos, 1996.

17.   Murray J, Lopez A. *Global Burden of Disease. Vol 1*. Harvard: Harvard University Press, 1996.

18.   National Institute of Public Health. *Determinants of Burden of Disease in the European Community*. Stockholm: National Institute of Public Health, 1997.

19.   Peterson S, Backlund I, Diderichsen F. *Sjukdomsbördan i Sverige – en Svensk DALY-kalkyl* (Burden of disease in Sweden. A Swedish DALY estimation). Stockholm: Karolinska Insitutet, Folkhälsoinstitutet, Epidemiologiskt Centrum, Stockholms Läns Landsting, 1999.

20.   Pless IB, ed. *The Epidemiology of Childhood Disorders*. New York: Oxford University Press, 1994.

21.   Bremberg S, ed. *Evidence-based Health Promotion for Children and Adolescents in Stockholm County*. Huddinge: CBU, 1999.

22.   University of York *Review of the Research on the Effectiveness of Health Service Interventions to Reduce Variations in Health*. York, 1995.

23.   Gepkens A, Gunning-Schepers LJ. *Interventions to Reduce Socioeconomic Health Differences*. Amsterdam: University of Amsterdam, Institute of Social Medicine, 1995.

24.   Gepkens A, Gunning-Schepers LJ. Interventions to reduce socioeconomic health differences: a review of the literature. *Eur J Public Health* 1996: 6: 218–26.

25.   Kehrer BH, Wolin CM. Impact of income maintenance on low birth weight: evidence from the Gary Experiment. *J Human Resources* 1979: XIV (4): 434–62.

26.   Department for Education and Employment (DFEE). *Sure Start: Making a Difference for Children and Families*. London: DFEE, 1999.

27.   HM Treasury. *Comprehensive Spending Review: Cross-departmental Review of Provision for Young Children, Supporting Papers, Volumes 1 and 2*. London: The Stationery Office, 1998.

28.   Piachaud D, Sutherland H. *How Effective is the British Government's Attempt to Reduce Child Poverty?* CASE paper 38. London: London School of Economics, 2000.

29.   Piachaud D. Progress on poverty. *New Economy* 1999: 6(3): 154–60.

30.   West P. Health inequalities in the early years: is there equalisation in youth? *Soc Sci Med* 1997: 44(6): 833–58.

31.   Lazarus RS. Coping theory and research: past, present, and future. *Psychosom Med* 1993: 55(3): 234–47.

32.   Lazarus R, Folkman S. *Stress, Appraisal, and Coping*. New York: Springer, 1994.

33.   Bosma H, van de Mheen D, Mackenbach JP. Social class in childhood and general health in adulthood: questionnaire study of contribution of psychological attributes. *Br Med J* 1999: 318: 18–22.

34.   Arborelius E, Bremberg S. It is your decision – behavioural effects of a student centred school health education model for adolescents. *J Adolesc* 1988: 11: 287–97.

35.   Arborelius E, Bremberg S. How do teenagers respond to a consistently student-centred programme of school health education at school? *Health Promotion in Action*, ESSOP Congress. Valencia, Spain: 1992: 69.

36. Back P. *Du bestemmer projektet, '– en anderledes form for sundhedsamtaler'* (*'It's Your Decision'* – *An Alternative Method for Communication about Health*). Ringkjøbing, Denmark: Ringkjøbing Amt, 1998.

37. Bisegger C, Bolliger-Salzmann, H. *Evaluation des 'Du seisch wo düre' (Evaluation of 'It's Your Decision')*. Bern: Institut für Sozial- und Präventivmedizin, Universität Bern, 1998.

38. Mackenbach JP, Gunning-Schepers L. How should interventions to reduce inequalities in health be evaluated? *J Epidemiol Commun Health* 1997: 51: 359–64.

39. Baker IA, Elwood PC, Hughes J, Jones M, Moore F, Sweetnam PM. A randomised controlled trial of the effect of the provision of free school milk on the growth of children. *J Epidemiol Commun Health* 1980: 34(1): 31–4.

40. James J, Lawson P, Male P, Oakhill A. Preventing iron deficiency in preschool children by implementing an educational and screening programme in an inner city practice. *Br Med J* 1989: 299(6703): 838–40.

41. Kowash MB, Pinfield A, Smith J, Curzon MEJ. Effectiveness on oral health of a long-term health education programme for mothers with young children. *Br Dent J* 2000: 188: 201–5.

42. Nicoll A, Mann N, Mann S, Vyas H. The child health clinic: results of a new strategy of community care in a deprived area. *Lancet* 1986: 1: 606–8.

43. Roberts H, Smith S, Bryce C. Prevention is better. *Sociol Health Illness* 1993: 15: 447–63.

44. Svanström L, Ekman R, Schelp L, Lindström Å. The Lidköping accident prevention programme – a community approach to injury to preventing childhood injuries in Sweden. *Injury Prev* 1995: 1(3): 169–72.

45. Rutter M, Maughan B, Mortimore P, Ouston J. *Fifteen Thousand Hours*. London: Open Books, 1979.

46. Rutter M. School effects on pupil progress: research findings and policy implications. *Child Dev* 1983: 54: 1–54.

47. Sharples PM, Storey A, Aynsley-Green A, Eyre JA. Causes of fatal childhood accidents involving head injury in northern region, 1979–86. *Br Med J* 1990: 301(6762): 1193–7.

48. Childs F, Aukett A, Darbyshire P, Ilett S, Livera LN. Dietary education and iron deficiency anaemia in the inner city. *Arch Dis Child* 1997: 76(2): 144–7.

49. Somerville SM, Rona RJ, Chinn S, Qureshi S. Family Credit and uptake of school meals in primary school. *J Public Health Med* 1996: 8(1): 98–106.

50. Andersson BE. Effects of day-care on cognitive and socio-emotional competence of thirteen-year-old Swedish schoolchildren. *Child Dev* 1992: 63(1): 20–36.

51. Broberg A, Wesselt H, Lamb M, Hwang C. Effects of care on the development of cognitive abilities in 8-year-olds: a longitudinal study. *Dev Psychol* 1997: 33: 62–9.

52. Zoritch B, Roberts I, Oakley A. Day care for pre-school children (Cochrane Review). *The Cochrane Library* 2000 (3).

53. Carmichael CL, Rugg-Gunn AJ, Ferrell RS. The relationship between fluoridation, social class and caries experience in 5-year-old children in Newcastle and Northumberland in 1987. *Br Dent J* 1989: 167: 57–61.

54. Cooper HM. Does reducing student-to-instructor ratios affect achievement? *Educ Psychol* 1989: 24: 79–98.

55. Pekurinen M. The demand for tobacco products in Finland. *Br J Addiction* 1989: 84(10): 1183–92.

56. Rugg-Gunn AJ, Carmichael CL, Ferrell RS. Effect of fluoridation and secular trend in caries in 5-year-old children living in Newcastle and Northumberland. *Br Dent J* 1988: 165(10): 359–64.

57. Smith LK, Thompson JR, Woodruff G. Children's vision screening: impact on inequalities in central England. *J Epidemiol Commun Health* 1995: 49(6): 606–9.

58. Zarod BK, Lennon MA. The effect of school dental screening on dental attendance. The results of a randomised controlled trial. *Community Dent Health* 1992: 9: 361–8.

59. Rona RJ, Chinn S, Smith AM. School meals and the rate of growth of primary school children. *J Epidemiol Commun Health* 1983: 37(1): 8–15.

60. Rona RJ, Chinn S. School meals, school milk and height of primary school children in England and Scotland in the eighties. *J Epidemiol Commun Health* 1989: 43(1): 66–71.

61. Schou L, Wight C. Does dental health education affect inequalities in dental health? *Commun Dent Health* 1994: 11(2): 97–100.

62. Winter GB, Holt RD, Williams BF. Clinical trial of a low-fluoride toothpaste for young children. *Int Dent J* 1989: 39: 227–35.

63. Hafstad A. Provocative anti-smoking appeals in mass-media campaigns. An intervention study on adolescent smoking (Thesis). Oslo: University of Oslo, 1997.

64. Lawson GR, Craft AW, Jackson RH: Changing pattern of poisoning in children in Newcastle, 1974–81. *Br Med J (Clin Res Ed)* 1983: 287(6384): 15–7.

65. Maimaris C, Summers CL, Browning C, Palmer CR. Injury patterns in cyclists attending an accident and emergency department: a comparison of helmet wearers and non-wearers. *Br Med J* 1994: 308(6943): 1537–40.

66. Olweus D. Bullying at school: basic facts and effects of a school based intervention program. *J Child Psychol Psychiatry* 1994: 35(7): 1171–90.

67. Sabey B. Engineering safety on the road. *Injury Prev* 1995: 1(3): 182–6.

68. Sowden A, Arblaster L. Community interventions for preventing smoking in young people (Cochrane Review). In: *The Cochrane Library*, Issue 1, 2000. Oxford: Update Software.

69. Webster DC, Mackie AM. *Review of Traffic Calming Schemes in 20 mph Zones*, TRL Report 215. Crowthorne, Berkshire: Transport Research Foundation, 1996.

70. Boom van den DC. The influence of temperament and mothering on attachment and exploration: an experimental manipulation of sensitive responsiveness among lower-class mothers with irritable infants. *Child Dev* 1994: 65: 1457–77.

71. Boom van den DC. Do first-year intervention effects endure? Follow-up during toddlerhood of a sample of Dutch irritable infants. *Child Dev* 1995: 66: 1798–816.

72. Clamp M, Kendrick D. A randomised controlled trial of general practitioner safety advice for families with children under 5 years. *Br Med J* 1998: 316: 1576–9.

73. Colver AF, Hutchinson PJ, Judson EC. Promoting children's home safety. *Br Med J (Clin Res Ed)* 1982: 285(6349): 1177–80.

74. Davies J, Evans F. The Newcastle Community Midwifery Care Project. In: Robinson S, Thomson A, eds. *Midwives, Research and Childbirth*. London: Chapman & Hall, 1991.

75. Fitzpatrick P, Molloy B, Johnson Z. Community mothers' programme: extension to the travelling community in Ireland. *J Epidemiol Commun Health* 1997: 51(3): 29–303.

76. Gordon J, Swan M. Springburn Primary Care Project. *Community Support Groups for High-dependency Families – a Pilot Study in One General Practice*. Glasgow: Interim Report. Health Promotion Department, Greater Glasgow Health Board, 1994 (cited from Ref. 22, pp. 75 and 151).

77. James J, Brown J, Douglas M, Cox J, Stocker S. Improving the diet of under fives in a deprived inner city practice. *Health Trends* 1992: 24(4): 161–4.

78. Johnson Z, Howell F, Molloy B. Community mothers' programme: randomised controlled trial of non-professional intervention in parenting. *Br Med J* 1993: 306: 1449–52.

79. Lee P. The effects of a nutrition intervention programme on the nutritional status of pre-school children in disadvantaged areas of Dublin. University of Dublin: PhD dissertation 1988 (cited from Ref. 22, pp. 92 and 153).

80. Marsh GN, Channing DM. Narrowing the health gap between a deprived and an endowed community. *Br Med J* 1988: 296: 173–6.

81. Oakley A, Hickey D, Lynda R, Rigby A. Social support in pregnancy – does it have long-term effects? *J Reprod Infant Psychol* 1996: 14: 7–22.

82. Puckering C, Rogers J, Mills M, Cox A, Mattsson-Graff M. Process and evaluation of a group intervention for mothers with parenting difficulties. *Child Abuse Rev* 1994: 3: 299–310.

83. Wood J. A review of antenatal care initiatives in primary care settings. *Br J Gen Pract* 1991: 342: 20–6.

84. Arborelius E, Bremberg S. Child health centre based promotion of a tobacco-free environment in children's homes – a national case study. *Health Promotion International* 2001: 16(3): 245–54.

85. Jones DA, West RR. Effect of a lactation nurse on the success of breast-feeding: a randomised controlled trial. *J Epidemiol Commun Health* 1986: 40(1): 45–9.

86. Papiernik E, Bouyer J, Dreyfus J *et al.* Prevention of preterm births: a perinatal study in Haguenau, France. *Pediatrics* 1985: 76(2): 154–8.

87. Murphy PA. Preterm birth prevention programs. A critique of current literature. *J Nurse Midwifery* 1993: 38(6): 324–35.

88. Reading R, Colver A, Openshaw S, Jarvis S. Do interventions that improve immunisation uptake also reduce social inequalities in uptake? *Br Med J* 1994: 308(6937): 1142–4.

89. Wennemo I. Infant mortality, public policy and inequality – a comparison of 18 industrial countries 1950–1985. *Sociol Health Illness* 1993: 15: 429–45.

90. Cooper P, Murray L. Postnatal depression. *Br Med J* 1998: 316: 1884–6.

91. Gilbert R. The changing epidemiology of SIDS. *Arch Dis Child* 1994: 70(5): 445–9.

92. IJzendoorn van MH, Juffer F, Duyvesteyn MG. Breaking the intergenerational cycle of insecure attachment: a review of the effects of attachment-based interventions on maternal sensitivity and infant security. *J Child Psychol Psychiatry* 1995: 36(2): 225–48.

93.   Ytterstad B, Smith GS, Coggan CA. Harstad injury prevention study: prevention of burns in young children by community based intervention. *Injury Prev* 1998: 4(3): 176–80.

94.   Schorr LB, Schorr D. *Within Our Reach: Breaking the Cycle of Disadvantage.* New York: Anchor Books, 1988.

95.   Durlak JA. *Successful Prevention Programs for Children and Adolescents.* New York: Plenum, 1997.

96.   Biener L, Aseltine RH Jr, Cohen B, Anderka M. Reactions of adult and teen-age smokers to the Massachusetts tobacco tax. *Am J Public Health* 1998: 88(9): 1389–91.

97.   Webster-Stratton C, Herbert M. *Troubled Families, Problem Children.* New York: John Wiley, 1994.

98.   Tremblay R, Vitaro F, Bertrand L *et al.* Parent and child training to prevent early on-set of delinquency: the Montreal longitudinal experimental study. In: McCord J, Tremblay R, eds. *Preventing Anti-social Behavior: Interventions through Birth to Adolescence.* New York: Guilford Press, 1992.

10 Equality of access to healthcare

Iain Paterson and Ken Judge

Introduction

There is growing evidence that health inequalities are not only a function of the maldistribution of economic and social resources that lie outside the health system but are also exacerbated by differential access to health services. Any comprehensive strategy to reduce avoidable inequalities in health must therefore try to improve equality of access to healthcare. Unfortunately, evidence about the existence of such inequality is easier to find than is detailed guidance about effective interventions that tackle the problem. This chapter therefore has two main aims, first, to summarize some of the most recent or compelling evidence about inequalities in access to healthcare, and second, to outline some of the approaches that have been advocated to improve it.

It is important at the outset to clarify certain key assumptions. We believe that equality of access to healthcare involves more than the simple utilization of services. Health needs cannot be defined solely in terms of medical conditions: they are conditioned by social circumstances. As a consequence, the equality imperative requires that all patients should be provided with timely and quality services appropriate to their particular needs and circumstances and their capacity to benefit. This means that judgements about equality of access to healthcare ought to be made in terms of the degree to which potentially achievable health outcomes associated with healthcare system interventions are actually realized for all social groups.

The evidence

There have been two recent major cross-national studies on healthcare access. The first of these, sponsored by the Commonwealth Fund, found striking differences between countries in the relative equality of healthcare experiences. The greatest inequalities in access to care were, not surprisingly, reported in those countries where there is a reliance on private insurance and patient user fees (the United States (USA), Australia and New Zealand). The effects of patient cost sharing are discussed in more detail in

Chapter 11. Within a health system providing universal coverage, such as in the United Kingdom (UK), the absence of financial concerns at the point of delivery facilitates access that reflects need more than ability to pay. As a result, little difference was reported in access to, or quality of, healthcare between income groups in the UK. It was also discovered that the lower income groups were far more likely than the higher to use general practitioners (GPs) more regularly (1). Van Doorslaer *et al.*'s (2) cross-European study of equality in access to care also indicated that lower-income groups are more intensive users of GPs and hospital and specialist services. Taking into account the tendency for relatively poor self-reported health status (and, by implication, the need for healthcare) to be more concentrated at the bottom end of the income distribution, little evidence of an inequitable overall healthcare distribution emerged. The actual distribution of GP and hospital care across income groups was very close to the needs-expected distribution: utilization was much higher among lower-income groups in all countries. However, in about half of the countries studied, more affluent people report significantly more physician contacts than would be expected on the basis of need (Belgium, Denmark, Finland, The Netherlands). Nevertheless, all of the universal healthcare systems in the European countries studied performed reasonably well in terms of horizontal equality in access to and utilization of healthcare in the late 1980s and early 1990s (2).

However, despite reducing inequalities, universal access to healthcare has not eliminated them. There is a large and growing body of European evidence that highlights persisting inequalities not simply along socioeconomic lines, but also in relation to gender, age, ethnicity and geography. The overall picture is not by any means unambiguously bad, but there are grounds for concern in many countries. Summarized below are some of the key research findings in relation to access to primary care and to hospital services.

Access to primary care

Access to primary care is important for two reasons. First, the GP is the initial point of contact with the healthcare system for most people. Second, inequalities in access to secondary care may originate in, and therefore need to be addressed in, the primary care sector. Whereas studies in the early 1990s concluded that there was a 'pro-poor' bias in access to local primary healthcare in the UK (3–5), more recent studies now indicate otherwise. Goddard and Smith's *Equity of Access to Health Care* (1998) reviewed many local studies that found inequalities in access and provision of care in different parts of the UK (6). Some key results are set out below.

- Although higher rates of consultation were associated with greater deprivation (after adjusting for need), the quality and length of time of consultation was poorer for lower income groups.

- Chinese, Africans and young Pakistanis had low consultation rates relative to need.
- The further away patients lived from their general practice, the less likely they were to consult (although differences were not that great for serious health problems).
- Women consulted more often than men, but it is unclear whether this represented a gender inequality for men or whether the differences (found mainly in the 15–44-year-old age group) represented appropriate responses to need during the main reproductive and child-rearing years for women.
- There was an inequitable distribution of GPs – the position had been worsening for those living in the most deprived parts of the country and improving in the least deprived.
- Deprived areas suffered increasing difficulty in recruiting GPs because of poor quality of primary care premises, large numbers of single-GP practices, GPs approaching retirement, and practices without training status.
- The 'inverse prevention law' existed, whereby communities most at risk of ill-health had the least access to a range of effective preventive services, including cancer screening programmes, health promotion and immunization.

De La Hoz and Leon (7) in Spain found self-perceived health status to be strongly linked with medical consultation. After adjustment for age, health service use decreased as socioeconomic level, measured by education and/or income, went up. However, as health status became worse, those in higher educational groups were more likely to consult a doctor than those in lower educational or income groups (7). Van der Meer *et al.* (8) demonstrated socioeconomic differences in the utilization of Dutch healthcare services. Although all services were used more frequently by the less educated, the differences in GP contacts were reduced when controlling for health status (8). Whitehead *et al.* (9) have shown how inequalities in the use of doctor consultations in Sweden favoured non-manual groups in relation to health status by 1993–4. In Germany, low social groups were found to make more use of medical services, demonstrated as a higher average number of visits to a doctor, though not necessarily enough to compensate for their higher needs (10). In Finland during the 1980s, the needs-adjusted physician utilization rates favoured those with higher incomes, mainly from the higher use of services in private practices and occupational healthcare by the affluent groups. The low-income groups more often used general practitioners' services in municipal health centres (11).

The overall picture in relation to equality of access to primary care across Western Europe is complex and varied. At best, however, there are no grounds for complacency. The risk continues in many healthcare systems that the most disadvantaged do not receive the services they require in relation to their needs.

Access to hospital care

UK evidence shows a strong positive relationship between levels of deprivation in an area and hospital admission rates. For outpatients, attendance is either higher among disadvantaged groups or similar to those who are better off, after adjusting for need (6). Socioeconomic differences in hospital utilization in The Netherlands were unclear (8). Whereas Borrell *et al.* (12) found no social class differences in hospital utilization in Barcelona, other recent Spanish studies found that waiting times for hospital admission were greater among people with lower educational levels. In Finland the overall use of short-term somatic inpatient care seemed to be distributed across socioeconomic groups more or less according to need (11).

Access to general services in European hospitals, therefore, appears largely equitable. However, this might not be true of access to and quality of care in specialist or intensive services. For example, there is strong evidence showing systematic inequalities in access to investigation and treatment for specialist cardiac services and in survival after cancer treatment in the UK (6). Keskimäki (11) has demonstrated 'inappropriate socioeconomic differences' in access to coronary bypass operations in Finland, as procedure rates favouring the better-off diverged clearly from the estimated need as indicated by Coronary Heart Disease (CHD)-related mortality and hospitalization. Hip replacement operations and cataract surgery also had procedure rates that favoured the more affluent. He concludes that surgical services in Finnish hospitals are under-utilized by low-income groups despite their high use of non-surgical hospital services (11).

Interventions to improve access to care

The provision of universal access to healthcare free at the point of delivery could itself be classed as a health intervention in tackling social and regional health inequalities. This is certainly the case in countries such as the USA. One quantitative study based on data from the health insurance experiment conducted by the Rand Organization (13) has estimated that between 47,000 and 106,000 lives could be saved each year in the USA as a direct consequence of improving access to healthcare (14). Yet the evidence indicates a clear need for further improvement in the uptake of primary and secondary health services among disadvantaged and 'hard to reach' groups in most universalist healthcare systems across Western Europe.

Reviews of health interventions that tend to focus on health or access problems among general populations in Europe, particularly the UK, are available from the Cochrane Library, the National Health Service (NHS) Centre for Reviews and Dissemination at the University of York, or the associated Database of Abstracts of Reviews of Effectiveness (DARE). Bunton *et al.* (15), Arblaster *et al.* (16) and Gepkens and Gunning-Schepers (17) have extensively reviewed the literature on interventions specifically aimed at reducing socioeconomic health inequalities. In all of these cases the majority of the interventions, whether rated effective or not, are from the United States. Although database and literature searches can yield a number of effective health interventions in Western Europe, the vast majority are found to have targeted the general population or a specific health problem. Although these will also include low socioeconomic status groups and health problems prevalent among such groups, this does not necessarily mean that such interventions are effective or suitable if they are not specifically tested among these groups. As Woodward and Kawachi (18) point out:

> strategies to reduce smoking, increased cholesterol, and high blood pressure, have been designed to achieve overall reduction in these risk factors. But any preventive strategy that relies on access to the healthcare system for delivery – such as the detection of high cholesterol or blood pressure – may worsen socioeconomic gradients in outcomes (such as stroke, heart disease) if there are disparities in access to primary care. (p. 926)

This is why it is important, for the purposes of this chapter, to include only those interventions aimed at low socioeconomic groups, or those which at least report separate results for them. Table 10.1 summarizes a literature review. This review limits itself to interventions that either target low socio-economic groups only, or else the general population but where results were reported in terms of socioeconomic status. Furthermore, all the interventions are aimed at improving the uptake of services, improving health outcomes or both. Specific details about how the review was conducted are incorporated in the Appendix.

Table 10.1 summarizes information from a total of 36 interventions in terms of their primary objective, the target population, the nature and effects of the intervention, the type of evidence or evaluation design employed, and the source. Approximately half of the studies ($n = 19$) report that interventions aimed at groups with low socioeconomic status were effective. The aims of these projects varied from various forms of cancer screening, to treating health risks such as hypertension or substance abuse, to improving maternal and child health outcomes. The interventions themselves were very diverse and included hospital-based education programmes, community outreach activities, and personalized contacts with target groups by healthcare personnel. The quality of the evidence also varies. For example, observational and case studies are mixed in with randomized controlled trials (RCTs). Nevertheless, good-quality studies based on RCTs report such desirable outcomes as increases in the uptake of cancer screening tests or reductions in antisocial behaviour and emergent substance abuse among adolescents in high-risk families.

Not all attempts to improve access to healthcare will prove to be effective. Table 10.1 (under Interventions aimed at low SES groups, reported to be

Table 10.1 Healthcare interventions

Objective	Target population	Intervention	Effect of intervention	Evidence	Reference
Interventions aimed at low SES groups, reported to be effective					
Tuberculosis control	LSES people (USA)	Tuberculosis control programme (health department regulations and services, charity organizations)	Although the programme provided enormous benefits, people often had concerns that took priority over eradicating tuberculosis	Case study	27
Breast screening	Women (50–64 years) multi-ethnic deprived area (UK)	Practice reception staff (telephone calls or letter from GP) to improve screening attendance	The intervention improved breast screening rates modestly	Quasi-experimental design	28
Cancer screening	Low-income Vietnamese-American women (USA)	Community outreach programme to promote recognition, receipt and screening interval (lay health workers)	The intervention increased recognition, receipt and maintenance of cancer screening tests	Observational study with pre/post tests and control group	29
Asthma	LSES patients (Hong Kong)	Hospital-based asthma education programme	Improvement in lung function, reduction in number of hospitalizations, visits to family physicians and accident and emergency department attendance	Observational study with pre/post tests. No control group	30
Breastfeeding	Low-income women (USA)	Breastfeeding educational programme	The programme significantly improved breastfeeding rates	Observational study	31
Cervical cancer screening	LSES women (USA)	Personal visit from lay healthcare worker with written information about importance of screening read out	More experimental women made a visit to the clinic for a pap smear	Observational study with pre/post tests and control group	32
Passive smoking	Low-income women with young children (USA)	Minimal advice and assistance from community health service + tailored self-help guide	The intervention did promote cessation	Observational study with pre/post tests. No control group	33

Topic	Population	Intervention	Results	Study type	Ref
Breastfeeding	Low-income black women (USA)	Health professional prenatal education (individual or classes)	Women in the intervention groups were more likely to breastfeed	RCT	34
Improvement of maternal and child outcomes	LSES pregnant women (primarily black) (USA)	Nurse home visitation programme	Intervention group women had fewer subsequent pregnancies, closely spaced pregnancies and longer intervals between children, fewer months of using Aid to Families with Dependent Children and food stamps	RCT	35
Breast and cervical cancer screening	Women (40–79 years) Low-income managed care programme (USA)	Physician reminder letter and telephone contact	Intervention group women were significantly more likely to receive all needed cancer screening tests	RCT	36
Cervical cancer screening	Women with abnormal pap smears (USA)	Three interventions 1. Personalized follow-up letter and pamphlet 2. Slide–tape programme 3. Transportation incentives	Transportation incentives was the dominant intervention for LSES women	RCT	37
Access to care	Deprived community (UK)	Mailing, health visitors, preventive care in patients' homes	Programme raised uptake of preventive care of its patients in a severely deprived area	Observational study	38
Access to care	Homeless (France)	Early medical social intervention in emergency department (regularize inadequate insurance coverage)	Intervention may be useful for avoiding overcrowding in hospital and repeated visits	Observational study	39
Hypertension management	Inner-city black hypertensive patients (USA)	Three interventions 1. Exit interview 2. Family support intervention (home visit) 3. Small group sessions	Significant differences were found in final blood pressure control status	Quasi-experimental design	40, 41

Table 10.1 (Cont'd)

Objective	Target population	Intervention	Effect of intervention	Evidence	Reference
Intendedness of pregnancy	Low-income women attending family planning clinics (USA)	Brief preconceptional health promotion programme	Introductory programme of preconceptional health promotion programme is associated with a higher rate of intendedness in subsequent pregnancies	Prospective study	42
Preterm birth prevention	LSES pregnant women at high risk for preterm delivery (USA)	Individual instruction by nurses	Preterm birth rate could be markedly decreased as a result of medical provider and patient education	RCT	43
Adolescents' antisocial behaviour	Adolescents and their biological mothers or custodial parents (USA)	Nurse prenatal and early childhood home visitation	The intervention can reduce reported serious antisocial behaviour and emergent use of substances of adolescents born into high-risk families	RCT	44
Access to healthcare (early detection of cancer)	Middle-aged to older adults (USA)	Cancer prevention clinic	Clinic provided comprehensive and effective cancer prevention, education and early detection services to the poor	Observational study	45
Substance abuse	Cocaine-addicted pregnant women (USA)	Pregnancy substance abuse programme delivered in urban, tertiary care hospital	Treatment retention was statistically and clinically improved	Retrospective cohort control study	46
Intervention aimed at low SES groups, reported to be non-effective					
Alcoholism	LSES women (USA)	Multifaceted outpatient treatment (home and hospital visits, cultural and recreational activities, employment counselling)	Attendance was not associated with increased abstinence or employment	Observational study with pre/post tests. No control group	47

Improve medical care utilization	Low-income families (USA)	Outreach workers' services	The outreach intervention had a positive effect on access to care, less successful in changing utilization patterns, no effect on appointment-keeping behaviour	Quasi-experimental design	48
Smoking cessation	Female smokers attending low-income planned parenthood clinics (15–35 years) (USA)	1. 9-minute video, 12–15 minutes of behavioural counselling, clinician advice to quit and follow-up telephone calls 2. Advice only	Six weeks post intervention (10.2% quit rate vs. 6.9%) Six months post intervention (6.4% vs. 3.8%, not significant)	RCT	49
Maternal health status	Uninsured pregnant women (USA)	State-wide health coverage programme	The provision of health insurance alone may not be associated with an improvement in maternal health. The rates of caesarean sections increased	Observational study	50
Access to care	Low-income pregnant women (USA)	State-wide provision of health coverage to uninsured low-income women	Expansion of health coverage to uninsured low-income women was not associated with an improvement in access to prenatal care or birth outcomes	Observational study	51
Access to care	Low-income children (USA)	Medicaid	Children on Medicaid receive less well care from a private practice or paediatrician, see the same health professional at each well visit less often	RCT	52
Access to care	Uninsured patients (USA)	Free access to physicians	This intervention fills important needs but is not sufficient for many uninsured patients to receive necessary preventive services	Cross sectional survey	53

Table 10.1 (*Cont'd*)

Objective	Target population	Intervention	Effect of intervention	Evidence	Reference
Access to care	Low-income uninsured women and children (USA)	Medicaid	Medicaid is an inadequate resource for uninsured families with children	Observational study	54, 55
Intervention aimed at general population, reported to be at least as effective in low as in high SES groups					
Access to primary healthcare	General population (UK)	National Health Service	The NHS has achieved equality in terms of access to primary healthcare. There is no consistent bias against the LSES groups	General Household Survey	56
Smoking cessation	Adult smoking patients of six GP practices (UK)	Four study groups: 1. Verbal and written advice from GP 2. Advice + demonstration of exhaled CO 3. Advice + further help from health visitor 4. Control group	Giving advice and demonstration of exhaled CO is the most effective intervention in the lower social classes (approximately 14.5% quitters after 1 year)	RCT	57
Detection and treatment of hypertension	Adults (14–61 years) (USA)	Insurance plans 1. Providing free care 2. Cost sharing	Blood pressures with free care were significantly lower than with cost sharing plans. With a larger difference for low-income hypertensives	RCT	58
Cardiovascular risk reduction (community intervention which involves among others medical care providers)	Adults (USA)	Mass media programmes Print media (delivered through direct mail and organizations: work sites, medical care providers)	In general, declines in smoking prevalence, blood pressure and cholesterol were stronger in the least educated group	Four cross-sectional surveys	59

Dental care (encouraging school children to visit a dentist)	School children (4–6 years) (UK)	School dental inspection	Attendances at both general dental practitioners and community dental clinics were increased. (effect seen particularly in LSES areas)	Quasi-experimental design	60
Intervention aimed at general population, reported to be less effective in low than in high SES groups					
Mammography screening	Women (50–69 years) (Australia)	Public and personal recruitment strategies	Lower attendance rate was associated with living in an LSES area	Observational study	61
Hypertension	Hypertensive adults (USA)	Two groups: 1. Treatment by existing resources of medical care) 2. Treatment at study clinical centre	For people in group 2 no gradient of mortality was observed. In group 1 people with lowest education had a 5-year adjusted death rate twice as high as those with highest education	RCT	62
Cardiovascular risk reduction (community intervention which involves among others medical care providers)	Adults (18–74 years) (USA)	10 types of CVD intervention materials and programmes	People in the highest education group are 3–5 times more likely to report use of materials than people in the lowest education groups	Cross-sectional survey	63
Access to care	General population (Finland)	In the 1990s municipalities were given more choice in providing services and possibilities to introduce cost sharing	This system does not guarantee equitable access to services	Observational study	64

non-effective) summarizes eight studies that failed to show improved outcomes for groups in low socioeconomic groups relative to others. At the same time, other studies shown in the table (under Intervention aimed at general population, reported to be at least as effective in low as in high SES groups) (*n* = 5) appear to indicate that interventions aimed at the general population can be just as effective for low socioeconomic groups as they are for those with high socioeconomic status. However, a cautionary note should be made at this point. Systematic searches for evidence about effective interventions, no matter how carefully they are conducted, can produce odd results. For example, the table includes a study by Collins and Klein (56) that satisfied the search criteria specified for inclusion, despite the fact that since it was published many other more sophisticated studies addressing exactly the same issues have been published (6). In this instance it is not a serious problem because, strictly speaking, the findings reported by Collins and Klein have been replicated, but the later studies have raised more serious concerns about the underlying assumptions implicit in the data analysis that was undertaken. Our own view is that this particular study is not a very reliable indicator of the equality of access to primary care in the UK. Despite this, the most important point is that studies of successful healthcare interventions have been published which have important implications for strategies to reduce inequalities in health.

The way forward: Improving equality of access

What role can the health system itself play towards reducing socioeconomic inequalities in health?

As Table 10.1 indicates, evidence about effective service-led interventions that have affected the health of disadvantaged groups in Western Europe can be identified. This implies that the role of healthcare in reducing socioeconomic health inequalities, despite appearing minimal, especially compared to other policy areas, should not be neglected. For example, influence can be exerted on the three major risk factors for coronary heart disease (CHD): the system can provide support for smoking cessation; can discover and treat high blood pressure; and can identify and treat high serum cholesterol levels. Indeed, a systematic approach to CHD prevention could be developed from within primary care services in deprived communities (19). At the very least, the healthcare system is ultimately responsible for establishing equal accessibility to effective healthcare, regardless of the socioeconomic status of the patient. This involves a policy of resource allocation geared to healthcare needs, in particular of groups with low socioeconomic status, and also the development of adequate facilities for these groups (20).

It is important to ensure that resources be distributed in proportion to the relative needs of local populations. Several countries are now seeking to develop equitable resource allocation. For example, the NHS in Scotland has implemented recommendations from the Arbuthnott Report, whereby the relationship between service utilization and morbidity and life circumstances will determine the relative need for healthcare resources of the population living in each Health Board area (21). Similarly, both Sweden and England have already developed resource allocation formulas for secondary care services based on weighted capitation. Both have tried to identify, using routinely available statistics, indicators of increased need for care over and above demographic factors. Both take into account the higher needs and use by lower socioeconomic groups, and build these factors into the weighted capitation. In England, these capitation methods, which offer 'equal opportunity of access to those in equal need', are currently under review to consider how they can now 'contribute to the reduction in avoidable health inequalities' (22). In Sweden, the 'Stockholm' model for resource allocation takes into account the extra costs incurred for services for people who are not employed or who live alone. These models need continual refining, but they do show that attempts at equitable resource allocation can and should be made (23).

Yet, even if healthcare services were distributed between areas in direct proportion to the relative needs of their populations, this would not automatically result in equal access for all. Services may not be arranged in a convenient way, and some social groups could face greater barriers to access than others. As Dixon (24) describes, the long-standing problems of primary care in deprived inner cities of the UK, particularly London, have been the subject of many reviews and subsequent initiatives by the Department of Health and other bodies. For example, between 1993 and 1999 the London Initiative Zone (LIZ) sought to address problems regarding recruitment, retention and training of GPs in areas where they were most needed. However, although improvements in the standard of premises occurred, the initiative did not have a major impact on accessibility and quality of care in large parts of the city. Nevertheless, the number of such initiatives over the past 20 years indicates that a large amount of effort and resources has been devoted not only to improving the quality of primary care in deprived areas but also to addressing the relatively low uptake of preventive care and the barriers to access for black and ethnic groups. There appears to be a great deal of consensus as to what needs to be done to improve access to and quality of care, but sustained resources, an overarching strategy and an ongoing coherent focus of activity and research at national and local level are lacking (24).

Better monitoring of who benefits from health services is also required. It is being increasingly recognized that there is a need to develop ways of assessing access to specific groups, using methodologies that can be routinely applied at the local administrative level. One useful instrument is the 'equity audit', which is used to review health services systematically on the basis of quantitative criteria to establish whether obstacles to accessibility occur during the various steps in the care process. Routinely available patient registration data can facilitate the study of socioeconomic differences in both the use of facilities and health outcomes in local health authorities throughout the country. Such investigation is certainly required within the private sector and mental health services, where existing evidence of inequalities in access and quality of care is sparse (19, 23).

A specific example

Many European countries are committed to health equality strategies. For example, reducing inequalities in health is one of two core aims in the National Plan for the NHS in Scotland (25). Among the many proposals to pursue this aim are plans to establish health demonstration projects on preventing heart disease, improving sexual health, and improving children's health in the early years. There are also plans to create a Scotland-wide learning network for these projects.

Starting Well in Glasgow is focused on improving the health and well-being of children up to 5 years in deprived areas. It aims to change the way in which primary care services operate in terms of targeting vulnerable families, involvement in community development, prioritizing workloads and establishing effective mechanisms to build and strengthen relationships with vulnerable families.

It is hoped that a programme of activities to support families, coupled with access to enhanced community-based resources for parents and their children, will significantly improve health and welfare outcomes. In order to achieve this, the programme offers intensive home support to families with a new baby, provides an improved network of community support services for families with children under 5 years, and stronger linkages between families and support structures and services. Importantly, Starting Well is based on a body of evidence which suggests that early intervention programmes based on a combination of home support and centre-based parenting and child development promotion can be an effective means of influencing maternal and child outcomes (26).

Conclusions

Improved access to effective healthcare interventions for disadvantaged groups may not be the most important way of reducing health inequalities but it has a very significant contribution to make. Poor health outcomes are often associated with problems of gaining timely and good-quality access to healthcare, even in countries that have long since adopted universalist systems. Demonstrating that inequitable access to care is problematic is not difficult. There are now many studies in a host of different societies showing that people in the most disadvantaged circumstances often (but not always) benefit less from what their health services have to offer than their needs imply they should.

The implications are clear: services should be targeted more effectively at those who would benefit most from them. If this could be achieved, then some part of the health inequalities that are an endemic feature of modern societies would be reduced. But in an information-orientated technocratic world, where healthcare investments are increasingly driven by an emphasis on high-quality evidence about what works, there is a real paucity of studies about the best ways to reach poorer people with appropriate and effective services. We have shown that some such studies are available but they are still relatively rare. Even where they do exist, they seem not to be widely recognized or acted upon. The challenge for the future, therefore, is not only to strengthen the evidence base about healthcare interventions that can improve outcomes for poorer people, but also to find better ways of disseminating such information to policy-makers and practitioners. At the same time, another problem has to be overcome. It may not be sufficient to demonstrate that a particular service has the potential to improve health for disadvantaged groups. What is needed is a willingness to learn more about the principles that underpin the effectiveness of reaching out to socially excluded groups in ways that better meet their needs, circumstances and aspirations. Perhaps one part of the problem associated with inequitable access to healthcare is that care organizations, and many of the professionals they employ, have been too passive in thinking that simple availability of services on the basis of need is sufficient. This view is mistaken. The poor social and economic circumstances associated with health inequalities also influence the use of health services. Simply saying 'We are here, come and use us' will not do. If healthcare systems are to make a serious contribution to reducing health inequalities then new approaches to service delivery have to be developed. There are signs in some countries that this is beginning to happen, but much remains to be done to change the predominant culture of healthcare.

References

1. Shoen C, Davis K, DesRoches C, Donelan K, Blendon R. Health insurance markets and income inequality: findings from an international health policy survey. *Health Policy* 2000: 51: 67–85.
2. van Doorslaer E, Wagstaff A, Van der Burg H, Christiansen T *et al.* Equality in the delivery of healthcare in Europe and the US. *J Health Econ* 2000: 19: 553–83.
3. Haynes R. Inequalities in health and health service use: evidence from the general household survey. *Soc Sci Med* 1991: 33: 361–8.
4. O'Donnell O, Propper C. Equality and the distribution of UK NHS resources. *J Health Econ* 1991: 1–19.
5. Evandrou M, Falkingham J, Le Grand J, Winter D. Equality in health and social care. *J Soc Policy* 1992: 21: 489–523.
6. Goddard M, Smith P. *Equity of Access to Health Care*. York: NHS Centre for Reviews and Dissemination, 1998.

7. De la Hoz K, Leon D. Self-perceived health status and inequalities in the use of health services in Spain. *Int J Epidemiol* 1996: 25(3): 593–603.

8. van der Meer J, van den Bos J, Mackenbach J. Socioeconomic differences in the utilization of health services in a Dutch population: the contribution of health status. *Health Policy* 1996: 37: 1–18.

9. Whitehead M, Evandrou M, Haglund M, Diderichsen F. As the health divide widens in Sweden and Britian, what's happening to access to care? *Br Med J* 1997: 315(7114): 1006–9.

10. Bormann C, Schroeder E. The influence of socioeconomic factors on morbidity and the utilization of medical services in the Federal Republic of Germany. In: Mielck A, do Rosario Giraldes M, eds. *Health Inequalities: Discussion in Western European Countries*. New York: Waxmann, 1994: 51–66.

11. Keskimäki I. *Social equality in the use of hospital inpatient care in Finland*. STAKES research report 84: 1997.

12. Borrell C, Rohlfs I, Parasin M, Dominguez-Berjon F, Plasencia A. Social inequalities in perceived health and the use of health services in a southern European urban area. *Int J Health Serv* 1999: 29(4): 743–64.

13. Brook RH, Ware JE Jr, Rogers WH *et al*. Does free care improve adults' health? Results from a randomised controlled trial. *N Engl J Med* 1983: 309: 1426–34.

14. Woolhandler S, Himmelstein DU. Free care: a quantitative analysis of health and cost effects of a National Health Programme for the United States. *Int J Health Serv* 1988: 18: 393–9.

15. Bunton R, Burrows R, Gillen K, Muncer S. *Interventions to Promote Health in Economically Deprived Areas: a Critical Review of the Literature*. NHS Executive North and Yorkshire Region, 1994.

16. Arblaster L, Lambert M, Entwhistle V *et al*. A systematic review of the effectiveness of health service interventions aimed at reducing inequalities in health. *J Health Serv Res Policy* 1996: 1(2): 93–103.

17. Gepkens A, Gunning-Schepers L. Interventions to reduce socioeconomic health differences: a review of the international literature. *Eur J Public Health* 1996: 6: 218–26.

18. Woodward A, Kawachi I. Why reduce health inequalities? *J Epidemiol Commun Health* 2000: 54: 923–9.

19. Mackenbach J. Healthcare and socioeconomic inequalities in health. Working paper. 2000.

20. Benzeval M, Donald M. The role of the NHS in tackling inequalities in health. In: Gordon D, Shaw M, Dorling D, Davey Smith G, eds. *Inequalities in Health*. Bristol: Polity Press, 1999: 87–99.

21. Fair shares for all: national review of resource allocation. *Scottish Executive* 2000.

22. Sheldon TA, Smith PC. Equality in the allocation of healthcare resources. *Health Econ* 2000: 9: 571–4.

23. Whitehead M. Where do we stand? Research and policy issues concerning inequalities in health and in healthcare. *Acta Oncol* 1999: 38(1): 41–50.

24. Dixon J. What is the hard evidence on the performance of 'mainstream' health services serving deprived compared to non-deprived areas in England? Report for the Social Exclusion Unit, 2000.

25. Our National Health: a plan for action, a plan for change. *Scottish Executive*, 2000.

26. Kendrick D, Elkan R *et al.* Does home visiting improve parenting and the quality of the home environment? A systematic review and meta analysis. *Arch Dis Child* 2000: 82: 443–51.

27. Abel EK. Taking the cure to the poor: patients' responses to New York City's tuberculosis programme, 1894 to 1918. *Am J Public Health* 1997: 97: 1808–15.

28. Atri J, Falshaw M, Gregg R, Robson J, Omar RZ, Dixon S. Improving uptake of breast screening in multiethnic populations: a randomised controlled trial using practice reception staff to contact non-attenders. *Br Med J* 1997: 315: 1356–9.

29. Bird JA, McPhee SJ, Ha NT, Le B, Davis T, Jenkins CN. Opening pathways to cancer screening for Vietnamese-American women: lay health workers hold a key. *Prev Med* 1998: 27(6): 821–9.

30. Choy DK, Tong M, Ko F, Li ST, Ho A, Chan J *et al.* Evaluation of the efficacy of a hospital-based asthma education programme in patients of low socioeconomic status in Hong Kong. *Clin Exp Allergy* 1999: 29(1): 84–90.

31. Hartley BM, O'Connor ME. Evaluation of the 'Best Start' breast-feeding education programme. *Arch Pediatr Adolesc Med* 1996: 150(8): 868–71.

32. Kegeles SS. A field experimental attempt to change beliefs and behavior of women in an urban ghetto. *J Health Social Behav* 1969: 10(2): 115–24.

33. Keintz MK, Fleisher L, Rimer BK. Reaching mothers of preschool-aged children with a targeted quit smoking intervention. *J Commun Health* 1994: 19(1): 25–40.

34. Kistin N, Benton D, Rao S, Sullivan M. Breast-feeding rates among black urban low-income women: effect of prenatal education. *Pediatrics* 1990: 86(5): 741–6.

35. Kitzman H, Olds DL, Sidora K, Henderson CR Jr, Hanks C, Cole R *et al.* Enduring effects of nurse home visitation on maternal life course: a 3-year follow-up of a randomized trial. *JAMA* 2000: 283(15): 1983–9.

36. Lantz PM, Stencil D, Lippert MT, Beversdorf S, Jaros L, Remington PL. Breast and cervical cancer screening in a low-income managed care sample: the efficacy of physician letters and phone calls. *Am J Public Health* 1995: 85: 834–6.

37. Marcus AC, Crane LA, Kaplan CP, Reading AE, Savage E, Gunning J *et al.* Improving adherence to screening follow-up among women with abnormal pap smears: results from a large clinic-based trial of three intervention strategies. *Med Care* 1992: 30(3): 216–30.

38. Marsh GN, Channing DM. Narrowing the health gap between a deprived and an endowed community. *Br Med J* 1988: 296(6616): 173–6.

39. Monsuez JJ, Fergelot H, Le Gall JR. Homeless in the emergency department (letter). *Lancet* 1995: 346: 55.

40. Morisky DE, Bowler MH, Finlay JS. An educational and behavioral approach toward increasing patient activation in hypertension management. *J Commun Health* 1982: 7(3): 171–82.

41. Morisky DE, Levine DM, Green LW, Shapiro S, Russell RP, Smith CR. Five-year blood pressure control and mortality following health education for hypertensive patients. *Am J Public Health* 1983: 73(2): 153–62.

42. Moos MK, Bangdiwala SI, Meibohm AR, Cefalo RC. The impact of a preconceptional health promotion programme on intendedness of pregnancy. *Am J Perinatol* 1996: 13(2): 103–8.

43.   Mueller-Heubach E, Reddick D, Barnett B, Bente R. Preterm birth prevention: evaluation of a prospective controlled randomized trial. *Am J Obstet Gynecol* 1989: 160(5 Pt 1): 1172–8.

44.   Olds D, Henderson CR Jr, Cole R, Eckenrode J, Kitzman H, Luckey D *et al.* Long-term effects of nurse home visitation on children's criminal and antisocial behavior: 15-year follow-up of a randomized controlled trial. *JAMA* 1998: 280(14): 1238–44.

45.   Renneker M, Lim N, Wheatley B *et al.* An inner-city cancer prevention clinic in West Oakland, California. *Cancer Prac* 1994: 2: 427–37.

46.   Weisdorf T, Parran TV Jr, Graham A, Snyder C. Comparison of pregnancy-specific interventions to a traditional treatment programme for cocaine-addicted pregnant women. *J Substance Abuse Treat* 1999: 16(1): 39–45.

47.   Bander KW, Stilwell NA, Fein E, Bishop G. Relationship of patient characteristics to programme attendance by women alcoholics. *J Stud Alcohol* 1983: 44: 318–27.

48.   Freeborn DK, Mullooly JP, Colombo T, Burnham V. The effect of outreach workers' services on the medical care utilization of a disadvantaged population. *J Commun Health* 1978: 3(4): 306–20.

49.   Glasgow RE, Whitlock EP, Eakin EG, Lichtenstein E. A brief smoking cessation intervention for women in low-income planned parenthood clinics. *Am J Public Health* 2000: 90(5): 786–9.

50.   Haas JS, Udvarhelyi S, Epstein AM. The effect of health coverage for uninsured pregnant women on maternal health and the use of cesarean section. *JAMA* 1993: 270(1): 61–4.

51.   Haas JS, Udvarhelyi IS, Morris CN, Epstein AM. The effect of providing health coverage to poor uninsured pregnant women in Massachusetts. *JAMA* 1993: 269(1): 87–91.

52.   Levey LA, MacDowell NM, Levey S. Healthcare of poverty and non-poverty children in Iowa. *Am J Public Health* 1986: 76: 1000–3.

53.   Mainous III AG, Hueston WJ, Love MM, Griffith III CH. Access to care for the uninsured: is access to a physician enough? *Am J Public Health* 1999: 89(6): 910–12.

54.   Rosenbaum S, Johnson K. Providing health care for low-income children: reconciling child health goals with child health financing realities. *Milbank Mem Fund Q* 1986: 64(3): 442–78.

55.   Rosenbaum S, Hughes DC, Johnson K. Maternal and child health services for medically indigent children and pregnant women. *Med Care* 1988: 26(4): 315–32.

56.   Collins E, Klein R. Equality and the NHS: self-reported morbidity, access, and primary care. *Br Med J* 1980: 281(Oct): 1111–15.

57.   Jamrozik K, Vessey M, Fowler G, Wald N, Parker G, Van Vunakis H. Controlled trial of three different antismoking interventions in general practice. *Br Med J* 1984: 288(6429): 1499–503.

58.   Keeler EB, Brook RH, Goldberg GA, Kamberg CJ, Newhouse JP. How free care reduced hypertension in the health insurance experiment. *JAMA* 1985: 254(14): 1926–31.

59.   Winkleby MA, Fortmann SP, Rockhill B. Trends in cardiovascular disease risk factors by educational level: the Stanford Five-City Project. *Prev Med* 1992: 21: 592–601.

60. Zarod BK, Lennon MA. The effect of school dental screening on dental attendance. The results of a randomised controlled trial. *Commun Dent Health* 992: 9(4): 361–8.

61. Hurley SF, Huggins RM, Jolley DJ, Reading D. Recruitment activities and sociodemographic factors that predict attendance at a mammographic screening programme. *Am J Public Health* 1994: 84: 1655–8.

62. A further analysis. Hypertension Detection and Follow-up Programme Co-operative Group. Five-year findings of the Hypertension Detection and Follow-up Programme: mortality by race–sex and blood pressure level. *J Commun Health* 1984: 9(4): 314–27.

63. Jackson C, Winkleby MA, Flora JA, Fortmann SP. Use of educational resources for cardiovascular risk reduction in the Stanford Five-City Project. *Am J Prev Med* 1991: 7: 82–8.

64. Koivusalo M. Decentralisation and equality of healthcare provision in Finland. *Br Med J* 1999: 318: 1198–200.

11 Patient cost sharing and access to healthcare

Fred Louckx

Introduction

In studies on equality in healthcare (see Chapter 10) the terms 'access to' and 'use of' services are often bracketed together, which would seem to indicate that one is an extension of the other. However, equal access to healthcare does not necessarily result in equal use (1): factors such as different attitudes to health and healthcare prevent one from crossing over into the other. In this chapter a clear distinction will therefore be made between these two concepts. The focus will be on healthcare accessibility and, to be more precise, on one aspect related to it: patient cost sharing.

Research studies usually differentiate between three major types of patient cost sharing (2): co-payment refers to a flat amount for each service used, which is paid by the patient when receiving the care; co-insurance denotes the percentage of the total charge of a service used that is payable by patients; the deductible is the out-of-pocket amount patients have to pay in order to be entitled to a refund from their health insurance. In this chapter, the overall effect of the various types of patient cost sharing will be discussed.

Patient cost sharing practices in Western European countries

A comparison of healthcare systems in different countries is difficult and presupposes a high degree of knowledge of the various systems in operation (3). As a result of differences in funding (insurance-based versus tax-based systems), in underlying institutional rules and procedures, and in the actual provision of the various services (4, 5), any comparison inevitably involves a simplification. This is equally true for a comparison of cost-sharing mechanisms, as these are part of a collection of measures peculiar to each country. Nevertheless, we may cautiously distinguish a number of common characteristics.

In an attempt to restrict growing healthcare expenses, nearly all Western European countries have introduced cost containment measures. Despite the differences between these countries, it is possible to adumbrate two broad categories of measure (6). On the one hand there are measures intended to influence the supply of healthcare provisions. In this respect, one may refer to the establishment of fixed or target budgets for expenditure on healthcare, controls on hospital beds and manpower controls. The second group comprises measures that are aimed more at deflecting demand for healthcare. Patient cost sharing is the most important example of a direct check on demand. Conversely, there are more indirect forms of control on demand, such as the promotion of prevention, and the provision of more and better information.

A number of Western European countries started using patient cost sharing from the 1980s in order to influence demand for healthcare. Whereas previously patient cost sharing had played a rather modest role in Western European healthcare systems, from then on it became standard practice in a range of care provisions. Data from the period 1970–91 reveal that this development did not take place at the same pace and to the same extent in all Western European countries (7). Sweden, Greece, Italy, The Netherlands, Denmark and Portugal were among those that witnessed a fairly strong percentage increase in cost sharing. Portugal and Austria have a high score viewed from the overall impact of cost sharing. Luxembourg has the lowest score in regard to both the increase in terms of percentage and the overall impact of patient cost sharing. Although these types of international comparisons should be treated with the greatest caution, they do reveal a number of elements regarding the presence of patient cost-sharing mechanisms.

Our survey of the current situation in Europe regarding patient cost sharing is based on an exhaustive study by Mossialos and Le Grand (8). Table 11.1 provides a summary of some of the findings. It is striking that patient cost sharing is more prevalent than is generally assumed. For each of the services examined, patient cost sharing predominates, with dental care being the absolute leader. The most frequently encountered types of cost sharing are co-insurance and deductibles. In dental care, patient cost sharing is often high (sometimes with ceilings), especially when it involves crowns, bridges, dentures and orthodontic treatments. Conversely, young people of 17, 18 or 20, depending on the country, often enjoy free dental care. In some countries this is also the case for certain social categories, and in some centres. Preventive treatment and regular checks are usually stimulated through lower cost sharing. As far as pharmaceutical care is concerned, the proportionate out-of-pocket amount paid by the patient varies with the type, class or pack size of a drug. Sometimes a flat rate is charged. In several countries a substantial part of the item is exempt from all cost sharing. For in-patient care, the daily amounts payable by patients are often linked to the duration of the stay. In a large number of countries the rates depend on the duration, as well as on the difference between acute and long-term bed occupancy. The cost-sharing amount is sometimes means-tested, or subject to certain maxima. In some countries a distinction is also made between

Table 11.1 Patient cost sharing for GP, specialist visits, pharmaceuticals, in-patient care and dental care in 1996

	GP	Specialist	Pharmaceuticals	In-patient care	Dental care
Austria	+	+	+	+	+
Belgium	+	+	+	+	+
Denmark	+	+	+	−	+
Finland	+	+	+	+	+
France	+	+	+	+	+
Germany	−	−	+	+	+
Greece	−	+	+	−	+
Ireland	+	+	+	+	+
Italy	−	+	+	−	+
Luxembourg	+	+	+	+	+
Netherlands	−	−	−	+	+
Portugal	+	+	+	−	+
Spain	−	−	+	−	+
Sweden	+	+	+	+	+
UK	−	−	+	−	+

Notes:
+ = patient cost sharing ; − = no patient cost sharing

Source: Mossialos and Le Grand 1999 (8)

first-class hospital beds and second-class beds, with the former being subject to additional charges for doctors' fees. In out-patient GP and specialist care, the extent of cost sharing is often linked to the social category of the patient. For GPs, there are differences depending on whether a consultation or a home visit is involved. In the case of specialists, the difference in cost sharing may be predicated on whether or not a practice-based or a hospital-based specialist is involved.

Effects of patient cost sharing on access to healthcare

The classic point of reference in research into the impact of patient cost sharing is the RAND Health Insurance Experiment (9). Over 2,000 families from six different cities in the United States took part in the study between 1974 and 1982. Both the health status and healthcare expenditures were recorded. The first important observation of this study is that the use of medical care declines as patient cost sharing increases. This applies to all services, albeit not always to the same extent, and to all socioeconomic categories. However, this does not mean that no differences were established between these socioeconomic categories. Lower income categories are more sensitive to cost sharing in out-patient care than higher income groups. For hospital services this is the other way round.

Another key finding of the RAND Health Insurance Experiment was that, with the exception of emergency room visits, patient cost sharing reduces appropriate and inappropriate services by the same proportion. Cost sharing was just as likely to lower use when care is thought to be highly effective as when it is thought to be only rarely effective (10).

In the RAND Health Insurance Experiment, the reduced use of healthcare as a result of cost sharing did not adversely influence the health of the average person. However, an adverse effect on health was found in the case of the sick poor people, who were defined as the most disadvantaged 6 per cent of the population. For this category of the population the introduction of patient cost sharing clearly had a negative impact on a number of health problems.

Although numerous studies were conducted in the wake of the RAND experiment, none of them contradicted its findings in any fundamental way. Often smaller-scale research was involved which was hardly ever carried out in an experimental setting (11). One notable exception here is a recent French study (12). When, as a result of the 'Veil Act' of July 1993, social security cost sharing for outpatient care and pharmaceutical goods dropped by 5 per cent in France, most non-profit and profit-making insurance companies reacted to this increase in out-of-pocket payments by increasing their premiums. However, they did not all proceed in the same manner. Researchers seized this opportunity to examine the so-called moral hazard in demand for medical care, that is the assumption that patients make more use of healthcare provisions if they do not have to pay for them. To this end, two of the supplementary insurance contracts were compared. The 'reference' contract – the control group – did not change after the 'Veil Act' and continued to offer almost full coverage of out-patient care. The other contract – the test group – introduced a co-payment rate of 10 per cent for all out-patient care expenses as from 1994. The researchers were interested in discovering the effect the different co-payment rates would have on the demand for physician services. The survey revealed that there were no indications of moral hazard in the demand for physician surgery visits. According to the researchers this may be explained primarily by the combination of a relatively small co-payment increase and the presence of non-monetary costs, such as transport time, waiting costs and as on. As a result of these non-monetary costs the relatively small co-payment increase is merely a fraction of the total cost perceived by the patient, and consequently has very little effect, if any, on patient behaviour. Researchers also remark that this is the reason why co-payments do have an influence on the demand for home visits, as here the non-monetary costs are lowest.

An important aspect of this study is that it qualifies the often simplistic views of moral hazard. It is not true that patients necessarily make increased use of healthcare when this is offered without cost sharing, just as patient cost sharing does not automatically result in less use of services. It often involves a complex interaction of factors that affect patient behaviour. The French study refers to the importance of the size of the out-of-pocket payments as well as to the role played by various non-monetary costs.

However, there are other factors that play a substantial role, such as the nature of the provision for which out-of-pocket payments are requested (13). Another important question is whether or not it involves a first-contact service, initiated by the patient, or a provider-initiated service, over which the patient has far less control. Furthermore, the effect of cost sharing will naturally vary with the extent to which the additional cost can be reinsured.

In a recent Dutch evaluation study (14) attention was drawn to a number of aspects related to patient cost sharing on which relatively little research has been conducted so far. The study was carried out on the occasion of the introduction in January 1997 of the General Co-insurance Scheme under the Dutch Sickness Funds Act. Under this scheme, people insured by sickness funds had to pay 20 per cent of the costs for services received, except for costs related to GP care, dentistry and obstetrics. For each day in hospital about 4 euros had to be paid. However, an out-of-pocket maximum was set for this new cost sharing. At the same time, the flat-rate premium for all those insured by sickness funds was cut by 50 euros.

The scheme was intended to trigger both a decrease in consumption and a shift in costs, but research findings reveal that neither objective was reached. There was hardly a consumption-limiting effect, which is ascribed not only to the relatively low out-of-pocket amounts, but also to the fact that they were related mainly to 'follow-up consumption', which was largely beyond patient control. Of particular relevance is the fact that the scheme costs considerably more than it generates. This is an extremely important point, as patient cost sharing is very often introduced without decision-makers questioning the potential financial result. The Dutch example taught a clear lesson in this respect, and appropriate conclusions were drawn: on 1 January 1999 the new measure was rescinded. The second major conclusion of this study is that the measure had given rise to a feeling of unrest regarding accessibility to healthcare among certain sections of the population. As a result of the real or suspected costs, patients have a tendency to postpone or cancel healthcare visits, even when they involve essential services. In the Dutch study, patients' concerns had an effect mainly on the use of medicines.

Two case studies

The complexity and impact of patient cost sharing may best be illustrated by some examples. We have chosen two countries with different healthcare financing systems (tax-based versus insurance-based) that have been faced with a similar development in patient cost sharing.

Sweden

In the 1990s, Sweden witnessed a number of important healthcare reforms which marked a major step towards a more market-orientated approach to healthcare (8, 15, 16). From 1991, county councils have been able to determine their own fee structures, and hence cost sharing, regarding out-patient care. This deregulation of fees meant that a key power was taken away from central government. In 1992, the Ädel reform was put into effect. As a result, the responsibility for long-term healthcare to the elderly and the disabled was transferred from the county councils to the municipalities. In early 1994, two measures were introduced in the area of primary care services which would have a very short lease of life: the Family Doctor Act and the Act on freedom to establish private, publicly funded practices. These measures were an attempt by central government both to improve the con-tinuity of care and accessibility in primary healthcare and to limit county councils' regulatory power in concluding agreements with private practi-tioners. After a change of government, both measures were withdrawn in the course of 1995. Finally, the 1990s also saw a number of shifts in the pharmaceutical area. In this respect it is worth mentioning the introduction of a reference price system in 1993, as well as the large increases in patient cost sharing.

Over six years (1988–94) patient fees in the pharmaceutical area doubled in real terms. It was only in the cost sharing for doctor services that the increase was higher in that period (8). Until the last reform, which dates back to 1997, patients were paying a flat-rate fee for each prescription and a second fee for each additional item on the prescription (17). Since June 1998, patients have been paying 100 per cent of the first 107 euros for their prescriptions, 50 per cent of the cost between 107 and 202 euros, 25 per cent of the cost between 202 and 391 euros, and 10 per cent of the cost between 391 and 510 euros. For a visit to their GP, patients pay about 12 euros, whereas a specialist consultation at a hospital is priced at between 24 and 30 euros, which may possibly be reduced by 12 euros if the patient has been referred by the primary care provider. As a result of the Ädel reform, new patient charges were introduced in old people's homes, nursing homes, and for recipients of home help services. Charges per day in hospital and those related to dental services have also increased considerably.

Sweden issued a number of compensatory measures with a view to cushioning the consequences of patient cost sharing. The first involved the setting of an annual out-of-pocket maximum of 214 euros for prescription drugs. Some categories of patients, such as asthma sufferers and diabetics, do not have to pay for their medicines. Under the second measure, the patient pays a maximum of 107 euros per year for health services. Young people below the age of 20 enjoy free health services in most counties.

For all of this, the Swedish healthcare system failed to preserve financial accessibility (18). The previously mentioned reforms were aimed mainly at improving the efficiency and productivity of the system and did not suffi-ciently achieve the old 'trade-off' between efficiency and equality (15). A number of surveys by the Stockholm county council in 1993, 1995 and 1996 showed that in the year prior to being questioned, between 20 and 25 per cent of the population had not used the healthcare system at least once for financial reasons. A survey commissioned by the National Board of Health and Welfare revealed that in 1997 about 8 per cent of all households that had been prescribed medicines failed to collect them from the pharmacy at least once for financial reasons. According to the same National Board of Health and Welfare, the decline in demand for services in elderly care is linked to the increase in user charges (17). Based on a comparative analysis of survey data, another study stated that in the period 1993–4 Sweden witnessed unequal access to healthcare for the first time since the 1960s (19).

Belgium

In the 1990s Belgium witnessed a steep increase in patient out-of-pocket payments. In the period between October 1993 and April 1997 alone there were no fewer than 16 increases in out-of-pocket amounts (20) for, among other things, GP consultations and home visits, specialist consultations, in-patient care, clinical biology, and medico-technical treatments. Patient out-of-pocket payments for drugs also increased substantially in the course of the 1990s.

In 1998, the total annual out-of-pocket payments by patients in Belgium was estimated at some 3.74 billion euros (20), which constitutes over 20 per cent of the total healthcare expenditure of the country. A recent survey conducted by the National Union of Socialist Sickness Funds (21) found that chronically ill patients spend on average 23 per cent of their disposable family income on care. The first Belgian Health Survey of 1997 revealed that, on the whole, one-third of the Belgian population claimed to experience difficulty in paying for medical care (22). The survey also showed that 8 per cent of the families questioned occasionally postponed medical care for financial reasons. Visits to the dentist were most likely to be sacrificed. One should also mention that the poverty percentage in families with a sick or invalid breadwinner doubled between 1985 and 1997, from 8.3 per cent to 16.4 per cent (23).

In Belgium, the increase in patient cost sharing is partly offset by five measures. The best-known of these is undoubtedly the system of social and fiscal deductibles (out-of-pocket maxima), which was introduced in 1994. The social deductible fixes the annual out-of-pocket maximum for one family at 372 euros for a number of socially vulnerable categories. Once the out-of-pocket maximum has been reached, all other out-of-pocket payments are fully refunded by the sickness funds. Those who are not eligible for the social deductible are nevertheless entitled to a fiscal deductible, under which the annual maximum out-of-pocket amount depends on the net family income before taxes. The second measure involves the extension, in 1997 and 1999, of the increased contribution by the sickness fund. As a result, the out-of-pocket payments by the socially vulnerable categories for most medical services, some types of medicines and hospital admission were lowered.

In early 1998 the national insurance reform came into effect, making it possible for those who, for various reasons, are no longer eligible to claim health insurance, to re-enter the system quickly and cheaply. As from 1998, an additional budget of 24.8 million euros was allocated for the chronically ill. Finally, the fifth measure enables a number of social categories to qualify for the so-called third-party payment agreement for consultations and visits to GPs and for various dental care treatments. During their contacts with these services they only have to pay the legally prescribed out-of-pocket amount, with the remainder of the cost being paid directly by the sickness fund.

Although these social compensatory measures have undoubtedly facilitated financial access to healthcare for some categories of patient, there are a number of lacunae which are linked primarily to their selective nature (24). Despite the complicated regulations, a sizeable part of patient cost sharing remains outside the remit of these compensatory measures. For instance, the cost related to medicines is not included in the deductible scheme. The out-of-pocket sum payable by the patient for a hospital admission is calculated in the social, but not in the fiscal deductible. Besides the question of what falls outside these selective measures, there is also that of *who* falls outside them. The delimitation of the social categories that are eligible for one of the above-mentioned compensatory measures sometimes results in rather arbitrary dividing lines. Individuals or families who, despite being in a similar social–financial situation, cannot be subsumed into one of the standard social categories are at risk of being excluded from access.

Belgian primary healthcare centres paid on a capitation basis

After listing the drawbacks to patient cost sharing, it seems politic to discuss a number of advantages to the non-application of patient cost sharing. The Belgian primary healthcare centres paid on a capitation basis are a particularly good example in this respect, as they developed within a primary care system based predominantly on fee-for-service payments (25). This example allows for a comparison between two different forms of payment within one and the same healthcare system.

In comparison with countries such as The Netherlands, Denmark and the United Kingdom (26), the capitation payment system was never applied on a large scale in Belgium. Under the Belgian capitation payment system in primary care each provider or providing group gets a monthly lump sum, the size of which depends on the number of patients on their books. This covers doctors' fees related to consultations and visits, but excludes technical services. For nurses and physiotherapists all services come under the lump sum payment. The capitation payment system means that care providers commit themselves to refraining from asking payments from patients registered with them. As a result, these services are free for the latter, provided they go to the same care provider. If they do not, they lose their entitlement to intervention by the health insurance for those services.

In 1999, some thirty centres used capitation payment, together accounting for about 60,000 registered patients. Both the number of centres and the number of registered patients increases year on year. The majority of these centres are located in underprivileged areas, that is, in poorer towns and in poorer areas of wealthier towns. Among the patients registered, the percentage of the socially vulnerable is markedly higher than in the population at large. It becomes apparent, for instance, that the number of minimum-income claimants among the patients registered is almost six times that of the total population (27). The proportion of widows, disabled, pensioners and orphans with an income below a certain (low) threshold in relation to those with incomes above this threshold is some 20 per cent higher among the patients registered than in the total population. The capitation payment system has undoubtedly improved financial accessibility of healthcare for these categories of the population.

It would nevertheless be wrong to think that capitation payment in these centres has improved only financial accessibility. By analogy with examples in other countries (28, 29), one observes that this payment system has also created room to change the approach to healthcare. These centres start from an integral approach to health, with an emphasis on the relationships between physical, mental and social health components. Multidisciplinary teams establish coordinated care strategies through formalized consultation. For certain frequently occurring problems, such as psychosomatic complaints, a systematic approach is developed. By establishing networks, the centres set up local collaboration frameworks. The capitation payment system encourages the centres to develop various initiatives related to prevention and health promotion. Finally, it is worth mentioning that these centres are also actively involved in the development of patient participation.

This example of good practice does not constitute a kind of panacea for all problems related to accessibility to healthcare. We are keenly aware that the capitation system also has a number of disadvantages. Furthermore, there is no such thing as an ideal healthcare system that suits every country and every situation. The intention here is simply to show that, even in a system firmly rooted in fee-for-service payment, there are ways of avoiding patient cost sharing while at the same time improving the services provided. Thanks to the capitation system, the previously mentioned centres have succeeded in improving the quality of their work. Although this would perhaps have been possible without this payment system, it would have involved more difficult working conditions and a higher financial accessibility threshold for the patient.

Conclusions

Since the 1980s, patient cost sharing has been introduced on a large scale in many European countries as a cost containment measure. Depending on factors such as the nature of the service, the contact initiator (provider or patient) and the possibility of reinsurance of the additional cost to the patient, it has often reduced demand for healthcare services. However, as an instrument of an evidence-based healthcare policy, patient cost sharing does not withstand scientific scrutiny. Patient cost sharing is clearly unsuitable for making qualitative adjustments to demand behaviour. Furthermore, this measure raises the financial accessibility threshold of healthcare, especially for those sections of the population who are most in need of it, as a result of which socioeconomic inequalities in health threaten to increase even further. These consequences of patient cost sharing can be offset only partly by *post hoc* corrective measures.

References

1. Whitehead M. The concepts and principles of equity and health. *Int J Health Serv* 1992: 3: 429–45.
2. Saltman R, Figueras J. *European Healthcare Reform: Analysis of Current Strategies*. Copenhagen: World Health Organization, 1997.
3. Van Mosseveld C, van Son P. *International Comparison of Healthcare Data: Methodology Development and Application*. Dordrecht: Kluwer, 1998.
4. Freeman R. *The Politics of Health in Europe*. Manchester: Manchester University Press, 2000.
5. Immergut E. *Health Politics: Interests and Institutions in Western Europe*. New York: Cambridge University Press, 1992.
6. Aventur J. *Les systèmes de santé des pays industrialisés* (The Healthcare Systems in Industrialized Countries). Paris: Editions L'Harmattan, 1995.
7. Dumont J-P. *Les systèmes de protection sociale en Europe* (The Systems of Social Protection in Europe). Paris: Economica, 1995.
8. Mossialos E, Le Grand J, eds. *Healthcare and Cost Containment in the European Union*. Aldershot: Ashgate, 1999.
9. Newhouse JP and The Insurance Experiment Group. *Free for All? Lessons from the RAND Health Insurance Experiment*. Cambridge: Harvard University Press, 1993.
10. Lohr KN, Brook RH, Kamberg CJ, Goldberg GA, Leibowitz A, Keesey J *et al*. Effect of cost-sharing on use of medically effective and less effective care. *Med Care* 1986: 24(Suppl): 31–8.
11. Starmans B. *The effects of Patient Charges on Medical Utilization, Expenditure, and Health: Dutch Investigations and International Evidence*. Maastricht: Universiteit Maastricht, 1998.
12. Chiappori P-A, Durand F, Geoffard P-Y. Moral hazard and the demand for physician services: first lessons from a French natural experiment. *Eur Econ Rev* 1998: 42: 499–511.
13. *Standpunt eigen betalingen in de gezondheidszorg* (Views on Patient Cost-sharing in Healthcare). The Hague: Vereniging voor Volkgezondheid en Wetenschap, 1992.
14. Delnoij DMJ, Hutten JBF, Ros CC, Groenewegen PP, Friele RD, van de Lisdonk E *et al*. Effecten van eigen bijdragen in het ziekenfonds in Nederland (Effects of patient cost sharing in the Dutch Sickness Fund). *Tsg/Tijdschr Gezondheidswetensch* 1999: 77: 406–12.

15. Whitehead M, Gustafsson RA, Diderichsen F. Why is Sweden rethinking its NHS style reforms? *Br Med J* 1997 Oct 11: 315: 935–9.

16. Ranade W, ed. *Markets and Healthcare: a Comparative Analysis.* London: Longman, 1998.

17. Anell A, Svensson M. User charges in healthcare: the Swedish case. *Eurohealth* 1999: 5: 25–6.

18. Diderichsen F. Devolution in Swedish healthcare: local government isn't powerful enough to control costs or stop privatisation. *Br Med J* 1999: 318: 1156.

19. Whitehead M, Evandrou M, Haglund B, Diderichsen F. As the health divide widens in Sweden and Britain, what's happening to access to care? *Br Med J* 1997: 315: 1006–9.

20. Peers J. *Gezondheidszorg in België: uitdagingen en opportuniteiten* (The Belgian Healthcare System: Challenges and Potentialities). Brussels: Ministerie van Sociale Zaken, 1999.

21. *Resultaten enquête chronisch zieken* (Results of the Survey of Chronically Ill Patients). Brussels: NVSM studiedienst, 1999.

22. *De toegang tot de gezondheidszorg voor patiënten met zware pathologische verschijnselen en chronische aandoeningen: verslag over de hoorzittingen namens de Commissie voor de Sociale Aangelegenheden* (Accessibility to Healthcare by Patients with Serious Pathological Disorders and Chronic Diseases: Report of the Hearings Ordered by the Commission for Social Affairs). Brussels: Belgische Senaat, 1999.

23. Vranken J, Geldof D, Van Menxel G. *Armoede en sociale uitsluiting: jaarboek 1999* (Poverty and Social Exclusion: Yearbook 1999). Leuven: Acco, 1999.

24. Louckx F, Van Wanseele C. *Sociale correcties in de ziekteverzekering: balans en toekomst* (Social Adjustments in Health Insurance: Appraisal and Prospects). Brussels: Vrije Universiteit Brussel, 1998.

25. Louckx F, Van Wanseele C, eds. *De eerste lijn in beweging: forfaitaire geneeskunde als structureel alternatief voor prestatiegeneeskunde?* (Primary Care on the Move: Capitation Payment as a Structural Alternative to the Fee-for-service System?) Brussels: VUB Press, 1998.

26. Roland M. Le forfait à la capitation pour les soins primaires: une revue de la littérature internationale (Capitation payment in primary care: a review of the international literature). *Santé Conjuguée* 1998: (3): 71–83.

27. *Maisons Médicales: un outil pour l'avenir* (Primary Health Centres : a Tool for the Future). Brussels: Fédération des Maisons Médicales et Collectifs de Santé Francophones, 1995.

28. Berwick DM. Payment by capitation and the quality of care. *N Engl J Med* 1996: 335: 1227–31.

29. Flood CM. *International Healthcare Reform: a Legal, Economic and Political Analysis.* London: Routledge, 2000.

Part III
National experiences

12 England

Michaela Benzeval

Introduction

Health inequalities have been the subject of both research and policy attention for over 150 years in England and are currently experiencing unprecedented political and policy attention, already alluded to in Chapter 2. The purpose of this chapter is to describe the current policy agenda and development in research against this background. It is important to note that although there are many parallels between the experience of England and the other countries of the United Kingdom (UK), devolution increasingly means that there is a growing gulf in their social policies. For this reason, this chapter focuses on the policy response in England rather than the UK as a whole.

The socioeconomic situation

The UK has experienced considerable social and economic change in the past few decades. A reduction in manufacturing industry and a growth in the service sector has led to a reduction in male employment, particularly among unskilled workers, and a growth in female, often part-time, employment (1). This, together with the increasing number of lone parent families over the same period, has led to a growth in the number of working-age households where no one is in paid employment. By the second half of the 1990s, such families accounted for a fifth of all working-age households (2). These trends, together with changes in benefit and taxation policies during the last Conservative government, contributed to a massive increase in the number of families living on low incomes, and consequently a dramatic growth in income inequality, of an unprecedented degree compared with other industrial countries. By 1998/9 14.3 million people (about one-quarter of the population) and 4.4 million children (approximately one in three) lived in households with less than half the average income (3).

Alongside these economic changes, which have increased poverty and social exclusion, there has also been a dramatic rise in owner-occupation of houses, which has marginalized social housing to the most disadvantaged sections of the community. For example, around two-thirds of heads of households in social housing are unemployed, compared with about one-third in other housing tenures (4). Together, the labour and housing market changes have exacerbated geographical inequalities in poverty and wealth (1). Overall, these trends show a rise in unemployment, people living on low incomes, lone parent families, and increasing social and geographical polarization. Such trends are reflected in the health statistics.

The extent of socioeconomic inequalities in health

Health inequalities have been documented in England for more than 150 years. However, by far the most significant event in recent history was the publication of the Black Report in 1980, which concluded that 'class differences in mortality are a constant feature of the entire human life-span' (5). Since then, a considerable body of evidence has accumulated that demonstrates the poor health experience of people living in disadvantaged circumstances, in terms of premature mortality and excess morbidity across a wide range of diseases and conditions. Inequalities in health exist between socioeconomic groups, geographic areas and men and women, and among members of different ethnic minority groups (6). Box 12.1 illustrates some of these statistics.

Box 12.1 Health inequalities

- Men aged between 20 and 64 from the bottom two social classes are three times more likely to die from coronary heart disease and stroke than those in the top social class.
- Children from manual households are more likely to suffer from tooth decay than those from non-manual households.
- Mortality rates for people aged 60–74 living in social housing are 16 per cent above the national average, compared with 14 per cent below for those in owner-occupied housing.
- Mortality from all major causes has been found to be consistently higher than average among unemployed men.
- Mortality rates in the United Kingdom are about twice as high in infants of mothers born in Pakistan and the Caribbean Commonwealth, compared with the national average.
- Teenage girls from poor neighbourhoods are more likely to become pregnant, and teenagers account for one in ten births in some inner-city areas.
- Women in the northwest of England have a 33 per cent greater chance of suffering from cervical cancer than the national average.

Source: Cm 4386 1999 (7); Department of Health 1999 (8)

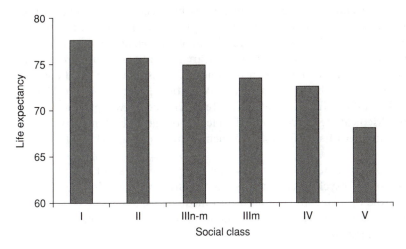

Figure 12.1 Male life expectancy at birth by social class, longitudinal study, England and Wales, 1992–6

Source: Hattersley 1999 (9)

The latest data on life expectancy at birth by social class for men are shown in Figure 12.1. Men born to professional parents can expect to live, on average, almost 10 years longer than those whose fathers have unskilled jobs (9). It has been estimated that if the death rate for all men of working age were the same as that for professional and managerial groups, 17,000 deaths would be avoided each year (7).

In many ways there is nothing especially remarkable about these inequalities: they are found in most if not all countries in Europe (see Chapter 1). What is particularly worrying is that a number of studies have begun to show that the health divide in England has widened sharply during the 1980s and 1990s (6). For example, in the early 1980s people under 65 living in the poorest income areas were 27 per cent more likely to die than the population as a whole. By the early 1990s the equivalent figure was 34 per cent (10).

Research

The United Kingdom has a long history of conducting research on health inequalities and has developed a significant multidisciplinary research community to undertake such work. Both medical and social research institutions, as well as a number of key welfare charities and the Department of Health, fund this research (11). As well as funding specific units and projects, a number of key datasets are supported which provide an invaluable foundation for health inequalities research (11).

Since the publication of the Black Report much research effort has focused on exploring the extent and nature of the problem in increasingly sophisticated ways. At the same time, considerable effort has been put into investigating the relative importance of the different explanations for health inequalities in what have often become quite acrimonious academic debates (12).

Recently, a number of major new research initiatives focusing especially on health inequalities have been established. These include the Economic and Social Research Council's Health Variation Programme, the Department of Health's Health Inequalities Research and Development initiative and the Medical Research Council's Health of the Public initiative. From these, a number of specific research themes are emerging (1), including:

- the role of circumstances across the life course for adult health;
- the role of psychosocial factors, particularly in the workplace;
- the role of 'place' in causing health inequalities; and
- how social policies and local public health interventions can reduce health inequalities.

Policies

The Conservative Government 1979–97

In spite of the massive accumulation of evidence on health inequalities, throughout most of the tenure of the last Conservative government action to tackle them was noticeable mainly by its absence (13). However, in their last few years in office, in response to considerable pressure, they did begin to take account of 'variations in health', at least in their health service policies. Key policies during this period are highlighted in Box 12.2.

The 'New Labour' government's first term 1997–2001

The Labour Party came to power in May 1997 with a massive majority and a commitment to reduce health inequalities. Within a month of taking office, the Prime Minister had acknowledged the link between poverty and health (something the previous government refused to do) and announced the government's intention to address it. In support of this he announced the establishment of an Independent Inquiry into Inequalities in Health (discussed later). A month later, the first-ever Minister for Public Health in England launched the development of a new health strategy that would have 'tackling inequalities at its heart'. When the new strategy was published for consultation in February 1998 (16) and as a final policy document in July 1999 (7), one of its two aims was 'to improve the health of the worst-off in society and to narrow the health gap'. It acknowledged the social causes of ill-health and inequalities and noted that 'tackling inequalities generally, is the best means of tackling health inequalities in particular' (16). The new health strategy was substantially criticized for not having a national target to reduce health inequalities. Therefore, in July 2000 a new strategy

---

Box 12.2 National policies to reduce health inequalities in England, 1977–97: highlights

1977   The Labour government commissions an independent inquiry into health inequalities chaired by Douglas Black.

1980   The Black Report is published but its recommendations are rejected by the incoming Conservative government as being too costly.

1985   The Conservative government signs up to the WHO Health for All strategy, which includes a target to reduce health inequalities.

1991   A Health Strategy for England – *Health of the Nation* – is published for consultation, which, despite having a welcome focus on health rather than healthcare, only mentions 'variations in health' in an appendix.

1992   The subsequent policy document is published, again only briefly referring to the issues of 'variations in health'.

1994   Substantial criticism led to a committee being set up to examine 'what steps the Department of Health and the National Health Service (NHS) should be taking to tackle variations'.

1995   The Committee report (14) is published alongside a government-funded systematic review of evidence about what works locally to reduce 'variations in health' (15).

1995–97   The priorities guidance for the NHS increasingly mentions the need for the health service to take account of 'variations in health' in its strategies.

Source: Benzeval 1999 (13)

---

setting out further reforms to the health service made a commitment to introduce a national target: 'to narrow the health gap in childhood and throughout life between socioeconomic groups and between the most deprived areas and the rest of the country' (17).

Independent inquiry into inequalities in health

Simultaneously with this rapidly moving policy agenda, Sir Donald Acheson was asked, in July 1997, to chair an Independent Inquiry into Inequalities in Health to 'identify priority areas for future policy development ... to reduce health inequalities' (6). The Inquiry's report, which was published in November 1998, is a comprehensive synthesis of the latest scientific evidence on a wide range of topics that affect people's health, with 39 main recommendations. From these, the Inquiry Committee argued that three were crucial:

1. All policies likely to have an impact on health should be evaluated in terms of their impact on health inequalities.
2. A high priority should be given to the health of families with children.
3. Further steps should be taken to reduce income inequalities and improve the living standards of poor households (6).

The general thrust of the Inquiry's recommendations is broadly consistent with those in the Black Report (5) and the King's Fund's Agenda for Action (18). The Inquiry therefore confirmed the main areas of policy development required to reduce health inequalities. Against this background, what has the Labour government done?

The government's strategy

The first articulation of the government's programme of work in this area was set out in *Reducing Health Inequalities: An Agenda for Action*, which it describes as 'the most comprehensive programme of work to tackle health inequalities ever undertaken in this country' (8). Although this document is simply a summary of the overall approach to tackling poverty and social exclusion in England, and does not contain any new policies, it is remarkable in that for the first time, the broad range of social policies that can influence health inequalities is acknowledged (see Box 12.3).

There is insufficient room here to undertake a critique of all of the policies the government emphasizes within this framework. Instead, two key strands are highlighted: tackling poverty through employment and social security; and making health inequalities a key priority for the health service. However, it is important to note that a key mechanism of the government's strategy to tackle social exclusion and poverty, both in these strands and in other policy fields, is area-based initiatives. In particular, they are investing significant sums of money in a range of initiatives in some of the most disadvantaged areas of the country (19).

Tackling poverty

The central theme of the government's welfare reform is 'Work for those who can, security for those who cannot' (2). The government emphasizes the need to tackle 'the *causes* of poverty and social exclusion, not just the *symptoms*' (8). Three sets of policies are therefore important to this endeavour: promoting employment; 'making work pay'; and increasing benefit levels.

The government has introduced a range of policies to reduce barriers to employment: for example, a national childcare strategy has been developed

---

Box 12.3 Reducing Health Inequalities: An Agenda for Action

The current government's strategy is organized into the nine themes set out below. Some of the specific policies it cites as action under each theme are also listed to illustrate its approach.

- *Raising living standards and tackling low income* by introducing a minimum wage and a range of tax credits and increasing benefit levels
- *Education and early years* by introducing policies to improve educational standards, creating 'Sure Start' – preschool services in disadvantaged areas, free to those on low incomes
- *Employment* by creating a range of welfare to work schemes for different priority groups
- *Transport and mobility* by setting targets to reduce road traffic accidents, developing safe walking and cycling routes, and standardizing concessionary fares for older people
- *Issues for the NHS* include working in partnership with local authorities to tackle the wider determinants of health, reviewing the resource allocation formula to local healthcare agencies, developing national service frameworks to standardize care across the country for particular conditions, and broadening the performance management framework for the NHS to include fair access and improving health
- *Building healthy* communities by investing in a range of regeneration initiatives in disadvantaged areas, including Health Action Zones
- *Housing* by changing capital financial rules to promote investment in social housing and introducing special initiatives to tackle homelessness
- *Reducing crime* by investing in range of community-led crime prevention schemes and tackling drug misuse
- *Public health issues* – the first-ever Minister for Public Health is overseeing a range of initiatives to encourage healthy lifestyles, strengthen the public health workforce and tackle specific problems such as fluoridation of water supplies

Source: Department of Health 1999 (8)

---

and additional investment has been made in areas of very high unemployment. However, its single biggest investment – £5.2 billion (€8.3 billion) – is on a range of initiatives known as New Deal, to promote employment for specific groups. The main focus has been on young people who have been unemployed for 6 months, lone parents, and people over 25 who have been unemployed for 2 years. The schemes are different for each population group, but basically involve three distinct components:

1. A single gateway for benefit claims and job advice, with intensive personalized support to find work.
2. A requirement to take up one of a range of options, including: a job subsidized for 6 months; training or full-time education; a job in the voluntary sector or as part of the Environmental Task Force.
3. Some groups, but not all, who refuse to take one of these options are faced with benefit sanctions.

Although many people have found work through these schemes, the extent to which this will have a long-term effect on their employment prospects is debatable. For example, the results of using simulation modelling suggest that many of those who have found employment during the gateway period would have done so anyway, representing a large dead-weight cost for the scheme (20). Moreover, given the lack of skills and work experience of many of the young people entering the scheme, six months' work experience is unlikely to improve their productivity sufficiently to enhance their long-term employability. As a result, 'it is likely that the effects of the policy will be far more modest than its proponents have hoped for' (20).

As well as trying to reduce 'worklessness', the government has also emphasized the need to 'make work pay'. First, in April 1999 the first-ever national minimum wage was introduced in Britain. Over 1.5 million workers were entitled to higher pay as a result, and an initial assessment suggests that the majority of them did have their wages increased to the minimum level (21). Moreover, despite fears that it would create unemployment, especially in the low-wage sector, there has been no evidence that this has occurred (21).

The government has also increased in-work income for low-paid workers by increasing a number of relevant tax credits, introducing a new 10 pence income tax rate and reforming the national insurance system (22). The combined effect of these changes and the introduction of the minimum wage has been estimated to increase average income by £7 (€11.2) per week for men and £4 (€6.4) per week for women, and to reduce the overall level of unemployment by 300,000 or 4 per cent (23).

Alongside measures to increase in-work income, the government has increased benefit levels for families outside the labour market and for pensioners. Figure 12.2 shows that, overall, the government has been successful in redistributing income towards the poorest. Families at the bottom of the income distribution have seen real increases in their income, whereas those in the top decile have experienced a modest fall. Families with children have experienced a real increase in their incomes, as have pensioners, whereas single people and couples without children have all seen a drop in their incomes (24).

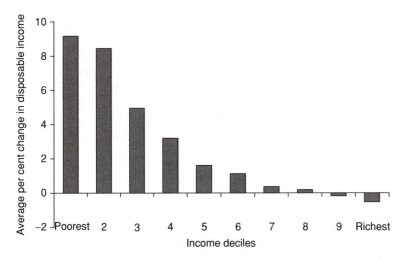

Figure 12.2 The redistributive effects of New Labour's first four Budgets
Source: Benzeval *et al.* 2000 (24)

Overall, therefore, the government appears to be making modest progress in reducing poverty. It estimates that by the end of this parliament they will have lifted 700,000 children out of poverty. In a detailed policy assessment, Piachaud (25) confirms that the government should achieve this target, and that more generally, the numbers of people experiencing poverty should be reduced from 14 to 12 million. This in itself would be a significant achievement, but to achieve their longer-term goal of eradicating child poverty in 20 years will require a significant acceleration in progress in the future (25). It is too early to see whether such reductions in poverty and income inequality are feeding through into the extent of health inequalities in England today.

The role of the health service

It has been argued that the National Health Service (NHS) needs to develop policies in two main areas to play its part in tackling health inequalities by:

- promoting equitable access to its services in relation to need;
- taking the lead in working with other agencies to tackle the broader determinants of health (26).

Again, the Labour government has made progress in these areas. For example, it is currently undertaking a major review of all resource allocation mechanisms across the healthcare sector, with the reduction of inequalities becoming a key criterion for allocation in the future (17). Reforms to the NHS have also taken place. These have introduced a much broader approach to performance management that emphasizes the importance of both fair access and health improvement alongside concerns about efficiency and effectiveness. In addition, standard service frameworks are being established in a number of significant policy areas – for example cancer, coronary heart disease, older people and mental health – to reduce variations in service provision and to improve standards of care around the country. Similarly, a National Institute for Clinical Excellence (NICE) has been set up to regulate new treatments, so that consistent rules are adopted across the country. Finally, and perhaps most importantly, the government has made tackling inequalities in health a key aim of the NHS.

There are a number of dimensions to this strategy. First, improving health and reducing inequalities has become a central part of the national priorities guidance for health and social care. Second, the health service reforms gave local health authorities the lead responsibility for working with other agencies to improve health and reduce inequalities. The key integrating device is the requirement to produce a three-year rolling strategy for health known as Health Improvement Programmes. The first wave was produced in April 1999, and they do have a much stronger focus than previous local plans in addressing a range of health determinants as well as improving access to care (27). However, many of them acknowledge the need for much more development work before they can really begin to address health inequalities locally. Moreover, the competing pressures on health authorities – for example to deliver on commitments to reduce waiting lists – means that reducing inequalities often remains in the second division as far as priorities are concerned.

Third, in 26 disadvantaged areas the government established new partnership organizations known as Health Action Zones (HAZs), to act as 'trailblazers in leading the way to tackle inequalities in health'. HAZs were initially given a 7-year life and additional support and resources to form partnerships between local statutory agencies and communities to develop innovative ways of working to reduce health inequalities. Action covers a broad spectrum of initiatives to provide training and job opportunities for local people, to promote educational attainment among the most disadvantaged, to improve housing conditions and local facilities, to promote social cohesion, and to improve access to healthcare (28). However, these places are the subject of a range of other partnership initiatives, which have overlapping but sometimes contradictory aims. In addition, HAZs have been subjected to considerable policy and priority changes since their inception, which has caused uncertainty about their future. Nevertheless, the local and national evaluations being undertaken offer the opportunity to produce real policy learning for future action (see Chapter 21).

Finally, the new health strategy for England has set up a number of initiatives to strengthen the public health agenda, with a particular emphasis on health inequalities. First, a Health Development Agency has been established to promote the development of an evidence base to improve health and reduce health inequalities. This is to be supported by the development of a public health research and development programme and the establishment of a public health development fund to provide seed funding for innovative approaches to tackling inequalities. Secondly, there is a commitment to produce a public health workforce national development plan and a public health skills audit to support the development of an effective multidisciplinary workforce. In particular, the public health role of health visitors, school nurses, midwives and occupational health specialists is to be strengthened. Finally, Public Health Observatories have been launched in all regions of England to strengthen the analysis of public health information locally.

Overall, the attempts by the government to reorientate the NHS to develop its role to promote health and to reduce health inequalities are welcome. Given time, the new local partnerships may be able to address some of the determinants of health as well as improve access to healthcare. However, the multiplicity of priorities and new strategies that health and local authorities are currently trying to address is in danger of undermining the stated importance of the public health agenda. In addition, the performance management incentives still emphasize waiting list and other health service priorities. The government needs to ensure that sufficient support is given to local initiatives to reduce health inequalities, and to learn from such activities to enhance subsequent policy development.

Possible lessons to be learned

It is difficult in a brief summary such as this to identify all of the complex factors that led to the development of a strategy to tackle health inequalities in England. It is also too early to judge how effective it will be. Nevertheless, a number of useful lessons emerge.

First, it is essential to have political will to encourage policy action. Even under the Conservative government, small changes in policy in this respect began to occur in response to the accumulation of pressure from charities and pressure groups, academics and, perhaps most importantly, the medical profession. Such pressure was underpinned and strengthened by the substantial multidisciplinary research evidence that exists on health inequalities. A new and more sympathetic government has resulted in a significant increase in the attention given to health inequalities.

Secondly, given that reducing health inequalities requires a broad social policy response, it will only be one of a number of legitimate goals being addressed at the same time. Within this framework, modest changes in poverty and income inequality can be achieved through a variety of employment policies, but improving living standards through the social security system is essential if substantial inroads are to be made into the numbers on low income. Such changes should reduce health inequalities in the future.

Finally, at the local level it is difficult to reorientate the health service to focus on health rather than healthcare issues. To achieve this, local agencies require consistent and clear messages, reinforced by a range of policy levers such as performance management systems. A multiplicity of initiatives and contradictory policy tools will, unsurprisingly, hinder progress. Nevertheless, there is evidence that local strategies to reduce health inequalities can be developed and innovative approaches and initiatives introduced. These need time to develop and to be evaluated in order to generate effective policy learning for the future.

References

1. Graham H. The challenge of health inequalities. In: Graham H, ed. *Understanding Health Inequalities*. Milton Keynes: Open University Press, 2000: 3–21.
2. Cm 4445. *Opportunity for All: Tackling Poverty and Social Exclusion. First Annual Report*. London: The Stationery Office, 1999.
3. Gordon D, Adelman L, Ashworth K, Bradshaw J, Levitas R, Middleton S *et al. Poverty and Social Exclusion in Britain*. York: Joseph Rowntree Foundation, 2000.
4. Rahman M, Palmer G, Kenway P, Howarth C. *Monitoring Poverty and Social Exclusion 2000*. York: Joseph Rowntree Foundation, 2000.
5. Townsend P, Davidson N, eds. The Black Report 1982. In: Townsend P, Whitehead M, Davidson N, eds. *Inequalities in Health: The Black Report and the Health Divide*. London: Penguin Books, 1992: 29–213.
6. Acheson D. *Independent Inquiry into Inequalities in Health Report*. London: The Stationery Office, 1998.
7. Cm 4386. *Saving Lives: Our Healthier Nation*. London: The Stationery Office, 1999.
8. Department of Health. *Reducing Health Inequalities: an Action Report*. London: The Stationery Office, 1999.
9. Hattersley L. Trends in life expectancy by social class – an update. *Health Statistics Q* 1999: 2: 16–24.
10. Shaw M, Dorling D, Gordon D, Davey Smith G. *The Widening Gap: Health Inequalities and Policy in Britain*. Bristol: Polity Press, 1999.
11. Graham H. Promoting research on inequality in health. In: Arves-Pares B, ed. *Proceedings from an International Expert Meeting in Stockholm, 24–25 September 1997*. Stockholm: Swedish Council for Social Research, 1998: 29–38.
12. Macintyre S. The Black report and beyond: what are the issues? *Soc Sci Med* 1997: 44(6): 723–45.
13. Benzeval M. Health inequalities: public policy action. In: Griffiths S, Hunter D, eds. *Perspectives in Public Health*. Oxford: Radcliffe Medical Press, 1999: 34–46.
14. Department of Health. *Variations in Health: What Can the Department of Health and the NHS Do?* (Variations Sub-Group of the Chief Medical Officers Health of the Nation Working Group). London: The Stationery Office, 1995.
15. Arblaster L, Entwistle V, Lambert M, Forster M, Sheldon T, Watt I. *Review of the Research on the Effectiveness of Health Service Interventions to Reduce Variations in Health. CRD report 3*. NHS Centre for Reviews and Dissemination, York. University of York, 1995.

16. Cm 3852. *Our Healthier Nation: a Contract for Health. A Consultation Paper.* London: The Stationery Office, 1998.

17. Department of Health. *The NHS Plan: a Plan for Investment, a Plan for Reform.* London: The Stationery Office, 2000.

18. Benzeval M, Judge K, Whitehead M, eds. *Tackling Inequalities in Health: an Agenda for Action.* London: King's Fund,1995.

19. Social Exclusion Unit. *National Strategy for Neighbourhood Renewal: a Framework for Consultation.* London: SEU, Cabinet Office, 2000.

20. Bell B, Blundell R, Van Reenen J. *Getting the Unemployed back to Work: the Role of Targeted Wage Subsidies.* Working Paper Series NO W99/12. London: IFS, 1999.

21. Low Pay Commission. *The National Minimum Wage: the Story So Far. Second Report of the Low Pay Commission.* London: LPC, 2000.

22. Benzeval M, Dilnot A, Judge K, Taylor J. Income and health over the lifecourse: evidence and policy implications. In: Graham H, ed. *Understanding Health Inequalities.* Milton Keynes: Open University Press, 2000: 96–112.

23. Gregg P, Johnson P, Reed H. *Entering Work and the British Tax and Benefit System.* London: IFS, 1999.

24. Benzeval M, Taylor J, Judge K. Evidence on the relationship between low income and poor health: is the government doing enough? *Fiscal Studies* 2000: 21(3): 375–99.

25. Piachaud D. Progress on poverty. *New Economy* 1999: 6(3): 154–60.

26. Benzeval M, Donald A. The role of the NHS in tackling inequalities in health. In: Gordon D, Shaw M, Dorling D, Davey Smith G, eds. *Inequalities in Health: the Evidence Presented to the Independent Inquiry into Inequalities in Health* (chaired by Sir Donald Acheson). Bristol: Polity Press, 1999: 87–99.

27. Benzeval M. HAs, HImPs, and tackling health inequalities. Paper presented at the *8th Annual Public Health Forum: Partnership, participation and power*, 28–29 March 2000, Harrogate, Harrogate Conference Centre.

28. Judge K, Barnes M, Bauld L, Benzeval M, Killoran A, Robinson R *et al. Health Action Zones: Learning to Make a Difference. Findings from a Preliminary Review of Health Action Zones and Proposals for a National Evaluation.* A report to the Department of Health. Canterbury: University of Kent, 1999.

13 France

Thierry Lang, Didier Fassin,
Hélène Grandjean, Monique Kaminski
and Annette Leclerc

Introduction

France is among those European countries where the differences in premature mortality, at least among men, are the highest (1), although the French healthcare system has been rated among those providing a high quality of care, as in a recent WHO report (2). In this context, it is not surprising that a sharp contrast exists between statistical data on socioeconomic inequalities in health and their perception by the population, the policy-makers and the health professionals.

The socioeconomic situation

In the last quarter of the twentieth century the situation in France was characterized by economic growth: from 1973 to 1996 gross national product increased continuously by 50 per cent. However, economic growth has declined in recent years and the financing of social services has become more constrained. In addition, economic growth has not benefited all sectors of the population equally. Unemployment increased from 5.7 per cent in 1979 to 9 per cent in 1991 and to 11.8 per cent in 1998. Not all social categories have been equally affected by unemployment: in 1982 and 1998, unemployment was 4 times higher among unskilled workers than among executives (3). Between 1984 and 1994, the purchasing power of unskilled workers decreased. The household income of a professional family was 2.9 times higher in 1984 and 4.2 times higher in 1994 than that of the family of an unskilled worker. The benefit of the national health insurance system has been extended to almost the entire population. However, because of exclusion and marginalization, many people are unaware of or unable to use these opportunities.

The extent of socioeconomic inequalities in health

With regard to health indicators, life expectancy has increased dramatically in France during recent decades. The differences between men and women

Table 13.1 Life expectancy, probability of death and occupational category

Occupational category in 1982	Life expectancy at 35 years		Probability of death between 35 and 64 years	
	Men	Women	Men	Women
Upper executives	44.5	49.5	13%	7%
Farmers	43.0	47.5	16%	8%
Middle executives	42.0	49.0	17%	7%
Craftworkers	41.5	48.5	19%	8%
Employees	40.0	47.5	23%	9%
Workers	38.0	46.0	26%	11%

Data from the INSEE cohort, 1982–96

Source: Mesrine, INSEE, 1999 (6)

are particularly large. For women, in 1997 life expectancy at birth was 82 years, as opposed to 74 for men. For women this was the highest in Europe, which is not the case for men.

In a comparative study involving 11 European countries, total mortality in France was 71 per cent higher among male manual workers aged 45–59 than among non-manual workers, whereas elsewhere this excess mortality ranged from 33 to 53 per cent. According to these data, in the 1980s this excess mortality concerned mainly cancer and gastrointestinal disease. Even considering the methodological limitations of international comparisons, it is clear that France is characterized by a high level of socioeconomic inequalities in mortality (4–6) (Table 13.1).

During the past decade, the decrease in mortality rates for most causes has been more pronounced in the upper than in the lower classes. Inequalities in mortality have thus increased. Among active men aged 25–54 years the decrease in total mortality between 1982 and 1990 is 16 per cent for the professionals and upper executives, compared to 7 per cent among employees and workers. The same trends were observed for cancer mortality (–21 vs. –1 per cent), cardiovascular mortality (–41 vs. –19 per cent) and violent deaths (–24 vs. –8 per cent). In 1990, in men of this age group total mortality was 2.9 times higher among employees and workers than among professionals and upper executives. Based on mortality data from 1982 to 1996, the probability of death between 35 and 64 years was 13 per cent among upper executives as opposed to 26 per cent among workers (1). Among pathologies for which morbidity data are available, results on incidence, case fatality and impairment have generally confirmed the existence of socioeconomic inequalities as large as could be expected from the mortality data. Although the data are more sparse, socioeconomic inequalities have been observed to concern those over 65 years of age, in relation to impairment or disabilities, but are less pronounced among women than among men. Infant mortality is one example of an inverse trend in inequalities, as this has been found to decrease. A synthesis of the data on inequalities in France was published in 2000 by Leclerc and colleagues (1).

Research

Socioeconomic inequalities in health have been demonstrated for many years in France. Researchers from the National Institute for Economic Studies and Statistics (INSEE) have produced statistics demonstrating important differences in mortality by occupational category. In 1965, a paper was published on mortality data from the period 1955–60, reporting that teachers and upper executives had an eight years longer life expectancy at 35 years than did unskilled workers (7). Such statistics have been regularly produced and published by INSEE since 1965 (5–7). Similarly, the same Institute, in 1981, published results from studies on morbidity by social class (8).

Since then, several research teams have been working on the subject. However, socioeconomic inequalities in health have rarely been their main research theme, although they have often been addressed as one theme for a limited period of time by various research groups (9, 10). Perinatal health and cardiovascular disease have been studied more often than other fields. Such studies were not coordinated and no scientific forums or public debates were held. Socioeconomic inequalities in health have thus been considered worthy of only minor research interest.

In the late 1980s and early 1990s, socioeconomic inequalities in health came back on the agenda, but were analysed primarily in terms of exclusion from and access to medical care (11, 12). Many sociological projects and local health initiatives, involving non-governmental organizations, were undertaken in order to understand the health issues among these groups and the way the healthcare system could deal with them.

In 1997, on the initiative of a National Health Research Institute (INSERM) committee, it was decided to promote research on this topic. There are probably two reasons for this. One is that social exclusion and its health consequences in France could not be ignored, leading to a concern with poverty but also to a new legitimacy for interest on socioeconomic inequalities in health. The other is the growing interest in this field, as evidenced in the international literature. In comparison with the United Kingdom, for example, very few data were available and few researchers were involved in the field, and France was absent from international conferences on the subject. In 1997, therefore, grants were offered in order to stimulate research. Most grant applications concerned precariousness and exclusion, with a sociological approach; few were concerned with the gradient approach to inequalities in health. At the same time, the publication of two books was encouraged by INSERM, the objective of which was to write a 'state of the art' critique on socioeconomic inequalities in France. One of these books deals with socioeconomic inequalities in health, using the gradient approach and trying to understand the social determinants involved (1); the other is devoted to disadvantaged groups (13). It is worth noting that few contacts were established between the two groups, the first consisting mostly of epidemiologists and the second mostly of social scientists, although the two books explore two facets of a common problem.

Policies

The situation with regard to socioeconomic inequalities in health should be interpreted in the broader context of the weakness of the public health system in France and the increase in socioeconomic inequalities in general.

Until the mid-1990s it would have been difficult to find a concern of public policy with this subject, as assessed by reports or defined priorities (14) (see Box 13.1), but this does not mean that socioeconomic inequalities were not a problem in France: the lack of debate concerns socioeconomic inequalities in health, but not other aspects of socioeconomic inequality. In the 1960s and 1970s, public reports (State Planning Commission; Commissariat Général au Plan) were published concerning inequalities in other domains, for

---

Box 13.1 Some important dates in France

1945 Establishment of the social security system

1946 Law on the objectives and organization of occupational medicine

1965 Statistics published by the National Institute for Statistics and Economic Studies demonstrating important differences in mortality by occupational category

1988 Law providing a minimum income and social security to people without jobs who no longer benefited from unemployment benefits

1994 First report on public health in France emphasizing inequalities in health as a priority

1997 Initiative of a National Health Research Institute committee to promote research into health inequalities and disadvantaged groups

1998 Two laws passed organizing the 'prevention of exclusion'

1998 Report of the High Committee on Public Health notes that socioeconomic inequalities have not been reduced

1999 Socioeconomic inequalities in health were not mentioned among the priorities of the Convention on Health Issues, a national forum where citizens were invited to debate health issues

2000 Publication of two books commissioned by INSERM on socioeconomic inequalities in health

example education, but it was not until the beginning of the 1980s that inequalities in health were noted in a report from the Commission.

In 1994, the first report on public health in France was published by the High Committee of Public Health (Haut Comité de la Santé Publique, HCSP) (15), a committee chaired by the Ministry of Health and co-chaired by a public health specialist. Inequalities in health were highlighted as a priority in the medium term, among three others: reducing avoidable deaths, reducing the burden of incapacity, and improving the quality of life of the disabled. In this report, it was pointed out that the increase in the difference in health indicators between social classes is a worrying and negative characteristic of France. It was also emphasized that this increase was observed despite the inequalities in healthcare utilization having been reduced in the previous 30 years, at least quantitatively. As a result, the following statement was made: 'This confirms the analysis according to which the healthcare system has a limited role to explain the health status of a population' (15). Another report relating to the health consequences of precariousness and exclusion was published in 1998 (16), noting that the social disparities in health had not been reduced. Interestingly, this 1998 report, in which all indicators are reviewed, does not include socioeconomic inequalities, although exclusion and disparity are discussed.

Socioeconomic inequalities in health were included among health priorities in several national and regional health conferences by health professionals and policy-makers. However, in these documents it was extremely uncommon to give priority to social and environmental determinants, access to care being the main topic discussed. This was largely the case in two recent workshops organized by a research unit of the Ministry of Employment and Solidarity (17, 18).

In a similar way, the French public has not been much concerned with socioeconomic inequalities in health. For example, in 1999 the Convention on Health Issues (Etats Généraux de la Santé) was organized, a forum where citizens were invited to debate health issues. It is interesting to observe that, unlike issues relating to access to care, inequalities in health were not mentioned.

Despite this clear lack of priority concerning interventions to reduce inequalities in health, some aspects of the French health system have implicitly addressed the problem. The national health insurance and occupational medicine systems are two examples of this.

The national health insurance system

Since the Second World War, the idea that healthcare should be accessible to all and medical expenses reimbursed by national health insurance has been widely accepted. The debate has focused on the level of reimbursement and the population that should benefit from such insurance (see Box 13.1).

In 1945, the aim of the generalization of the social protection system 'Edict on the French Public Welfare System' (Ordonnances sur la Sécurité Sociale), was to 'reduce the uncertainty of existence' and to provide security and protection for workers and their families against any risk that might reduce or suppress their earning capacity. Access to care and prevention, and the reduction of workplace accidents, were part of this plan.

During the past 20 years, as the number of persons insured by the French Public Welfare System (Sécurité Sociale) increased, so did the percentage of out-of-pocket health expenditures, owing to a reduced reimbursement of ambulatory care. The contrast between the general principles and the reality of access to care is exemplified by various studies dealing with the actual utilization of health services. For example, in 1997, 16 per cent of those interviewed stated that they had forgone medical care at least once during the previous year for financial reasons (low reimbursement of dental care, lack of resources, etc.). Among the unemployed this percentage was 50 per cent (1).

Although 84 per cent of the population has voluntary complementary insurance (mutual benefit societies or private companies), this percentage varies according to social category and is lower among the lower classes. It is also likely that the content of these insurances will be very different.

This policy approach considers people as clients of the health services. In keeping with the weakness of public health in France, this was not a population approach, dealing with determinants of health, but rather an individual approach which, combined with confidence in the progress of medicine, has suppressed the need for a debate on inequalities in health. It is a paradox that a health insurance system based on the idea of solidarity has provided the basis for an individual approach to health.

Since the late 1980s the political debate and action have been concerned primarily, if not exclusively, with exclusion. In line with the idea of reducing the uncertainty of existence through access to rights, in 1988 a law providing a minimum income and social security to those without a job and who no longer benefited from unemployment benefits (minimum welfare payment, *revenu minimum d'insertion*), was adopted. Combating exclusion was a major political issue for the 1995 government, and in 1998 two laws were passed regarding the 'prevention of exclusion', a very important aspect of which was to provide social protection, access to care and health insurance coverage. This universal medical coverage (*couverture médicale universelle*), which provides health insurance to any person with residency papers, including complementary insurance, became applicable in 2000. This protection is offered in certain conditions below a certain level of financial resources. However, a threshold effect might thus be expected, as a significant proportion of families characterized by incomes just above the level fixed by the law do not benefit from complementary insurance.

Overall, this policy probably had some effects on the level of inequalities. It was not, however, specifically designed for this purpose and was limited to access to care. Unfortunately, its impact on socioeconomic inequalities in health has not been assessed.

Occupational health

Despite the fact that occupational medicine is not viewed as part of a policy to reduce inequalities in health, its activity is potentially important in this respect. As set out by the 1946 law on occupational medicine, in France, as in a few other countries (and in contrast to the Nordic and Anglo-Saxon countries, where occupational medicine is a branch of public health that deals with workers' health as a whole), occupational medicine is exclusively preventive and takes a global approach to health in the workplace, including interventions on working conditions. Its goal has been to adapt working techniques and conditions to human physiology (19). Many occupational hazards have been shown to be more prevalent among manual workers than among other social categories. As an example, if around 5 per cent of cancers are estimated to be related to work, this percentage is estimated to be 20 per cent among manual workers (16). Because one major objective of occupational medicine is to improve working conditions, one might think that in its absence working conditions might have been more detrimental to health than they are.

France and Belgium are the only European countries where an annual medical examination is mandatory for every employee. This is an opportunity to introduce preventive activities to those who otherwise have few medical contacts (19), and interventions aimed at improving hypertension control or reducing smoking habits have been performed and evaluated (20, 21).

Because smoking, high alcohol intake and poor hypertension control under treatment have been shown to be more frequent among lower classes and lower educational groups, there is indirect evidence that occupational medicine has contributed to reducing inequalities in health. However, few interactions between occupational physicians and public health with regard to socioeconomic inequalities in health have been observed. In particular, no assessment has been performed in this respect.

Possible lessons to be learned

Health has not been considered a major issue in France, in either the public and political arenas or by trade unions. Instead, the debate has focused on access to care and the level of reimbursement of medical expenses. The idea that the healthcare system was theoretically accessible to all, even the poorest, has probably lessened the concern with health itself. Two consequences of this can be highlighted.

First, healthcare has been considered a fundamental right and thus the focus for interventions in relation to health. In contrast, health determinants, such as living, housing, working and socioeconomic conditions, other than individual behaviours (alcohol, tobacco consumption, etc.), have seldom been discussed and no intervention has been undertaken in this regard with health as an end-point. Some of the public policies implemented in recent decades might have influenced the situation in relation to health inequalities, for example occupational health, social policies such as the minimum welfare payment, or housing policies. However, these were not designed with health in mind, and their effects on health inequalities have not been assessed. None the less, it can be hypothesized that as the aim of such policies was to provide a minimum income and housing for the poorest sectors of society, without them their health would have been worse. In this respect, on the action spectrum proposed by Whitehead (22), France might be described as being in the denial/indifference phase, as the lack of concern cannot be ascribed to a lack of data.

Secondly, a strongly implicit idea is that the main issue for public policies is to provide formal, theoretical access to healthcare and services, and to a large extent the actual utilization of such care has not been a matter for concern. The data comparing theoretical access to care and its actual use have thus shown important discrepancies.

This approach to health has been encouraged by the lack of epidemiological and surveillance systems on health inequalities, as well as by the weakness of the public health movement. In this respect, the national health insurance system has probably helped to reinforce the idea that health is an individual concern and not a collective issue.

References

1. Leclerc A, Fassin D, Grandjean H, Kaminski M, Lang T, eds. *Les inégalités sociales de santé* (Inequalities in Health). Paris: La Découverte, 2000.
2. OMS/WHO. *Rapport sur la santé dans le monde 2000* (World Health Report 2000). Geneva: 2000.
3. Bihr A, Pfefferkorn. *Déchiffrer les inégalités* (Reading Inequalities). Paris: Editions Syros, 1998.
4. Mackenbach JP, Kunst AE, Cavelaars AE, Groenhof F, Geurts JJ. Socio-economic inequalities in morbidity and mortality in Western Europe. The EU Working Group on Socioeconomic Inequalities in Health. *Lancet* 1997: 349: 1655–9.
5. Desplanques G. *La mortalité masculine selon le milieu social. Données sociales* (Mortality in Relation to Social Status in Men. Social data). Paris: INSEE, 1984: 348–58.
6. Mesrine A. *Les différences de mortalité par milieu social restent fortes. Données sociales* (Differences in Mortality according to Social Class are still Important. Social data). Paris: INSEE, 1999.
7. Calot G, Febvay M. La mortalité différentielle selon le milieu social. (Differences in mortality according to social class). *Etudes et Conjoncture* 1965: 11: 75–159.
8. Anon. *Morbidité et appartenance sociale. Données sociales* (Morbidity and Social Belonging. Social data). Paris: INSEE, 1981: 75–81.

9. Drulhe M. Santé et société. *Le façonnement sociétal de la santé.* (Health and Society). Paris: Presses Universitaires de France, 1996.

10. Aiach P, Carr-Hill R, Curtis S, Illsley R. *Les inégalités sociales de santé en France et en Grande-Bretagne.* (Socioeconomic Health Inequalities in Health in France and in Great Britain). Paris: La Documentation Française, 1988.

11. Chauvin P, Lebas J, eds. *Précarité et Santé.* (Precariousness and Health.). Paris: Flammarion, 1998.

12. Paugam S. *L'Exclusion: L'état des savoirs* (Exclusion: State of the Art). Paris: La Découverte, 1996.

13. Joubert M, Chauvin P, Facy F, Ringa VS, Iwek P, Deschamps JP *et al.*, eds. *Précarisation, risques et santé* (Precariousness, Risks and Health). Collection 'Questions en santé publique'. Paris: Editions de l'Inserm, 2001.

14. Berthod-Wurmser M, Boiteux A, Henrard JC, Letourmy A, Lenoir N, Meyer C *et al. La santé en Europe* (Health in Europe). Paris: La Documentation Française, 1994.

15. Haut Comité de la Santé Publique. *La santé en France. Rapport général* (Health in France. Global Report). Paris: La Documentation Française, 1994.

16. Haut Comité de la Santé Publique. *La santé en France 1994–8* (Health in France, 1994–8). Paris: La Documentation Française, 1998.

17. Daniel C, Le Clainche C, eds. *Réduire les inégalités. Quel rôle pour la protection sociale?* (Reducing Inequalities. What Role for Social Welfare?). Paris: Ministère de la Santé et de la Solidarité, 2000.

18. Daniel C, Le Clainche C, eds. *Mesurer les inégalités. De la construction des indicateurs aux débats sur les interprétations* (Measuring Inequalities. Constructing and Interpreting Indicators). Paris: Ministère de la Santé et de la Solidarité, 2000.

19. Fouriaud C, Jacquinet-Salord, Mahé I, Ravelonanosy MJ, Lang T, et le groupe des médecins du travail de l'APSAT. Médecine du travail et prévention générale. Résultats d'une enquête épidémiologique auprès de 8203 salariés (Occupational medicine and prevention. Results of an epidemiologic study among 8303 employees). *Arch Mal Professionnelles* 1991: 52: 333–7.

20. Lang T, Nicaud V, Slama K, Hirsch A, Imbernon E, Goldberg M *et al.* and the worksite physicians from the AIREL group. Smoking cessation at the workplace. Results of a randomized controlled intervention study. *J Epidemiol Commun Health* 2000: 54: 349–54.

21. Lang T, Nicaud V, Darné B, Rueff B and the members of the WALPA group. Improving arterial hypertension control among excessive drinkers. Results of a randomised trial. *J Epidemiol Commun Health* 1995: 49: 610–16.

22. Whitehead M. Diffusion of ideas on social inequalities in health: a European perspective. *Milbank Q* 1998: 76: 469–92.

14 Greece

Yannis Tountas, Panagiota Karnaki and Dimitra Triantafyllou

Introduction

Only a few studies have examined the extent of health inequalities in Greece. This means that there has been no overall assessment of this phenomenon, which explains the lack of state interest in reducing such inequalities. However, as is discussed in this chapter, strong social policies are exercised in Greece, many of which contribute to the reduction of health inequalities.

The socioeconomic situation

Greece is a southeastern European country which has been a member of the European Union (EU) since 1981. The country has a mixed economy, with a large agricultural and tourist sector; it has one of the lowest gross national products (GNP) in Europe and a high unemployment rate that reaches over 10 per cent (1). Public health expenditure has increased from 3.7 per cent of GNP in 1980, to 4.8 per cent in 1990 and to 5.3 per cent in 1998. Nevertheless, this is still one of the lowest in Europe (2).

Although the health system in Greece has improved since the establishment of the National Health System in 1983, many of the planned initial reforms have not been implemented. There is no public primary healthcare system in urban areas; there is no organized referral system; the private health sector is growing with increasing private health expenditure (3.4 per cent of GNP); and there is considerable inequality in access to healthcare related to existing inequalities among the provisions of the numerous social funds (1, 3, 4).

The extent of socioeconomic inequalities in health

In general, Greece has quite satisfactory health indicators. Life expectancy in 1997 was 75 years for men and 81 years for women; total population mortality per 100,000 people for 1996 was 684.6. This is attributed more to the relatively high standard of living, the good climate and the healthy nutrition than to the healthcare system, which is poor in both quality and productivity (3).

Table 14.1 Standardized mortality (1991) and infant mortality (1996) in Greece

Region	Standardized mortality (per 100,000 population)	Infant mortality (per 1,000 births)
Athens region	753.51	6.91
Central Greece and Euboea	719.40	6.87
Peloponnese	675.32	7.22
Ionian Islands	760.73	3.80
Epirus	671.23	6.48
Thessalia	752.30	8.81
Macedonia	798.91	7.59
Thrace	894.79	10.76
Aegean islands	747.59	4.21
Crete	645.12	8.36
Total	727.20	7.27

Source: Center for Health Services Research (2000)

The lack of comprehensive statistical data on the socioeconomic status of different segments of the Greek population and of information on the socioeconomic distribution of health indices makes the examination of socioeconomic inequalities in health a difficult task (5). Because of this, relevant activities on a national scale are limited to the examination of differentiations by geographical region in the main, and to a lesser extent by type of social security and occupational status.

Concerning socioeconomic inequalities by geographical area, regions that are socially and economically disadvantaged show worse health indices than other areas of the country (Table 14.1). Thus, the region of Thrace in northern Greece, which has one of the lowest GNP per capita, had in 1996 higher infant mortality and in 1991 higher general standardized mortality rates than all other regions of Greece. Higher mortality and morbidity rates are observed in socioeconomically underprivileged groups such as the unemployed, refugees, illegal residents, migrants of Greek origin who have settled back in Greece, gypsies and, in general, people who are vulnerable to social exclusion, many of whom live in the greater Athens area, which because of this has a comparatively high mortality rate compared to other areas (2).

Regarding the social security system, people who are insured in the 'poor' insurance funds which cover those working in agriculture and the private sector (73.3 per cent of the total population) tend to have higher morbidity rates than those who are insured in wealthier funds (2, 6).

Health inequalities in Greece are also observed according to occupational status. Manual workers (farmers, technicians and agricultural employees) are more susceptible than other occupational categories to communicable and musculoskeletal diseases and accidents. According to national statistics data from patients in Greek hospitals, office workers and employees of the services sector more often experience diseases of the digestive, circulatory and respiratory systems, and are more often victims of traffic accidents (6).

Research

Only a limited number of research projects on health inequalities have been carried out, mainly by the departments of social medicine of the Universities of Athens and Crete. Research has focused on examining the relationship between specific socioeconomic groups and particular diseases. Between 1958 and 1982 the mortality rates for leukaemia, lymphoma and cancer of the liver were higher in rural than in affluent urban populations (7). Two case-control studies provided important evidence of the positive relationship between low socioeconomic status and higher incidence of breast and lung cancer in women living in Greece (8). Studies have also indicated that people from lower socioeconomic categories have a poor perception of their health and believe they suffer more from chronic illnesses than those in higher social categories (9). In other studies it has been found that children of low socioeconomic family background had a higher number of hepatitis A antibodies (10), and that 86.6 per cent of children from high socio-economic status families had good oral health compared to only 21.8 per cent of children of low socioeconomic status (11).

A recent study conducted in hospitals belonging to the Hellenic Health Promoting Hospital Network found that people belonging to lower occupational categories had poorer self-perceived health status, reported more chronic illness, and were exposed to more risk factors than doctors and administrative staff (12).

Research-related intervention activities to alleviate health inequalities have been few and are attributed mainly to the initiatives of non-governmental organizations or academic institutions. Few of them have been evaluated, and among these the most important concern nutrition and addiction.

The Preventive Medicine and Nutritional Clinic of the Medical School, University of Crete, conducted a 6-year health and nutritional education programme to promote healthy dietary and lifestyle habits in primary school children who belonged mostly to deprived families of the island. Evaluation indicated the positive effect of the intervention on obesity indices and physical activity, by increasing knowledge of the benefits of a healthy diet among deprived families with limited access to health-related information (13).

The Greek Gerontological and Geriatric Society carried out a two-year project to promote healthy nutrition among elderly underprivileged populations as a way of preventing or minimizing the risk of cardiovascular disease. With the help of elderly volunteers, teaching material was developed and distributed to recreation centres across the country, an action evaluated as positive in reducing health inequalities (14).

The Centre for the Care and Treatment of Addicted People has implemented a school-based intervention programme in the city of Piraeus, with the objective of promoting healthy lifestyles, creative leisure activities, teamwork and the development of social skills in order to prevent antisocial behavior and delinquency in adolescents who are members of deprived families, the families of economic refugees and the offspring of mixed marriages. An evaluation of the ongoing programme has indicated that this model project is suitable to be incorporated in the health education activities of school curricula (15).

Policies

Even though Greece does not have an official policy to tackle health inequalities, several reforms have been made to the country's social policy in the direction of relieving families and individuals of the burden of poverty, unemployment, inadequate housing, inequality in healthcare access and social exclusion, factors that influence the health status of underprivileged populations.

In 1983 a new Act (no. 1397/83, Act 2519/1997) acknowledged the elderly as a group with special care needs vulnerable to social exclusion. The measures taken to tackle this problem were a monthly benefit for low-paid pensioners, and the coverage of balneotherapy and summer holidays. Special economic measures have also been taken to support families with more than three children in the hope that economic support will improve their living conditions.

The issue of unemployment has been addressed through vocational and continuous training, and by employment and self-employment programmes with a special emphasis on young people, women, the long-term unemployed, gypsies, migrants, returning migrants of Greek origin, ex-prisoners and economic refugees.

Housing is also an area of priority in the social policy of Greece. Labourers in low-income families are entitled to enrol for low-interest-rate loans to acquire their first house. People who suffer from physical disabilities, mental or physical disorders or chronic diseases receive support and benefits from the state. These include free transport facilities, monthly benefits, vocational training, social and psychological support, and access to treatment facilities such as speech therapy, physiotherapy and occupational therapy. State support is also provided to the 1.5 million economic immigrants who present important health problems.

In November 2000, the Minister of Health and Welfare proposed a new bill for the reform of the National Health System. Many of the proposed changes aim to alleviate socioeconomic inequality in healthcare through the regional organization of the National Health System, and the introduction of new services within the public sector, such as the family doctor, home care and special rehabilitation services, which until now were available only to those who could afford private health services.

Although these social policies have a considerable effect in alleviating health inequalities, they have not been planned as such, as in Greece socio-economic inequalities in health have not yet been recognized as a priority in public policy. Greece, according to the action spectrum of Margaret Whitehead (16), is still in the first phase, that is, 'measurement'. Such measurements, as already mentioned, are still inadequate and recognition of the problem is only indirectly assumed by public authorities. The reasons for this delay are due to the lack of the necessary statistical data and limited research, mainly due to the fact that the Ministry of Health was until now mostly preoccupied with the operation of the health system at the expense of other public health issues. In addition, in Greece the National School of Public Health is a professional school and not an academic institution, and the six medical schools of the country have small departments of social medicine which are preoccupied mainly with traditional epidemiology and hygiene.

Possible lessons to be learned

As already mentioned, in Greece the need for specially designed policies to tackle health inequalities cannot be satisfied as long as the relevant research and concern are restricted to academic institutions and are not a priority on the agenda of public authorities. Measurements and research on a national scale are certainly a prerequisite for more concrete action. On the other hand, social policies can have an important positive effect, even if they are not designed specifically to act in the framework of health inequalities.

Greece is also indicative of the limited influence of free access to health services on alleviating inequality in their use. For this reason, free access to the National Health System needs to be enhanced by specific organizational measures taking into consideration the social factors that influence the use of health services.

From what we have discussed, it might be concluded that within the action spectrum described by Whitehead (16), Greece still seems to be in the measurement stage.

References

1. World Health Organization. *Highlights on Health in Greece*. Geneva: World Health Organization, Regional Office for Europe, 1998.
2. Kentro Meleton Ipiresion Ygeias (Center for Health Services Research). *Oi ipiresies ygeias stin Ellada* (Health Services in Greece). Athens: Ministry of Health and Welfare, 2000.
3. Tountas Y, Stefansson H, Frissiras S. Health reform in Greece: planning and implementation of a National Health System. *Int J Health Planning Mgt* 1995: 10: 283–304.
4. World Health Organization. *Healthcare Systems in Transition*. Copenhagen: World Health Organization, Regional Office for Europe, 1996.

5. Tountas Y, Frissiras S. The relationship between socioeconomic status and health. *Iatriki* 1996: 69(3): 270–6.
6. Karagiorgas S. *Diastasis tis Ftohias stin Ellada* (Dimensions of poverty in Greece). Athens: EKKE, 1990.
7. Linou A, Kiamouris H, Tsoukas A. The relationship between agricultural occupations and the incidence of leukemia and lymphoma in the Greek population. *Iatriki* 1988: 54: 431–6.
8. Katsouyanni K, Trichopoulos D, Boyle P, Xirouchaki E, Trichopoulou A *et al.* Diet and breast cancer: a case-control study in Greece. *Int J Cancer* 1986: 38: 815–20.
9. Alamanos Y, Tsamandouraki K, Tountas Y. Assessing health status and service utilization in Athens: the implications for policy and planning. *Health Promotion Int* 1992: 8: 263–9.
10. Xristofillea-Georgoulia E. Oro- epidimiologikes parametroi tis loimoxis apo Ipatitida-A se paidia kai enilikous stin Ellada (Epidemiological parameters of infection with hepatitis-A in children and adults in Greece). Doctoral dissertation, University of Athens, 1983.
11. Koletsi-Kounari E. Odondiatriki frontida ston elliniko plithismo (Dental care in the Greek population). Doctoral dissertation, University of Athens, 1984.
12. Pavi E, Tountas Y, Arkadopoulos N *et al.* Health risk behaviors among the hospital personnel of the Hellenic Network of Health Promoting Hospitals. Proceedings of the 8th International Conference on Health Promoting Hospitals, Athens, Greece, 14–16 June 2000.
13. Manios Y, Kafatos A, Mamalakis G. The effects of a health education intervention initiated at first grade over a 3-year period: physical activity and fitness indices. *Health Educ Res* 1998: 13: 593–606.
14. Komitopoulos N, Ioannidis I, Sourtzi P, Velonakis E, Varsamis E. A health promotion programme may affect attitudes and modify behaviours in the elderly with cardiovascular risk factors. Proceedings of the 8th International Conference on Health Promoting Hospitals, Athens, Greece, 14–16 June 2000.
15. Kiritsi I, Tsiotra S. Prevention in primary school: a holistic approach. Presented at the 38th International Council on Alcohol and Addictions (ICAA), Vienna, Austria, 16–20 August 1999.
16. Whitehead M. Diffusion of ideas on social inequalities in health: a European perspective. *Milbank Q* 1998: 76: 469–92.

15 Italy

*Giuseppe Costa, Teresa Spadea and
Nerina Dirindin*

Introduction

Socioeconomic inequalities in health have been only scantily documented in
most Mediterranean countries; consequently, the issue has not been raised
on the public agenda for social, health and research policy until recently.
Nevertheless, compared to northern Europe these Mediterranean countries
show some peculiarities in socioeconomic inequalities which are interesting
to analyse and discuss. In this chapter we will first describe health inequalities in Italy, and then summarize current progress in the field of research and
of reporting evidence on this subject. As for policies, the first attempts to
address the problem of reducing socioeceonomic inequalities will be illustrated; unfortunately, the effectiveness of such policies has not been evaluated and their impact on health cannot be determined.

The socioeconomic situation

Living conditions in Italy have improved over the past decade. General
economic recovery stabilized in 1996 and is reflected in the growth of gross
domestic product, although limited by the burden of public debt. The educational level has risen, with nearly total coverage (99 per cent) for compulsory schooling and an increase in high-school enrolment from 82 per
cent in 1987 to 94 per cent in 1997. Life expectancy at birth in 1997 was
75 years for males and 82 years for females; health expectancy in 1994 was
50 and 48 years, respectively.

The labour market in Italy did not benefit from the economic recovery:
the unemployment rate stood at 12 per cent in 1997, with rates as high as 25
per cent in some areas of the south. Women are the most affected, representing 52 per cent of the total unemployed population and twice the unemployment rate of men. Moreover, social welfare is still based on a model
of full employment and on the role of the family, assuming that each family
has at least one member/worker covered by social security, whereas most
poverty concerns single adults without a job. The social security system is
now slowly changing, expanding its coverage to particular groups of disadvantaged people, such as lone mothers and children in poverty. The

prevalence of households below the poverty line is substantially stable at around 11 per cent; poverty varies widely according to geographical area in terms of both prevalence and intensity (poverty gap).

Access to the healthcare system is formally universal and inexpensive or free of charge (particularly for the poor), but some evidence indicates that cultural and socioeconomic disadvantages may make access more difficult.

The extent of socioeconomic inequalities in health

In the 1990s mortality at a municipality level increased linearly with the score of a composite deprivation index (1). This direct correlation is evident in both genders, with a steeper gradient among adults than among the elderly (Figure 15.1). On an individual basis, a census-based record linkage study during the early 1980s highlighted very regular inequalities by education (2). Preliminary results of a similar study conducted in the early 1990s show increasing inequalities among men (3). Reproductive outcomes also indicate inequalities of the same type: children born to Italian women with a low education systematically show an excess of unfavourable events compared to those of educated mothers (4).

More detailed data on mortality are available from local longitudinal studies. Specifically, in Turin, Florence and Leghorn, mortality increases linearly with social disadvantage for any chosen indicator at both the individual level (education, unemployment, social class, quality of housing) and the geographical level (deprivation index) (5). The causes of death most highly associated with socioeconomic inequalities are those correlated to addiction and exclusion (drugs, alcohol, tobacco), to very poor life histories (respiratory disease and stomach cancer), to low prevention in the workplace and on the streets (accidents), and to the quality of healthcare (avoidable deaths). Italy, like most countries in southern Europe, shows few inequalities in the distribution of ischaemic heart disease, especially among men, as already indicated by comparative studies (6).

We observe an analogous picture of inequalities in cancer incidence (7), self-reported morbidity and health-damaging lifestyles (8). The only exception is smoking among women, where rates increase along with socioeconomic status; however, because women in the upper classes have a greater tendency to stop smoking, differences in this case are declining (9).

As for the health system, there is evidence of a social gradient both in access to primary prevention and in early diagnosis and in the results of early and appropriate care (10–14).

These relative differentials in health are the premise for a deeper impact on health of absolute poverty, which in Italy concerns marginal groups of the native population and broader classes of immigrants. The latter still present a healthy epidemiological profile stemming from the 'healthy migrant effect', but dangerous signs of a deteriorating heritage are becoming evident as time since migration elapses (15).

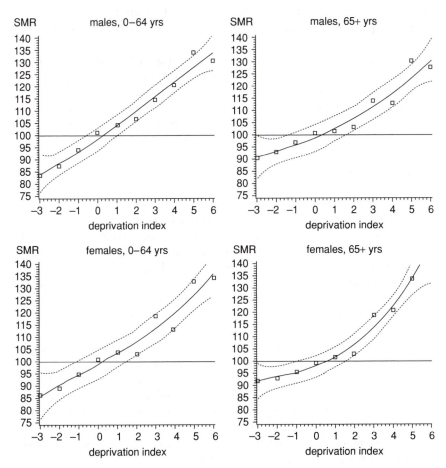

Figure 15.1 All-cause mortality and deprivation in Italian municipalities, 1990–2.
Standardized mortality ratios (SMR) and their 95% confidence
intervals plotted against deprivation index, by gender and age band

Source: Cadum *et al.* 1999 (1)

Research

The epidemiology of health inequalities is a fairly recent field of research
in Italy. Early interest in related issues can be found in essays on social
medicine from the 1970s (16), which reflect a strong leftist spirit and a
confrontational approach.

At the beginning of the 1980s occupational epidemiologists focused great
attention on the development of surveillance systems of occupational mortality, using routine administrative data. In accordance with recommendations by the National Institute for Prevention and Safety at Work, the Turin
Longitudinal Study was implemented (17). Early results on unemployment

and mortality (18) confirmed the usefulness of these kinds of data in monitoring inequalities in health (in fact, it proved even more useful than for occupational purposes in the strict sense).

At the same time in the statistical and demographic domain, the National Institute of Statistics (ISTAT), favourably impressed by the model of the British Longitudinal Study, introduced a pilot study based on record linkage as a six-month mortality follow-up of the 1981 census (2). This study showed an unsatisfactory level of completeness owing to the limited co-operation by the municipalities, which own record linkage keys.

Within such a scanty framework of the knowledge and skills involved in the investigation of health inequalities, in 1991 the Health Department and the Piedmont Region started a national research programme intended to test possible procedures using record linkage techniques for monitoring socioeconomic and occupational inequalities in health in Italy. The programme achieved two main results. First, it demonstrated that it is possible to study health inequalities in Italy through record linkage between health information systems (mortality at the national level and morbidity at the local level) and administrative sources containing socioeconomic information (population census, income registers, pension fund archives, work accidents database). Secondly, it resulted in the creation of a network of researchers, epidemiologists and statisticians, as well as health and research institutions at both the national and local level, which pooled their resources to modify the structure and the operational functioning of information systems for inequality monitoring purposes. As a direct outcome of these efforts, the first Italian report on health inequalities was published, following a national conference organized by the Smith Kline Foundation and co-promoted by the National Department of Social Affairs and ISTAT (19).

Four recommendations offered by the report have led to significant advances in research (see Box 15.1 for details).

Two new programmes have been funded by the National Health Department, aimed at accomplishing the objectives of the 1998–2000 National Health Plan (20). The first is to write a second report on the status of health inequalities at the end of the 1990s and to develop new models for monitoring and explaining inequalities on a cross-sectional and geographical basis, as well as a longitudinal and individual one. The second aims to evaluate the role of healthcare and health system organization in generating inequality. The two projects involve six research units from the National Health Service and four from the universities with a total funding of about 1,100,000 euros.

Furthermore, inequalities have begun to be analysed within the framework of several important epidemiological studies planned for different purposes. A special issue of the Italian epidemiological journal *Epidemiologia e Prevenzione* was dedicated to this topic in 1999 (21) and the 2000 annual conference of the Italian Epidemiological Association once again concentrated on health inequalities.

Box 15.1 The first Italian report on inequalities in health (1994): recommendations and consequences

Recommendations	Consequences
1. *Research*	
• from descriptive to explanatory research, looking at every critical point for inequality across life courses	• two new regional (1999–2001) and national (2000–2) programmes for research and monitoring (based on administrative data)
• advocacy role of medical research on the issue of health inequalities	
2. *Policies*	
• including a measure of health inequalities in the algorithm for financing local health authorities	
• mitigating the potentially iniquitous impact of rationing healthcare (tickets, new technology, market competition)	• a new instrument ('sanitometro') to measure wealth and allow the poor to be exempted from paying for healthcare
• high priority towards most disadvantaged (the handicapped, immigrants, etc.)	• 1997 social security reform: differentiating retirement age according to occupational inequalities in life expectancy
	• 1998–2000 National Health Strategy: tackling health inequalities as a key issue in every national health priority and particular attention to disadvantaged groups
	• 1999 healthcare regulation for immigrants: full and free access to emergency and essential care for illegal poor immigrants
	• 2000–2 National Programme for the development of health and healthcare in more deprived metropolitan areas
	• sporadic experiences following action zone model (Emilia Romagna, Turin)

3. *Monitoring inequalities in health*

- aggregate (census tract) measures of deprivation for local and national studies
- record-linkage studies (longitudinal at local level, cross-sectional at national level)
- simple (as opposed to composite) covariate to describe differences

- aggregate deprivation analyses at local (census tract) and national (municipality) level
- new record linkage studies: 1991–2 Italian cross-sectional; Turin, Florence and Leghorn longitudinal

4. *Health professional training and health education*
inducing people and institutions at local level to:

- identify inequalities and
- ask for interventions

- no systematic initiative in training and education

Overall, the recommendations of the first Italian report on health inequalities had little impact on social and economic research, with the exception of the field of demographic research and among the researchers who helped create the document. None the less, the Italian National Council of Research did decide to participate in the ongoing interdisciplinary research programme of the European Science Foundation on Social Variations in Health Expectancy in Europe, and this is an encouraging sign.

Policies

Socioeconomic inequality in health has never been a key issue in Italy. At first glance this is no surprise, as the geographical distribution of health in this country is in indirect relation to the indicators of wealth and healthcare supply: southern regions that are poorer in resources and services have always had lower mortality rates than the richer northern regions. As a consequence, before 1990 there was no policy explicitly addressing the issue of health inequalities.

The health reform of 1978 (Law 23/12/78 n. 833), which reorganized healthcare from an insurance model to a national system, was based on the principle of promoting equality in the distribution of health and healthcare services, although mostly this meant a homogeneous geographical distribution of the healthcare supply. There has been no formal evaluation of its effects, but some clues can be derived from trends in avoidable mortality. Between 1980/5 and 1986/90, rates for most avoidable deaths decreased; the decline in both sexes (27 per cent) was higher than that for overall mortality in the corresponding years (12 per cent). The regions with higher avoidable mortality were in the south in both periods, but the gap between that and the north tended to decrease (22).

In the 1990s, following the first evidence about health inequalities, political initiatives were taken in both the health and non-health sectors, including policies for information systems (see Box 15.1).

Health policies

The most significant health interventions were the National Health Plan, the 'sanitometro' (a meter for access to healthcare) and the programme for metropolitan areas.

The 1999–2000 National Health Plan (20) marked the first time that the Italian government and parliament had ever established a national strategy for health based on an agreement among the different players involved in reaching health objectives. Reducing health inequalities is one of the nine qualifying points of this strategy. In particular, the plan explicitly states that one important way to reach each specific target (cancers, cardiovascular diseases, accidents, etc.) is to improve the health of disadvantaged groups, reducing the differences relative to healthier ones. The Health Department is trying to disseminate information concerning actions for reducing inequalities at every level of regional and local planning, but penetration of this issue in the medical community is still quite moderate and there has been no significant attempt at professional communication or education. The development of local screening programmes for breast and cervical cancers is the only action that has appeared effective in reducing health inequalities (23), despite not having been aimed explicitly at this, contrasting the previous tendency of a major access to early diagnosis by more educated women (8).

The emphasis on equality in the National Health Plan has also influenced two other national initiatives. The first is the 'sanitometro' ('healthcare meter'), which offers a method of measuring individuals' economic means in order to establish who is exempt and who should pay for healthcare, so as to guarantee free access to all services for the more disadvantaged. Trials will be made to evaluate problems or undesirable effects, such as stigmatization, in the application of the 'sanitometro'.

The second initiative is the special programme in metropolitan areas, which will offer €750 million between 1999 and 2001 for the restyling of healthcare supply in big cities (Law 23/12/98 n. 448; art. 71). These areas have a high rate of new health problems (for example, immigrants, single parents, lone elderly, addicts, etc.) as well as problems of inadequate health structures and difficult access to healthcare. Combating the causes of health inequalities is a key factor in the ongoing evaluation of the grant proposals submitted. For the first time the criteria for the acceptance and financing of programmes include the presence of an appropriate evaluation protocol.

Policies regarding foreign immigrants lie half-way between the health and the social sectors. In 1998 a national strategy on immigration was approved (DL 25/7/98 n. 286). This was founded on the principles of equality in access to services, the defence and appreciation of individual differences, and the inclusion of immigrants in the targets of policies for professional education, housing and healthcare. Based on these principles, a 1999 law (DPR 31/8/99 n. 394) regulated the procedures of enrolment to the national health service for legal immigrants. Moreover, it has made it possible for illegal immigrants to access preventive services and emergency healthcare (with the opportunity for long-term care). Access is free for the self-reported poor and does not imply compulsory notification of identity to the police.

Non-health policies

In sectors other than health we cannot document policies explicitly aimed at reducing health inequalities. Some general policies, such as those on employment or income support, or specific ones such as those on housing, education and the environment, may be beneficial but are not designed to have an impact on health. Following the action zone model, some instances of the inclusion of health outcomes in local policies are being implemented in Turin and Emilia Romagna.

The only significant example of a change in social policy in response to data on health inequalities has been the reform on pensions (Law 8/8/95 n. 335). At the beginning of the 1990s, owing to a financial crisis, Italy initiated a social security reform centred on extending working life and postponing the retirement age. This proposal assumed that life expectancy was uniform across the population, but trade unions called general attention to data on occupational inequalities in life expectancy that showed disadvantages for blue-collar workers (24). This led to a one-year reduction in the retirement age for manual workers (Law 27/12/97 n. 449), and the government is currently identifying a list of 'particularly wearing jobs' that will benefit from a further reduction. The impact on health of this policy cannot be determined. However, unfavourable signs seem to come from the Turin Longitudinal Study (17), where retirement in men belonging to the working class or to the middle classes appears to be associated with excess mortality of 60 per cent and 90 per cent, respectively, compared to those who continue to work in the same classes and independently of their health status before retirement.

As far as information systems are concerned, the development of deprivation indexes was one of the first consequences of the recommendations (see Box 15.1) to study inequalities at municipality level for national data and at a lower level (census tract) for local data (1, 25). However, the suggestion of collecting routine health data on the census (for example, mortality, birth origin, hospital admission, etc.) is meeting with difficulty from the national statistical system. Second, within the National Statistical Plan a number of studies based on record linkage have been designed; concurrently, the health interview surveys (1994 and 1999–2000) have been improved in their ability to measure the social characteristics of people and families by analysing lifestyles, reported morbidity and self-perceived health.

It is impossible to evaluate empirically to what extent these political initiatives were affected by the results of research on health inequalities. In the case of social security reform the relationship was manifest: the data on occupational health inequalities were used effectively by unionists to impose the idea of differentiating pension schemes. In the case of health policies, financial constraints leading to rationing choices coincided with a reforming government that was open to evidence-based planning. At the same time, a number of health, social science and economics professionals involved in the field of health inequalities were called on to interpret these requirements, thereby suggesting that research was a good stimulus for the penetration of equality objectives.

Nevertheless, health inequalities have so far caused little public comment. On the one hand this is because it is difficult to transform anti-news such as 'the poor are worse off than the rich' into a communicable piece of information; on the other hand, it is because health inequalities risk being perceived as an issue of one political side, rather than a collective responsibility, particularly among health professionals.

Possible lessons to be learned

In the action spectrum on health inequalities (26) Italy has moved quite rapidly from not measuring health inequalities at all (through the late 1980s) to showing a significant commitment to health inequalities in the National Health Plan, and implementing strong national programmes of monitoring and research involving several centres (that is, half-way between 'will to take action' and 'isolated initiatives'). This appears to be a preamble for more structured developments, such as the newest policies concerning healthcare for immigrants and on reductions in the retirement age.

The main drawbacks are that these processes have not yet stabilized and the results cannot yet be proved, either in the ongoing process or in their impact. Moreover, the dissemination of information, the perception of the importance of health inequalities and of the possibility of reducing them have remained elitist and probably factious; this could endanger the success of processes whenever, as at present, the political balance in the country is in flux. Also, from the point of view of scientific research, the results obtained are still insufficient to ensure a significant development of investigation into causes and evaluation. The main reasons for delay are related to the lack of collaboration between different fields of research (epidemiology, social science, demography and economics), also reflected in the division of research funding; and the lack of common information sources (particularly longitudinal studies) that give rise to combined research initiatives.

What can we learn from this scenario to promote equality in health? Explicit information campaigns need to be designed to bring this issue and potential solutions to public attention. Communication within the medical community should be prioritized, as its advocacy role may be the key for lending authority to the issue. The creation of a network of experts has successfully led to specific policies based on their results; promoting greater integration and cooperation between various research fields should thus be a priority. As new sources of data for analytical research are developed, renewed attention and effort in the area of health inequalities are likely to follow.

References

1. Cadum E, Costa G, Biggeri A, Martuzzi M. Deprivation and mortality: a deprivation index suitable for geographical analysis of inequalities [Italian]. *Epidemiol Prev* 1999: 23: 175–87.
2. ISTAT. *La mortalità differenziale secondo alcuni fattori socioeconomici 1981–2* (Differential Mortality by Socioeconomic Factors). Note e Relazioni No. 2. Roma: ISTAT, 1990.
3. ISTAT. *La seconda indagine sulla mortalità differenziale secondo alcuni fattori socioeconomici.* Anni 1991–2. (The Second Survey on Differential Mortality by Socioeconomic Factors. Years 1991–2.) Collana Informazioni. Roma: ISTAT (in press).
4. Faggiano F, Versino E, Lemma P. Decennial trends of social differentials in smoking habits in Italy. Cancer Causes Control 2001: 12: 665–71.
5. Cardano M, Costa G, Demaria M, Merler E, Biggeri A. Inequalities in mortality in the Italian longitudinal studies [Italian]. *Epidemiol Prev* 1999: 23: 141–52.
6. Kunst AE, Groenhof F, Andersen O *et al.* Occupational class and ischemic heart disease mortality in the United States and 11 European countries. *Am J Public Health* 1999: 89: 47–53.
7. Faggiano F, Partanen T, Kogevinas M, Boffetta P. Socioeconomic differences in cancer incidence and mortality. *IARC Sci Publ* 1997: 138: 65–176.
8. Vannoni F, Burgio A, Quattrociocchi L, Costa G, Faggiano F. Social differences and indicators of perceived health, chronic diseases disability and lifestyle in the 1994 ISTAT national health interview survey [Italian]. *Epidemiol Prev* 1999: 23: 215–29.
9. Faggiano F, Crialesi R, Costa G, Buratta V. Trends in social distribution of smoking habits in Italy. In: Abstracts. 9th World Conference on Tobacco and Health. Paris: 10 14 October 1994.
10. Angelillo IF, Anfosso R, Nobile CG, Pavia M. Prevalence of dental caries in schoolchildren in Italy. *Eur J Epidemiol* 1998: 14: 351–7.
11. Faggiano F, Zanetti R, Rosso S, Costa G. Social differences in cancer incidence, fatality and mortality in Turin [Italian]. *Epidemiol Prev* 1999: 23: 294–9.
12. Rapiti E, Perucci CA, Agabiti N *et al.* Socioeconomic inequalities in healthcare efficacy. Three examples in Lazio Region [Italian]. *Epidemiol Prev* 1999: 23: 153–60.
13. Materia E, Spadea T, Rossi L, Cesaroni G, Arcà M, Perucci CA. Healthcare inequalities: hospitalization and socioeconomic position in Rome [Italian]. *Epidemiol Prev* 1999: 23: 197–206.
14. Ciccone G, Lorenzoni L, Ivaldi C, Ciccarelli E, Piobbici M, Arione R. Social class, mode of admission, severity of illness and hospital mortality: an analysis

with 'All Patient Refined – DRGs' of discharges from the Molinette hospital in Turin [Italian]. *Epidemiol Prev* 1999: 23: 188–96.

15. Marceca M. *La salute degli stranieri* (The Health of Foreigners). In: Ministero della Sanità. Relazione sullo stato di salute della popolazione, 2000. Rome: Ministero della Sanità, 2000.

16. Berlinguer G. *Malaria urbana* (Urban Malaria). Milan: Feltrinelli, 1976.

17. Costa G, Demaria M. Un sistema longitudinale di sorveglianza della mortalità secondo le caratteristiche socioeconomiche, come rilevate ai censimenti di popolazione: descrizione e documentazione del sistema (A longitudinal surveillance system of mortality by socioeconomic characteristics as recorded at population censuses: description and documentation of the system). *Epidemiol Prev* 1988: 36: 37–47.

18. Costa G, Segnan N. Unemployment and mortality. *Br Med J* 1987: 294: 1550–1.

19. Costa G, Faggiano F, eds. *L'equità nella salute in Italia. Rapporto sulle diseguaglianze sociali in sanità* (Equity in Health in Italy. Report on Social Inequalities in Health). Milan: Fondazione Smith Kline, Franco Angeli, 1994.

20. Ministero della Sanità. *Piano Sanitario Nazionale 1998–2000. Un patto di solidarietà per la salute* (National Health Plan 1998–2000. A Solidarity Agreement for Health). Rome: Ministero della Sanità, 1998.

21. Costa G, Perucci CA, Dirindin N. Health inequalities and the national health strategy [Italian]. *Epidemiol Prev* 1999: 23: 133–40.

22. Barchielli A, Salomoni A. 'Avoidable mortality' in the Italian regions, 1980–90 [Italian]. *Epidemiol Prev* 1996: 20: 318–27.

23. Segnan N. Socioeconomic status and cancer screening. *IARC Sci Publ* 1997: 138: 369–76.

24. Costa G, Faggiano F, Lagorio S. *Mortalità per professioni in Italia negli anni '80* (Occupational Mortality in Italy in the Eighties). Rome: ISPESL (Collana quaderni Ispesl 2), 1995.

25. Michelozzi P, Perucci CA, Forastiere F, Fusco D, Ancona C, Dell'Orco V. Inequality in health: socioeconomic differentials in mortality in Rome, 1990–5. *J Epidemiol Commun Health* 1999: 53: 687–93.

26. Whitehead M. Diffusion of ideas on social inequalities in health: a European perspective. *Milbank Q* 1998: 76: 469–92.

16 Lithuania

Vilius Grabauskas and Zilvinas Padaiga

Introduction

Lithuania is a small country on the Baltic coast with a population of 3.7 million, of whom 81 per cent are of Lithuanian descent, 8 per cent Russian, 7 per cent Polish and 3 per cent other. Lithuania became independent from the former Soviet Union in 1990. Rapid economic change, with the transition from a planned towards a market economy, has severely affected all sectors of society, including the research community. Since independence there have been frequent changes of government (ten in ten years).

The socioeconomic situation

The economy of Lithuania is based on industry, which produces nearly 25 per cent of gross domestic product (GDP), supported by agriculture, construction and services. In 1990 GDP decreased significantly but started to recover in 1994. In 1997 real gross domestic product, adjusted for purchasing power parity, was €4,627 per capita. According to the labour force survey, unemployment in 1998 was 13.5 per cent (people are considered unemployed when they are within the working age limits, are not registered as a full-time student, and are registered at the Labour Exchange by place of residence, being ready for professional training or retraining or actively seeking employment).

Mandatory social insurance encompasses the largest proportion of the social security system. In 1998, total social insurance expenditure (without health insurance) was more than €1 billion (8.4 per cent of GDP). Pensions insurance made up the greatest proportion of this. The main source of income for social insurance is mandatory contributions from workers and their employers, which constitutes more than 96 per cent of social insurance revenues. The system is therefore extremely dependent on the number of workers and their wages. For many reasons, social insurance expenditure exceeded revenues in 1998 and 1999, and the budget deficit of the State Social Insurance Fund continued to grow (1).

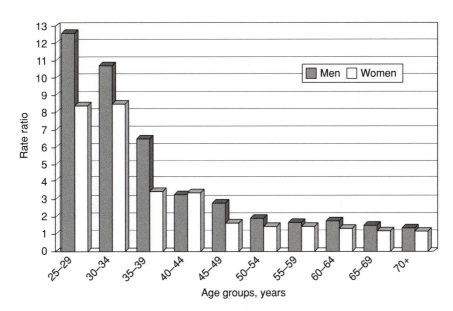

Figure 16.1 Comparison of age-specific mortality between population groups with university and primary education (Lithuania) (mortality of university education group equals 1)

Source: Equity in Health and Healthcare in Lithuania. A situation analysis, p. 32 (2)

The extent of socioeconomic inequalities in health

The extent of socioeconomic inequalities in health in Lithuania varies depending on the health and socioeconomic indicators selected. Data from the mortality register indicate that education, socioeconomic group and marital status were significant predictors of health inequality. A higher level of education, higher income and an urban place of residence were strongly positively related with self-reported health status and health behaviour, especially for smoking and alcohol abuse for men, and for more healthy nutrition. Large inequalities in neonatal health by the mother's level of education and marital status were discovered, with maternal smoking, alcohol and drug abuse accounting for a large proportion of the observed differences. Finally, socioeconomic inequalities were found for healthcare accessibility, lower socioeconomic status predicting worse access to services (2–4).

According to the data from the national mortality register, the Lithuanian population experiences large mortality inequalities by different educational groups, especially when comparing between university and primary education (Figure 16.1). In both men and women the largest mortality differences were observed for the 25–35-year age group. The differences

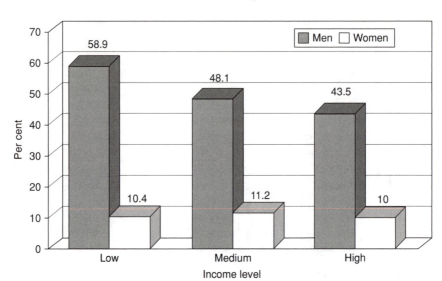

Figure 16.2 Proportion of daily smokers by family income (Lithuania)

Source: Health Behaviour among Lithuanian Adult Population, 1996 (5); National Public Health Institute, Helsinki, 1998 (6)

observed are rather high; however, numbers of deaths are substantial and the mortality register has been validated (4).

To a large extent inequalities in mortality might be explained by inequalities in health behaviour. Up to 50 per cent of all-cause mortality in Lithuania can be attributed to alcohol abuse and smoking, with a smaller proportion contributed by traffic accidents. According to Health Behaviour Monitoring among Adult Population surveys in Lithuania (5, 6), an urban place of residence, a higher level of education and income correlated with a better health behaviour profile. Despite nearly 70 per cent of all expenditure being on food, lower-income groups had a higher prevalence of smoking (Figure 16.2), thereby further reducing the amount they could spend on education, health or housing (2).

Research

The research institutions had to share a greatly reduced budget and are urgently trying to raise money from international grants and searching for possibilities to start projects with Western institutions. However, the limited capacity for high-level research and fund-raising led to protracted financial difficulties and a subsequent 'brain drain', lowering the prestige of research and reducing career possibilities. Research potential inherited from the past had to be evaluated and firm decisions as to its reduction or transformation be made without delay, in order to maintain centres of excellence with technologies and personnel of international standards. However, many research institutions had a fixed annual budget and the possibility of competing for only a small national research grant. Although it faced the same problems, the public health research sector, owing to its international cooperation with the World Health Organization (WHO)-led projects, maintained its capacity. From the year of independence in 1990, public health researchers were the driving force in the formulation of a national health policy and healthcare reform, backing it up with research results.

Prior to the 1990s researchers had demonstrated socioeconomic inequalities in health in Lithuania, which is a relatively homogeneous country. However, it was only through the stimulating role of WHO that a systematic research effort into health inequalities began in 1997. Under the auspices of this collaboration, Lithuania joined the Health Inequalities project. The data from the National Health Information Centre, the Ministries of Education, Health, Social Welfare and Labour, combined with the datasets from a number of research projects – Countrywide Integrated Noncommunicable Disease Intervention Programme (CINDI), Health Behaviour Monitoring among the Adult Population (within the Finnish–Baltic Health Monitoring Programme), Health Behaviour Monitoring in Schoolchildren, National Household Survey, Newborn Register, Accessibility of Healthcare Project – constituted the database for this project.

Current national health research priorities formulated by the Ministry of Health focus on the areas of maternal and child health, healthcare reform management, environmental health and health policy development. Research on health inequalities in Lithuania is not defined as a priority, but is strongly advocated within health policy development. The Health Inequalities programme has created eleven research projects, the majority of finance for which comes from national sources, whereas some projects (for example, health behaviour monitoring in adults and schoolchildren, MONICA, CINDI) are partially supported by international research grants.

As mentioned earlier, a substantial amount of information on health inequalities was collected before 1990, that is the regaining of independence. For instance, the WHO Kaunas–Rotterdam Intervention Study, carried out in 1971–2, demonstrated large inequalities in self-reported health by level of education in middle-aged men (7), and mortality of middle-aged men by educational level of their spouses (8).

During the past 5 years, two Ph.D. theses (9, 10) and one habilitation thesis (11) dealing with health inequalities have been defended, and over 30 national and international papers have been published. One Ph.D. thesis analysing inequalities in neonatal health is in progress. Numerous Ph.D. research plans include parts aimed at measuring socioeconomic inequalities in health and healthcare.

On the basis of a combined analysis by Kaunas University of Medicine, in collaboration with and funded by the European Bureau of the World Health Organization and the Swedish International Development Agency, the report *Equity in Health and Healthcare in Lithuania: A Situation Analysis* was published (2).

Policies

The research activities and major steps in policy addressing health inequalities in Lithuania are summarized in Box 16.1.

Research data on health inequalities accumulated through WHO coordinated projects prior to 1990 have been used extensively in health policy formulation and implementation since independence.

The Lithuanian Health Programme (12), adopted by parliament in July 1998, set three major objectives aiming to reduce mortality and increase average life expectancy, equality in health and healthcare, and quality of life. The programme contains a separate target on equality which states that 'By the year 2010 differences in health and healthcare between various socioeconomic population groups should be reduced by 25 per cent.' The first step in the strategy to achieve this is defined as follows: 'By the year 2000 inequalities in health and healthcare between different socioeconomic groups should be assessed and indicators for monitoring proposed.' Further on, the problems of health inequalities have to be revised as stated: 'By the year 2005, to supplement health policy by measures aimed at the reduction of inequalities in health and healthcare'. The strategy includes intersectoral collaboration and systematic evaluation of the impact of all legal Acts on health inequalities. The National Board of Health is responsible for monitoring progress in this area. Following the adoption of the Health Programme the National Board of Health prepared its first annual report, in which it undertook to bring health inequalities and actions to the attention of parliament in December 1998 (13). The report was distributed, presented and discussed on several occasions at international, national, regional and municipal levels. Following the presentation of the report, parliament adopted a resolution requesting that action should focus on ensuring equal rights of access to health for all (by decreasing health differences among the rural and urban populations, and populations with different education, income level and age groups) by active cooperation of the state, local self-government institutions and non-governmental organizations. In 1999 the Health Minister issued an order certifying the programme for competence assessment by heads of healthcare institutions involving socioeconomic health inequalities among other major topics.

Referring to the schematic approach proposed by Whitehead (14) for action on health inequalities on a national level, the activities in Lithuania have passed the phases of measurement, recognition and awareness-raising, and are approaching the phase of action. In spite of being high on the list at the national level, policies regarding health inequalities have not yet been translated into concrete action. Formally, politicians still have time, as the National Health Programme requests, to formulate measures aimed at reducing health inequalities by the year 2005.

Box 16.1 Research activities and health policy formulation addressing health inequalities in Lithuania during 1970–2000

Time period	Activities undertaken
1970–90	• Research on health inequalities available, but inequalities not considered a problem
1990–6	• Increasing amount of data on health inequalities; re-analysis of ongoing projects and initiation of new projects
1996–8	• Preparation of Lithuanian Health Programme, including a section on equity, accessibility, acceptability and appropriateness
1997	• World Health Organization/Swedish International Development Agency project 'Health Inequalities' initiated
1998	• Lithuanian Health Programme, which includes specific objectives and targets on equality in health and healthcare, adopted by parliament
	• World Health Organization/Swedish International Development Agency project published: *Equity in health and healthcare in Lithuania. A situation analysis*
	• First annual report of the National Board of Health tackling health inequalities published and presented to parliament
1999	• Parliament resolution on the principles of health policy; equal access to healthcare and reduction of health differences between social groups
	• First Health Policy Forum focusing on reducing health inequalities by joint intersectoral action taking cardiovascular health as an example. Low participation of partners for intersectoral action
	• Project of the National Board of Health to present report to regional and municipal administrations fails owing to severe economic recession. Negotiations with potential donors in order to renew activities
2000	• During his Annual Address to the Parliament (Vilnius, April 2000), the President of the Republic of Lithuania stated that 'It is time to raise awareness that health problems due to difficult living conditions are increasing. Therefore, healthcare reform should be in line with social policy. Special attention should be paid to the most vulnerable layers of society' (http://www.president.lt/).

Possible lessons to be learned

Successes

The major success in Lithuania was the identification of a solid database on inequalities in health and healthcare and the publication of the first report on such inequalities without the need for a specifically designed research project. The ongoing projects provide an opportunity to monitor regional and socioeconomic inequalities at the national level. Additional indicators which are essential for monitoring health inequalities (including the accessibility of healthcare) might be collected through targeted surveys.

Another success was the quick translation of national research data into health policy formulation. These approaches might be recommended for other countries of the former Eastern Bloc, the identification of potential data being the first step. The collection of additional data should be avoided, as it would take extra time and resources and in many instances result in duplication. Collaboration with WHO and other international organizations is essential in exchanging experience, especially for the translation of policy into action.

Failures

The inability to involve all partners in intersectoral cooperation for comprehensive coordinated policy formulation might be considered a failure. Frequent changes of government have not been conducive to the creation of long-standing committees for a more structured development at a national level. Simultaneously, other major problems in healthcare reform (the development of public health legislation and institutional reform, healthcare management and financing, etc.) are considered of higher priority for the current policy-makers.

In order to avoid similar failures, and aiming at a translation of policy into action, stable intersectoral partnerships should be created.

Recommendations and conclusions

Attempts should be made to introduce health inequality issues into the election programmes of the major political parties, and aim at receiving their joint agreement on long-standing and continuous dialogue, irrespective of elections and changes of government.

In order to reduce the research–policy–formulation–action gap, the academic community should increase its efforts to advertise research results, participate further in policy formulation, and be willing to constantly evaluate its implementation. This is closely connected with the development of a critical mass of human resources and capacity, necessary for building a new public health policy, and its implementation at both national and regional level.

Currently, health policy in Lithuania is implemented largely via state health programmes. However, criteria for the preparation, adoption, financing and evaluation of these programmes lack the equality dimension and should be included in formal requirements to monitor progress in health inequalities during programme implementation.

Research into health inequalities should be intensified at a regional and municipal level, aiming to strengthen health information to back up policy formulation and action. Currently, only four administrative regions (out of ten) have formulated a health policy, and health inequalities are not addressed. According to 'Health 21', until the year 2010 Health for All policies should be created and implemented, not only nationally, but at regional and local levels as well. Therefore, intervention from the National Board of Health and the Ministry of Health would be helpful for the inclusion of the equality dimension in this process.

Far more active efforts by the health sector to involve partners from other sectors is required. A first step might be a review of existing and planned programmes of the Ministries of Education, Health, Finance, Social Welfare and Labour, to identify areas of common interest, possible joint action and the potential for additional research, if needed. Following that, interest should be solicited from the stakeholders on their involvement in preparing a joint action plan aimed at reducing health inequalities, which would include a time-scale and quantitative targets. Further, corresponding changes should be made in each sector's policy formulation activities, involving regional and municipal administrations. Similarly, the interests of industry and trade unions, community services, non-governmental organizations and the mass media should also be explored. An assessment of all new and planned programmes within these sectors should be undertaken to evaluate their impact on health inequalities.

International collaboration with countries that have already started co-ordinated intersectoral action aimed at reducing health inequalities should be further strengthened.

References

1. United Nations Development Programme. *Lithuanian Human Development Report – 1999*. Vilnius, 1999: 85–6.
2. WHO, National Board of Health, Kaunas University of Medicine. *Equity in Health and Healthcare in Lithuania. A Situation Analysis*. Copenhagen: WHO, 1998.
3. Kalediene R. *Demographic, social and territorial inequalities in health of Lithuanian population* [Dissertation]. Kaunas: Kaunas University of Medicine, 2000.
4. Kalediene R, Petrauskiene J. Inequalities in life expectancy in Lithuania by level of education. *Scand J Public Health* 2000: 28: 4–9.
5. Grabauskas V, Klumbiene J, Petkeviciene J, Dregval L, Nedzelskiene I, Prättälä R *et al. Health Behaviour among Lithuanian Adult Population, Spring 1996*. Kaunas

Medical Academy, Lithuania and National Public Health Institute, Finland. Helsinki: 1998.

6. Grabauskas V, Klumbiene J, Petkeviciene J, Dregval L, Saferis V, Prättälä R et al. *Health Behaviour among Lithuanian Adult Population*, 1998. National Public Health Institute, Finland. Helsinki: 1999.

7. Appels A, Bosma H, Grabauskas V, Gostautas A, Sturmans F. Self-rated health and mortality in a Lithuanian and a Dutch population. *Soc Sci Med* 1996: 42(5): 681–9.

8. Bosma H, Appels A, Sturmans F, Grabauskas V, Gostautas A. Educational level of spouses and risk of mortality: the WHO Kaunas–Rotterdam Intervention Study (KRIS). *Int J Epidemiol* 1995: 24(1): 119–26.

9. Bankauskaite V. *Health inequities and their causes within two administrative regions* [Ph.D. thesis]. Kaunas: Kaunas University of Medicine, 1999.

10. Jankauskiene D. *Evaluation of healthcare reform in Lithuania during 1990–8* [Ph.D. thesis]. Kaunas: Kaunas University of Medicine, 2000.

11. Kalediene R. Demographic, social and territorial inequalities in health of Lithuanian population [Habilitation thesis]. Kaunas: Kaunas University of Medicine, 2000.

12. Ministry of Health. *Lithuanian Health Program, 1997–2010*. Vilnius: 1998.

13. National Board of Health. *Nacionalines sveikatos tarybos metinis pranesimas* (Annual Report of the National Board of Health, 1998). Vilnius, 1998.

14. Whitehead M. Diffusion of ideas on social inequalities in health: a European perspective. *Milbank Q* 1998: 76: 469–92.

17 The Netherlands

Karien Stronks

Introduction

In The Netherlands, interest in socioeconomic inequalities in health has grown enormously over a relatively short period. Two national research programmes on socioeconomic inequalities in health, the first focusing on explanation and the second on interventions, illustrate the fact that Dutch policy-makers and researchers have made a systematic effort to come to grips with this issue.

The socioeconomic situation

For a small country with a small population, The Netherlands has a powerful economy. Its gross domestic product (GDP), for example, is the 14th-highest in the world. High economic growth has gone hand in hand with a significant rise in the number of employed people. This is generally considered to be a success of the so-called Dutch 'poldermodel', referring to the economic order characterized by a high degree of cooperation and consensus between government, employers and trade unions. For example, with the support of the employers and unions, since 1983 the government has cut public spending as a share of GDP from 60 to 50 per cent. The unemployment rate now equals approximately 5 per cent.

The Netherlands has an extensive social welfare system. Approximately 10 per cent of the working population is dependent on social security benefits because of chronic illness. In The Netherlands, a person is eligible for long-term disability benefit if he is unfit to do his job after a waiting period of 52 weeks. The amount of benefit is usually about 80 per cent of the person's last wage. Supplemental to the provision of benefits, a specific poverty policy is pursued in The Netherlands, primarily at the municipal level. The core of the education policy is the emphasis on equality in access to (higher) education.

Almost 100 per cent of the population is insured for healthcare costs. People with an income below a certain level (some 60 per cent of the population) are compulsorily insured with the Health Insurance Fund, and almost

Table 17.1 Prevalence of self-reported health problems in The Netherlands by educational level, 16 years and older, Central Bureau of Statistics Health Interview Survey, 1995, adjusted for age and sex

Health indicator	Educational level (1 = highest, 4 = lowest)				
	1	*2*	*3*	*4*	*Total*
Per cent of people reporting a chronic condition	36	38	38	43	39
Per cent of people with less-than- 'good' self-perceived health	15	19	22	32	22
Average number of minor health complaints	3.0	3.3	3.8	4.6	3.6
Per cent of people with a physical disability	7	12	14	23	14

Source: Van de Water *et al*. 1996 (2)

all people above that level are privately insured. For long-term care and nursing (approximately 45 per cent of the healthcare budget), The Netherlands has a compulsory taxation scheme to which everyone makes an income-linked contribution.

The extent of socioeconomic inequalities in health

Despite the extensive social welfare system, and despite the fact that there seem to be no serious financial barriers to healthcare, socioeconomic inequalities in health do exist in The Netherlands. The difference in life expectancy, for example, for men from higher and lower socioeconomic groups equals approximately 3.5 years, and the corresponding difference in healthy life expectancy 12 years (1). Also, the prevalence of morbidity indicators varies between socioeconomic groups. Table 17.1 summarizes some of the descriptive evidence on morbidity differences.

As in many other Western European countries, the prevalence of health problems in The Netherlands varies not only between socioeconomic groups but also, for example, between men and women, between people living in different regions, and between people from different ethnic groups (3). This chapter, however, focuses specifically on inequalities in health associated with socioeconomic status.

Research

First national research programme

Before 1980, socioeconomic inequalities in health were a non-issue in public health research. This has changed since the publication in 1980 of a study on inequalities in health between neighbourhoods in Amsterdam. This showed that inequalities in health were still present, despite the extensive social welfare and healthcare services that had been set up since the Second World War. Until the 1990s, this neighbourhood study was one of the few describing socioeconomic inequalities in health. This has changed radically since the introduction of a 5-year national research programme in 1989, sponsored by the government. The political developments that led to this programme are described in the section on policy developments.

The aim of that (first) research programme (1989–93) was to generate more knowledge about the size and nature of socioeconomic inequalities in health and their determinants (4). It included 40 studies, most of which were small-scale secondary analyses of the available data, and a large follow-up study (the so-called GLOBE study), aimed at unravelling the causes of socioeconomic inequalities in health. The programme also aimed to improve conditions for future research, for instance by developing a standardized operationalization of socioeconomic status, and improving conditions for the application of this measurement instrument in registration systems. Efforts were made to involve a large number of researchers in the programme, not only from the field of epidemiology, but also from (medical) sociology, psychology and as on. An independent committee, consisting of established researchers, a representative from the ministry, and several people familiar with (but not representing) other policy areas, developed and implemented the research programme. The committee was chaired by a senior politician of the Dutch Conservative Party (5). This renewed interest in socioeconomic inequalities in public health research has led to an increase in the number of publications on this issue in international journals, from approximately 60 in 1985–8 to 100 in the 3 years between 1993 and 1996 (6). The results of the programme were made available to a broad public (7) and show socioeconomic inequalities in health for almost all indicators studied (7). As in many other countries, the causation mechanism (that is, effect of socio-economic position on health status) appeared to be more important in the explanation of these inequalities than the selection mechanism (that is, effect of health status on socioeconomic position). Within the causation mechanism, structural factors (living and working conditions, etc.) seem to be as important as behavioural factors (smoking, physical exercise, etc.) (8, 9).

Second national research programme

Following the recommendations of the steering committee, in 1995 a second research programme was launched, steered by an independent committee chaired by a senior politician of the Dutch Christian-Democratic Party. The main aim of this second programme was to generate more knowledge on the *effectiveness* of interventions and policies to reduce socioeconomic inequalities in health. In addition, the earlier longitudinal study on the *explanation* of socioeconomic inequalities in health was continued during the second programme.

The committee steering the second national research programme identified four possible strategies to reduce inequalities in health:

1. improving the socioeconomic position of people in the lower strata;
2. diminishing the effect of health problems on the individual's socioeconomic position;
3. diminishing exposure to health-damaging conditions and behaviours; and
4. offering extra curative healthcare to people in lower socioeconomic groups.

An attempt was made to identify for evaluation possible interventions or policies for each of these strategies. As Box 17.1 shows, the programme finally consisted of 12 evaluation studies, most of which looked at interventions and policies pertaining to strategies 3 and 4. We will briefly describe some examples.

Several studies investigated the effectiveness of workplace interventions. One example involved the introduction of a lifting device and several other improvements for bricklayers. The evaluation showed that the new working method was less physically demanding. As a result of the intervention, absence due to sickness decreased, despite the fact that the level of physical complaints remained the same (10). A review, commissioned by the Programme Committee, of interventions to diminish exposure to physically demanding work indicates that these have been evaluated on a much larger scale than interventions in most other policy areas. Most of the interventions that had been evaluated in this field appeared to be successful in improving the health status of people in lower occupational groups (11).

Several other studies investigated the effectiveness of interventions to promote healthy behaviour. These included a school-based programme intended to prevent children (12–13 years old) starting to smoke, based on a strategy of providing information and teaching social skills to resist peer pressure, and a group statement on not to start smoking as a group (12). After the intervention, the percentage of pupils who had started smoking appeared to be lower in the experimental group than that in the control group, although the difference appeared not to be statistically significant in the long term. There also appeared to be a positive change in the extent of peer pressure experienced by the pupils in the intervention group.

Extra efforts within the healthcare sector might also contribute to a further decrease in socioeconomic inequalities in health. General practice in particular may be a useful setting to promote healthy behaviour and to offer extra care for the chronically ill, for instance, people with diabetes. One of the projects in the research programme focused on the effect of the introduction of a practice nurse on the health status of people in lower socioeconomic groups with a chronic disease, particularly asthma (13). The

Box 17.1 Overview of projects within second research programme in the Netherlands

Improving socioeconomic position in itself
- Process evaluation of an intervention aimed at reducing the number of children living in poverty, by providing a benefit supplement to the household income for children whose health is likely to be damaged by poverty.
- Evaluation of the effect of a strategy of counselling secondary school pupils who are frequently absent because of illness on the level of absence among pupils in lower socioeconomic groups in particular.

Interventions in the workplace
- Study on the effect of self-regulating teams in industrial organizations on the psychosocial health status of the employees, in particular those at lower occupational levels.
- Evaluation of the effect of another type of work organization – specifically job rotation – in a specific occupational group (dustmen) on exposure to physical strain and the health status of the employees involved.
- Evaluation of the effect of a new method of working among a specific occupational group (bricklayers) on exposure to physical strain, perceived health status and absence because of illness.

Promoting healthy behaviour
- Evaluation of the effect of a regional campaign encouraging the use of pre- and periconceptional folic acid supplements, in addition to a mass media campaign, on the use of folic acid among women in lower educational groups in particular.
- Evaluation of the effect of toothbrushing in primary schools on the prevalence of tooth decay among schoolchildren from lower socioeconomic groups.
- Evaluation of a healthy cities/community development project on health determinants among people in deprived neighbourhoods.
- Evaluation of the effect of an anti-smoking intervention among children in secondary schools (see main text)

Providing extra healthcare
- Evaluation of the effect of the introduction of local care networks on the health status of people suffering from psychiatric problems.
- Evaluation of the effect of counselling in general practice on the health status of Turkish people suffering from diabetes.
- Evaluation of the effect of the introduction of a practice nurse in general practice on the health status of people in lower socioeconomic groups with asthma (see main text).

results of that project indicated that the special attention and counselling given by the practice nurse to people with a lower education resulted in better compliance and, as a result, better health.

Most of the studies in the programme finished at the end of 2000. At the beginning of 2001, the steering committee made recommendations as to how to reduce socioeconomic inequalities in health in The Netherlands (14). These were based not only on the knowledge obtained from the programme, but also on knowledge and experience from outside, both national and international. Possible recommendations were discussed with representatives from several policy areas (education, housing, health promotion, healthcare, etc.) during a series of conferences, thereby increasing awareness of possibilities for the reduction of socioeconomic inequalities in health among those involved in these specific policy fields. The outcome of these conferences as well as the underlying papers is included in a handbook for those who are involved in the reduction of socioeconomic inequalities (policy-makers, healthcare workers, etc.) (15).

The 26 recommendations are briefly reviewed in Chapter 2. They cover the four strategies to reduce socioeconomic inequalities in health and focus on the implementation of measures that have been shown to be effective, as well as on further research and development to increase the range of policy options. Examples of measures that were recommended for implementation include specific interventions in the workplace, an anti-smoking intervention among children in secondary schools, and local care networks in deprived neighbourhoods for people suffering from psychiatric problems. The programme committee also recommended the formulation of (quantitative) targets, for example in the field of income inequality ('no increase beyond the level observed in the late 1990s') and in the field of smoking ('reduction by 50 per cent of the difference in smoking rates between upper and lower socioeconomic groups, by differential decrease in smoking rates in the lower socioeconomic groups').

Policies

Policy documents

As mentioned earlier, the renewed interest in the issue of socioeconomic inequalities in health began in 1980, with the publication of the results of a study showing large differences in mortality rates between neighbourhoods in Amsterdam. This study was given political follow-up in 1985, as in that year the Dutch government adopted the WHO Health for All policy targets (see Box 17.2). In 1986, this resulted in the publication of the so-called Health 2000 Report (16) by the Ministry of Welfare, Health and Cultural Affairs, which included a paragraph on inequalities in health. This important policy document was followed by a conference, organized by a prestigious advisory council of the national government, the Scientific Council

Box 17.2 Summary of policy developments in the Netherlands from 1980 to 2000

1985 The Dutch government adopted the WHO Health for All policy targets

1986 Publication of the Health 2000 Report (15) by the Ministry of Welfare, Health and Cultural Affairs, including a paragraph on socioeconomic inequalities in health

1987 National conference on socioeconomic inequalities in health, organized under the aegis of the Scientific Council for Government Policy, resulting in a proposal for a national research programme (1989–93) funded by the Ministry of Welfare, Health and Cultural Affairs

1991 National conference, again organized under the aegis of the Scientific Council for Government Policy, resulting in an agreement among several parties involved to implement activities to reduce inequalities in health

1994 Results of the first national research programme were reported to the Minister of Public Health

1995 Publication of an important policy document by the Ministry of Public Health, Welfare and Sport (*Health and Wellbeing*). Reduction of socioeconomic inequalities in health was mentioned as one of the policy goals. Initiation of second national research programme (1995–2000)

1996 Publication of a second document on *Public Health Status and Forecasts*, by the National Institute of Public Health and Environmental Protection. Socioeconomic inequalities in health were stressed as a major public health problem

2000 Report of the Lemstra committee on the enforcement of public health. The reduction of socioeconomic inequalities was mentioned as an important policy aim.
Growing demand by the Ministry of Public Health and parliament for information on effective interventions to reduce inequalities in health

2001 Results of the second national research programme, and recommendations based on these results, reported to the Minister of Public Health

for Government Policy (17), the outcome of which was a recommendation for the (first) national research programme, described earlier.

The first research programme finished in 1994, and in that same year the results were reported to the minister. In 1995, the reduction of socioeconomic inequalities in health was again mentioned as a major policy goal in an important policy document of the Ministry of Health (*Health and Well-being*). In 1997, the National Institute of Public Health and Environmental Protection published a second document on *Public Health Status and Forecasts*. This was a nationwide effort to review the available scientific data on the health status of the Dutch population. Its intention was to provide a scientific basis for health policy. In that document, socioeconomic inequalities in health were stressed as a major public health problem. Moreover, the report concluded that inequalities in health had not diminished since the 1980s (18). (Also, in the recent report of a national advisory committee on the enforcement of public health (so-called Lemstra Committee, 2000 (19)) the reduction of socioeconomic inequalities was mentioned as an important policy aim. From many sides, the demand for interventions that have been proved to be effective increases (for example, as indicated by the number of questions by the parliament members to the Minister of Public Health), which seems a reflection of a growing willingness to tackle inequalities in health.

Since the second half of the 1990s, the attention paid to the issue of inequalities in health in policy seems to increase not only in the public health area, but also in other policy areas. Examples include the network of parties involved in the 'Major Cities' policy, including the Minister of that department, and the attention paid to the consequences of the future healthcare reforms for the accessibility of care to people from lower socioeconomic groups (17). At the beginning of 2001, the results of the second research programme were reported to the Minister. At the time of writing, the policy response by the Dutch government is not yet known.

Interventions and policies

From this review, it can be concluded that in The Netherlands the process of putting equality in health on the political agenda has been successful. There is a broad consensus that such inequalities are unfair, and that avoidable inequalities should be reduced (18, 20).

To what extent has this (political) awareness and concern been followed by initiatives to reduce socioeconomic inequalities in health? In other words, which interventions and policies have been set up to reduce socioeconomic inequalities in health? The second national research programme, described earlier, is part of the answer to this question, but the interventions and policies evaluated in this programme all had an experimental character. They should, however, be seen within the context of a longer tradition of policies to reduce socioeconomic inequalities generally, and socioeconomic inequalities in health specifically.

Inequalities in income are relatively small in The Netherlands compared to other European countries. As a consequence, those participating in debates on socioeconomic inequalities in health have typically refrained from advocating further reductions in income inequality. An exception should probably be made for the policy debate on poverty. In this debate attention is sometimes drawn to the consequences for health of people living below the poverty line (21). Even without regard to health consequences, however, the Dutch national and local governments have pursued active anti-poverty policies, including income support (for example, supplementary benefits in the case of high medical expenses), measures to reduce recurrent expenses such as rent, costs of electricity and gas, and local taxes (for example, Rent Subsidy Act), and measures to reduce the non-use of services (22).

As mentioned in the introduction, a large proportion of the working population, almost 10 per cent, is entitled to a long-term work disability benefit. In the 1990s, many policy measures were taken to reduce this number by restricting the criteria for entitlement (1993) and, more recently, by measures aimed at the reintegration of people with a disability into the workforce. Whether this kind of measure might have led to a reduction of socioeconomic inequalities in health (through a reduction of the number of people without a paid job) depends of course on whether people with a (chronic) illness are better off in or outside the labour market. Whereas not having a paid job might have negative health consequences, working also involves health risks. Further studies are needed to empirically evaluate the effect of this kind of measure on the size of socioeconomic inequalities in health.

In public health policy, much emphasis is placed on promoting healthy behaviour. Nationwide interventions focus mainly on dietary habits and smoking (23). These initiatives have had at least some success, given, for example, the decrease in the number of smokers since the 1960s. Many people now realize, however, that most of these measures are less effective among people from lower socioeconomic groups. For this reason, there is growing interest in developing health-promoting activities aimed at these groups, particularly at the local level (municipal health services). Examples include community-based interventions and providing personal support to those who want to change their health behaviour (23, 24). The lack of evidence on the effects of these interventions, as well as on determinants of health behaviour in lower socioeconomic groups, however, is striking. Experts in the field seem to agree that we are in great need of further research on both aspects, in order to be able to develop interventions that actually change the behaviour of people in the lower socioeconomic groups. A few evaluation studies were carried out within the second research programme (mentioned earlier), but it is clear that further work needs to be done. This should address not only 'individualistic' determinants of health behaviour, but also more 'structuralist' factors, such as social pressure and price policies.

In regard to health-damaging conditions, risk factors in the work environment seem to contribute most to socioeconomic inequalities in health in The Netherlands (7). Over recent decades, the Dutch government has pursued an active policy to improve physical working conditions, among other things by introducing the Working Conditions Law (1980, revised in 1998). As indicated earlier, many effective interventions to, for example, diminish exposure to physically demanding work, are available, yet not all of them have been implemented nationwide. Therefore, the main challenge to this policy field is a further implementation of effective interventions.

A recent study found no evidence for a substantial contribution of healthcare services to the worse health status in lower socioeconomic groups, because the healthcare system appeared to be equally accessible to both lower and higher socioeconomic groups. Those services for which differences were found – for instance, the well known pattern of higher consumption of general practitioner's care and lower consumption of specialized care was also observed in this study – could not account for socioeconomic inequalities in the prognosis of a disease (25). In recent years, the Dutch government has on several occasions considered financial measures (for example, introduction of patient cost sharing) which could lead to an increase of inequalities in healthcare access. Although some of these measures have indeed been introduced, there has been a lot of opposition, mainly on the grounds of a possible increase in socioeconomic inequalities in health, and many of them have been withdrawn (26).

Possible lessons to be learned

From this review, it might be concluded that the position of The Netherlands within the action spectrum described by Whitehead varies by the government level considered. At the national level, that is, at the level of the Minister of Public Health, there is certainly concern about socioeconomic inequalities in health. Moreover, the will to take action seems to be growing. However, so far only a few initiatives have been aimed explicitly at reducing socioeconomic inequalities in health. In contrast, at the local level many initiatives have been taken, especially in the area of preventive healthcare, which is largely the responsibility of municipal health services.

There seem to be at least three elements in the Dutch approach that have worked well: consensus building, the step-by-step approach, and the fact that the issue of inequalities in health is dealt with separately from other public health issues.

Many authors have already drawn attention to the element of political consensus building, which seems crucial in the Dutch process of putting equality in health on the political agenda (5, 6, 27). The problem was defined in politically neutral terms, and the responsibility for reducing inequalities was shared by all parties concerned. Most of the time the public health argument was used as a rationale for the policy of reducing inequalities in health ('diminishing inequalities will improve the average health status of the population'), instead of the more political argument of 'unfairness'. This process seems to fit perfectly well within the so-called Dutch 'poldermodel', which was mentioned in the introduction. Consensus lies at the heart of this model, and the same is true for the way inequalities in health have been tackled so far. Conversely, this might imply that the strategy of consensus building might not work in other countries, with a different political culture.

Another important feature of the Dutch strategy is the systematic way in which the issue of socioeconomic inequalities in health was studied by two national research programmes. The first programme in particular relied to a large extent on secondary data analyses, which led to an enormous increase in our knowledge in a relatively short period of time. The decision of the Minister to focus the second programme on research into the effectiveness of interventions, was a good stimulus for researchers not only to study the way in which inequalities arise, but also how they can be tackled effectively. It is beyond doubt that this step-by-step approach has contributed to the enormous growth in our knowledge on socioeconomic inequalities in health in a relatively short period of 10 years.

A final characteristic of the Dutch approach relates to the fact that, so far, the issue of socioeconomic inequalities has been dealt with separately from other public health issues, such as the increase in unhealthy habits such as physical inactivity. In the stage of knowledge production, such an approach is likely to have contributed to the enormous growth in awareness of and attention given to this issue. However, as the emphasis shifts towards actually tackling inequalities in health, integrating this problem into current public health policies, such as the anti-smoking policy or the policies to improve working conditions, seems to be necessary. On the other hand, there remains a need to give special attention to the issue of inequalities in health, in order to prevent it from fading away from the political agenda in the near future.

References

1. Water HPA van de, Boshuizen HC, Perenboom RJM. Health expectancy in The Netherlands 1983–90. *Eur J Public Health* 1996: 6: 21–8.
2. Stronks K, Mheen H van de, Mackenbach JP. *Sociaal-economische gezondheidsverschillen* (Socioeconomic Inequalities in Health). Volksgezondheid Toekomst Verkenning. II Gezondheidsverschillen. RIVM Elsevier/De Tijdstroom, 1997.
3. Mackenbach JP. Inequalities in health in The Netherlands according to age, gender, marital status, level of education, degree of urbanisation, and region. *Eur J Public Health* 1993: 3: 112–18.
4. Gunning-Schepers LJ, Spruit IP, Krijnen JH. *Socioeconomic Inequalities in Health. Questions on Trends and Explanations.* The Hague: 1989.
5. Mackenbach JP. Socioeconomic inequalities in health in The Netherlands: impact of a five year research programme. *Br Med J* 1994: 309: 1487–91.
6. Whitehead M. Diffusion of ideas on social inequalities in health: a European perspective. *The Millbank Quarterly* 1998: 76: 469–92.
7. Mackenbach JP. *Ongezonde verschillen* (Unhealthy Inequalities). Assen: Gorcum, 1994.
8. Stronks K, Mheen H van de, Looman CWN, Mackenbach JP. Behavioural and structural factors in the explanation of socioeconomic inequalities in health: an empirical analysis. *Sociol Health Illness* 1996: 18: 653–74.

9. Schrijvers CTM, Stronks K, Mheen H van de, Mackenbach JP. Explaining educational differences in mortality: the role of behavioral and material factors. *AJPH* 1999: 89: 535–40.

10. Bongers P, Luijsterburg P, Miedema M, Heuvel F van den, Vroome E de. *Evaluatie van een nieuwe werkmethode voor de metselploeg: opgehoogd metselen en mechanisch opperen* (Evaluation of a New Working Method for Bricklayers). Hoofddorp: TNO Arbeid, (in preparation).

11. Dijk F van, Kuijer P. Interventies op de werkplek ter vermindering van sociaal-economische gezondheidsverschillen, toegespitst op lichamelijk belasting (Interventions at the workplace to reduce socioeconomic inequalities in health, with a specific focus on physically demanding working conditions). In Stronks K, Hulshof J, (eds). *De kloof verkleinen. Theorie en praktijk van de strijd tegen sociaal-economische gezondheidsverschillen* (Reducing the Gap. Theory and Practice of the Struggle against Socio-economic Inequalities in Health). Assen: Koninklijke Van Gorcum, 2001.

12. Crone MR, Reijneveld SA, Leerdam FJM van. *Preventie van (het beginnen met) roken bij jongeren uit het VMBO* (Prevention of (Starting with) Smoking among Adolescents at Vocational Schools). Leiden: TNO preventie en gezondheid, 2000.

13. Sorgdrager J, Groothoff JW, Matthesius DM, Haan J de, Post D. De praktijkverpleegkundige. Implementatie en evaluatie van een praktijkver-pleegkundige in een sociaal-economisch achterstandsgebied (The Practice-nurse. Implementation and Evaluation of a Practice-nurse in a Socioeconomic Deprived Neigbourhood). *Eindrapport voor de Programmacommissie Sociaal-Economische Gezondheidsverschillen.* (Final report for the programme committee socio-economic inequalities in health). Groningen: Gezondheidswetenschappen, Sociale Geneeskunde 2000.

14. *Programmacommissie Sociaal-Economische Gezondheidsverschillen-tweede fase. Sociaal-economische gezondheidsverschillen verkleinen. Eindrapportage en beleidsaanbevelingen van de Programmacommissie SEGV-II* (Reducing Socio-economic Inequalities in Health. Final Report and Policy Recommendations of the Programme Committee SEIH-II). Den Haag: ZorgOnderzoek Nederland, maart 2001.

15. Stronks K, Hulshof J, (eds). *De kloof verkleinen. Theorie en praktijk van de strijd tegen sociaal-economische gezondheidsverschillen* (Reducing the Gap. Theory and Practice of the Struggle against Socio-economic Inequalities in Health). Assen: Koninklijke Van Gorcum, 2001.

16. Ministry of Public Health. *Nota 2000.* Rijswijk: Ministry of Public Health, 1986.

17. Wetenschappelijke Raad voor het Regeringsbeleid (Scientific Council for Governmental Policy). *De ongelijke verdeling van gezondheid* (The Differential Distribution of Health). Verslag van een conferentie gehouden op 16–17 Maart 1987. Voorstudies en achtergronden V58. Den Haag: SDU, 1987.

18. Mackenbach JP, Verkleij H, eds. *Gezondheidsverschillen* (Inequalities in Health). VolksgezondheidsToekomstVerkenning 1997, deel II. RIVM: Elsevier/De Tijdstroom, 1997.

19. Platform Openbare Gezondheidszorg (Public Health Platform). *Spelen op de winst. Een visie op de openbare gezondheidszorg.* Den Haag: Ministerie van Volksgezondheid, Welzijn en Sport, 2000.

20. Stronks K, Gunning-Schepers LJ. Should equity in health be target number 1? *Eur J Public Health* 1993: 3: 104–111.

21. Stronks K, Mackenbach JP. Tweeledige ongelijkheid in levenskansen: de effecten van armoede op de gezondheid. In: Engbersen G, Vrooman JC, Snel E, eds. *Effecten van armoede*. Amsterdam: AUP, 1998.

22. Stronks K. Income-related policies and their possible impact in inequalities in health in The Netherlands 1993–9. In: Mackenbach JP, Droomers M, eds. *Interventions and policies to reduce socioeconomic inequalities in health. (Proceedings of the Third Workshop of the European Network on Interventions and Policies to Reduce Socioeconomic Inequalities in Health)*. Rotterdam: Department of Public Health, Erasmus University, 1999.

23. Droomers M, Mackenbach JP. Interventions and policies on socioeconomic differences in health-related behaviour in The Netherlands, 1993–8. In: Mackenbach JP, Droomers M, eds. *Interventions and policies to reduce socioeconomic inequalities in health. (Proceedings of the Third Workshop of the European Network on Interventions and Policies to Reduce Socioeconomic Inequalities in Health)*. Rotterdam: Department of Public Health, Erasmus University, 1999.

24. Gepkens A, Gunning-Schepers LJ. Interventions to reduce socioeconomic health differences: a review of the international literature. *Eur J Public Health* 1996: 6: 218–26.

25. Meer JBW van der. Equal care, equal cure? (Dissertation). Rotterdam: Erasmus University Rotterdam, 1998.

26. Foets M, Stronks K, Rijken M, Weide M, Mackenbach J. Armoede en gezondheidszorgbeleid (Poverty and healthcare policy). In: Engbersen G, Vrooman C, Snel E. *Armoede en verzorgingsstaat. Vierde jaarrapport armoede en sociale uitsluiting*. Amsterdam: Amsterdam University Press, 1999.

27. Gunning-Schepers LJ. How to put equity in health on the political agenda? *Health Promotion* 1989: 4: 149–50.

18 Spain

*Joan Benach, Carme Borrell and
Antonio Daponte*

Introduction

Spain is an example of a country that has moved rapidly from having no monitoring of socioeconomic inequalities in health to one which has made limited but remarkable progress in the 1990s to understand socioeconomic inequalities. Regular airing of health inequalities, however, has not been followed by specific national or regional policies or interventions aiming to reduce them. Although a number of social policies are likely to have had an impact on reducing health inequalities, the most crucial policy issue today is to put both research and policy on the government agenda.

The socioeconomic situation

After four decades of a Fascist regime, in 1977 a political transition began in Spain which in 1978 established a democratic constitution. At that point, wealth and social spending were low in comparison to more developed European Union (EU) countries, social services were financed under a social insurance scheme and available only to workers and their dependants (1), and research and policies to tackle socioeconomic inequalities were non-existent. In recent decades, political, economic and social developments have greatly changed the country (2). A decentralization process created 17 autonomous regions with their own political institutions having varying degrees of legislative and executive power, the Spanish economy was linked more strongly into the European and international economies, and stable welfare policies increased social spending, establishing universal access to educational and health services and expanding social security, employment and social protection benefits.

In spite of these remarkable changes, Spain still shows worse socioeconomic indicators than more developed EU countries, and large social and spatial inequalities still persist (3). Today, wealth is less than 80 per cent of the EU average, one in every five households is considered poor, and surveys have consistently estimated at about 20 per cent the number of people living below the poverty line. Income is more unequally distributed than in most EU countries, and regional differences within Spain are large. Since the mid-1980s unemployment has consistently been about twice the EU average and the country still suffers severe unemployment, with high levels of long-term, female and youth unemployment and large regional and local differences (4). Moreover, Spain has the highest percentage of precarious employment within the EU, a new research topic that deserves to be investigated. Although education consistently improved during the 1980s and 1990s, and over the past 15 years the number of illiterate people reduced substantially and those in tertiary education more than doubled, differences in educational opportunities still persist.

The extent of socioeconomic inequalities in health

The majority of studies on socioeconomic inequalities in health have been based on mortality statistics, most research is descriptive, there are very few investigations into trends, and no studies have attempted to investigate the specific reasons for such inequalities (5). Individual-based mortality studies are few, owing to the absence or poor quality of information on socioeconomic characteristics in death certificates. Thus, research has been done in a few cities where it is possible to link local census information with the death register, and in a study conducted in eight provinces where occupation was more consistently available from death certificates. This study has evidenced the higher mortality in males between 30 and 64 years of age among the more disadvantaged social classes for most causes of death, differences which have increased over the period from 1980/2 to 1988/90 (6). There is a greater abundance of ecological studies using provinces, regions or small areas, all finding associations between mortality and socioeconomic level. The analysis of deprivation-related mortality in 2,220 small areas of Spain found the worst deprivation and mortality zones concentrated in southern regions such as Extremadura or Andalusia; these regions have one-fifth of Spain's population and account for one-third of excess deaths due to area deprivation levels. Annual excess mortality in more deprived areas of Spain was estimated at 35,000 deaths (7). Recently, small-area health inequalities have been studied for the top 10 leading causes of death, showing that increasing levels of deprivation are differently associated by both cause and gender (8), with an excess mortality of more than 225,000 deaths for the period 1987–95 (9).

The more deprived social classes present poorer perceived health status, more chronic illness and more health-related behaviours, which are summarized here. It has been found that 40 per cent of those in manual occupations and 27 per cent in professional classes in 1995 reported deficient perceived health status, and these differences increased in the period 1987–95 (10). Inadequate perceived health status increased in the low-income regions in the period 1987–93 (Figure 18.1). Health inequalities in chronic

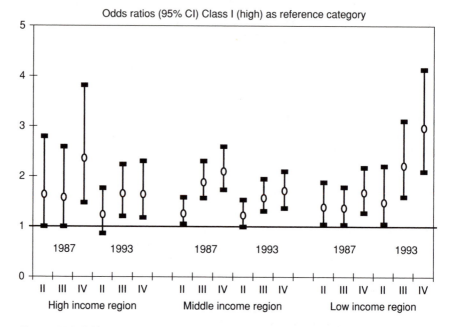

Figure 18.1 Self-perceived poor health in Spain by occupational social class and region by income level in men (National Health Surveys 1987 and 1993)

Source: Navarro *et al.* 1996 (14)

conditions according to educational level have been reported in Spain (11). Regional variations in the prevalence of long-term disability in the poorest people according to income are higher than those of the most affluent individuals (12). Inequality in the risk of obesity, according to educational level and occupational class, has been reported (10, 13, 14) as showing an increase in the past few years. Smoking differences between social classes are not so marked as in northern countries among men, but among women the privileged classes smoke the most (14). In addition, smoking among women has been increasing in recent years (15), fuelled by high social acceptance and low prices. Moreover, inequalities in smoking cessation have increased in males and females in all educational groups (Table 18.1) (16). The percentage of women heavy drinkers is still low, the privileged classes being the heaviest drinkers. In men the opposite occurs: they drink more heavily than women, and it is the disadvantaged classes who do so (14). A recent study has found that between 1987 and 1997 the more deprived population has obtained no benefits, nor has it opted for healthier behavioural choices, whereas the opposite has occurred in the better-off groups (17). Finally, the lack of suitable and timely prevention policies has caused the prevalence of AIDS in Spain to be the highest in Europe.

Table 18.1 Smoking cessation. Age-standardized quit ratios (and 95 per cent confidence intervals) by sex and educational level in Spain, 1987–97. Spanish National Health Interview Surveys, 1987, 1993, 1995 and 1997

	1987 Quit ratio[a] (per cent)	(95 per cent CI)	1993 Quit ratio[a] (per cent)	(95 per cent CI)	1995 Quit ratio[a] (per cent)	(95 per cent CI)	1997 Quit ratio[a] (per cent)	(95 per cent CI)
Males								
Total	26.5	(25.7–27.3)	32.8	(31.3–33.4)	33.1	(31.3–35.0)	34.1	(32.3–36.0)
Level of education								
Less than primary	24.9	(23.2–26.6)	28.9	(25.6–32.2)	27.8	(22.7–32.8)	30.4	(20.8–40.0)
Primary	25.7	(23.3–28.2)	30.7	(29.3–32.1)	29.6	(27.2–32.1)	31.0	(28.7–33.4)
Secondary	26.2	(23.7–28.6)	31.7	(28.6–34.8)	36.9	(31.9–41.9)	36.4	(31.5–41.2)
University	29.1	(26.0–32.2)	37.1	(34.2–40.0)	34.9	(28.8–40.9)	43.7	(37.3–50.2)
Relative Index of Inequality	1.47	(1.22–1.77)	1.58	(1.27–1.96)	1.68	(1.15–2.46)	1.95	(1.31–2.91)
Females								
Total	31.3	(29.0–33.2)	28.5	(26.4–30.7)	25.8	(22.2–29.4)	28.4	(25.0–31.9)
Level of education								
Primary and less than primary	31.0	(29.1–34.0)	27.0	(24.3–29.7)	25.0	(20.4–29.5)	26.7	(22.0–31.4)
Secondary	33.2	(27.0–39.3)	28.6	(23.5–33.7)	26.1	(18.0–34.2)	28.9	(21.5–36.3)
University	32.6	(26.4–38.9)	32.2	(26.8–37.6)	29.5	(19.3–39.6)	31.2	(23.8–38.6)
Relative Index of Inequality	0.78	(0.56–1.05)	1.68	(1.21–2.34)	1.12	(0.64–2.00)	1.68	(0.99–2.87)

Notes:
a Quit ratios and 95 per cent confidence intervals (CI) were computed as the proportion of former smokers who were ever smokers, for males and females separately, and according to educational level, with direct standardization for age, based on the 1991 Spanish population.

Source: Fernández *et al.* (16)

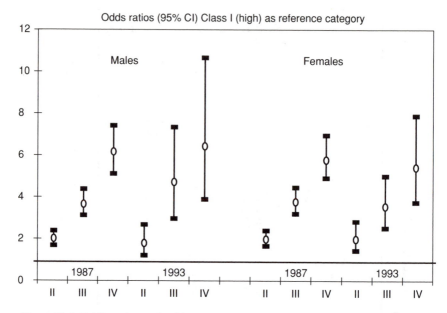

Figure 18.2 Public primary healthcare service use in Spain by occupational social
class and gender (National Health Surveys 1987 and 1993)

Source: Navarro *et al.* 1996 (14)

In regards to access to and utilization of health services, before the
healthcare reform, inequalities in the use of primary healthcare and hospital inpatient services were reported in Spain (18). However, the establishment of a National Health System (NHS) in 1986, with universal coverage,
improved access to services for all social classes. Since then no such inequalities have been found. Nevertheless, inequalities still remain in the use
of those health services provided only partially by the NHS, and when
quality of care is taken into account. Public primary care service use follows
a social class pattern: about 60 per cent of the higher social class use a
public health centre when visiting a doctor, whereas more than 90 per cent
of the working classes use public centres. For example, in both men and
women the probability of attending this type of service in the two weeks
prior to the survey was about six times higher for class IV than for class I
(Figure 18.2). This fact leads to some health inequalities in the type of care
received, such as waiting times at medical offices and to be admitted to
hospital (19, 20), or in preventive practices such as access to dentistry services or breast cancer screening. Although most healthcare needs are covered
by the NHS, adult dental needs are in general not covered. Because of this
situation there is a clear gradient according to class in the use of dental
services (19) that seems to be increasing (14).

Research

Spain exemplifies a country that has moved rapidly from having no monitoring of socioeconomic inequalities in health to one that has a small but active research programme in some centres. Whereas in the 1970s and early and mid-1980s socioeconomic inequalities in health were a non-issue, an increase in the number of studies took place in the late 1980s and remarkable progress has been made since then (Box 18.1). A comprehensive literature

---

Box 18.1 Main research and policy activities undertaken in Spain addressing health inequalities during the period 1970–2001

1970–80	• No research on socioeconomic inequalities in health
	• Health inequalities are a non-issue
1980–7	• Increasing amount of data on health inequalities
	• Initiatives at the legislative level and implementation of a National Health System
1983	• First health survey at the local level (Barcelona)
	• First sociological book on social inequality and disease[a]
1986	• The General Health Service Act establishes a National Health Service with 17 autonomous health services, universal coverage and public financing through taxation
1987	• First health survey at the regional level (Basque Country)
	• First health survey at the national level
	• First intervention to reduce health inequalities (Barcelona city)
1988–96	• Remarkable progress in health inequalities research
	• Quasi-universalization of many healthcare services
	• Macro-level socioeconomic policies have the potential to reduce socioeconomic inequalities
	• Implementation of regional policies on poverty
	• Publication of the 'Spanish Black Report'
1988	• First monographic congress to address health inequalities
1989	• First Spanish adaptation of the British occupational social class[b]
	• First regional social programme to reduce poverty (Basque Country)
1993	• The Spanish Ministry of Health appoints a Commission to study socioeconomic inequalities in health following the model of the Black Report

1994	• First comprehensive book on health inequalities in Spain[c]
1995	• New proposal on occupational social class[d]
1996	• Publication of the 'Spanish Black Report'[e]
1997–2000	• Findings of the 'Spanish Black Report' are not considered, conclusions and recommendations are dismissed
	• There is no administration sponsored research
	• Small research groups regularly document health inequalities
	• Regular airing of health inequalities is not translated into discussion or interventions to reduce health inequalities
1997	• Neither debate nor action follows the publication of the 'Spanish Black Report'
	• A statutory minimum wage is set in Spain
2001	• Health inequalities research and policy are not on the government's agenda

Notes:

a Durán MA. Desigualdad social y enfermedad. (Social inequality and disease). Madrid: Tecnos, 1983.

b Domingo A, Marcos J. Propuesta de un indicador de la clase social basado en la ocupación. (A proposal of an occupation-based social class indicator). Gac Sanit 1989: 3: 320–6.

c Regidor E, Gutierrez-Fisac JL, Rodríguez C. Diferencias y desigualdades en salud en España. (Differences and inequalities in health in Spain). Madrid: Díaz de Santos, 1994 (11).

d Alvarez-Dardet C, Alonso J, Domingo A, Regidor E. Grupo de Trabajo de la Sociedad Española de Epidemiología. La medición de la clase social en Ciencias de la Salud. (The measurement of social class in health sciences). Barcelona: SG Editores, Sociedad Española de Epidemiología, 1995.

e Navarro V, Benach J and the Scientific Commission for the study of health inequalities in Spain. Desigualdades sociales en salud en España (Social Inequalities in health in Spain). Madrid: Ministerio de Sanidad y Consumo, 1996 (14).

search looked for all available investigations on health inequalities for the period 1980–94 (21); the majority of the 233 studies located were empirical, published in the grey literature, and mostly conducted in two regions (Catalonia and Valencia). A clear increase in the number of studies, as well as in their formal publication as articles, was observed from 1988 onward.

In 1993 the Ministry of Health of the Spanish socialist government appointed a scientific commission to study socioeconomic inequalities in health, as well as to make recommendations for improving Spanish health through the implementation of public policies to reduce existing inequalities (22). The final report extensively reviewed class, gender and geographical health inequalities, documenting marked inequalities in mortality, health status, health behaviours and utilization of health services (14). It also showed various examples of social and health policy interventions on health inequalities, and made specific recommendations to tackle them. The report emphasized the urgent need to monitor health inequalities; the development of both social and health data to monitor and study health inequalities; the establishment of a scientific commission to study health inequalities on a permanent basis; and to implement interventions to tackle health inequalities in all social groups, rather than only in the worst-off population. Similarly to the Black Report or the Health Divide in the United Kingdom (UK), the new conservative government did not show much enthusiasm, and the report, finally published in February 1996, was 'buried', its findings were not considered, and the conclusions and recommendations were dismissed. No additional funding was established to support a permanent commission to study socioeconomic inequalities in health, and research came to an end. Currently, government-sponsored research into health inequalities at the national level has ceased. In spite of the progress achieved in recent years, the number of research groups focusing on health inequalities, as well as the public health institutions and funding to support them, are very limited. From a policy perspective there has been little reaction with regard to health interventions and actions.

Policies

Through the 1980s and early 1990s, several macro-level policies, including the reform of the social security system, an increase in public funds for social protection, or the implementation of more progressive taxation policies, are likely to have reduced socioeconomic inequalities (3), with a potential positive impact on health inequalities. Public funds for social security increased, reaching about 22 per cent of gross domestic product (GDP) in 1995. The pensions paid by the social security system, together with illness and unemployment benefits, are the main lines of social protection, accounting for 75 per cent of total social expenditure. The implementation of other national public policies, including the enlargement of protection for the unemployed, or public policies on key sectors such as the extension of mandatory education from 6–14 to 6–16 years, or the universalization of healthcare services, may have had a positive impact on reducing health inequalities as well. In 1986 the General Health Service Act established a National Health System (23) that covered about 99 per cent of the population by 1995. By that year seven regions (covering 62 per cent of the population) had taken over healthcare provision and now all of them have dene so. The principles of the system are universal coverage and free access, public financing, integration of existing health service networks, political devolution of health services to regions, and a new model of primary care with multidisciplinary teams based in health centres throughout the territory and, finally, territorial planning of hospitals and other health centres to provide access (24).

Specific policies on poverty have been implemented in Spain, primarily at the regional level. Between 1989 and 1994 all autonomous regions had implemented social programmes known as 'social salaries', which had as their main goal to alleviate the worst cases of extreme poverty or social exclusion (25). The three main types of programme were: (1) the provision of a minimum income, including financial help and social support; (2) social employment programmes, providing temporary employment; and (3) economic programmes provided by social services. In spite of the many differences across regions, common features of those programmes included the following: the unit of reference was the family (housing benefit) instead of the individual; the main eligibility criterion was to earn less than a specific income level; people entitled to rent subsidy had to have been resident in the region for between one and ten years; the rent subsidy was provided for a specific period of time; and, finally, all income policies were related to the need to make specific actions of reinstatement (under some circumstances people are entitled to get a subsidy if they meet and accept specific requirements). Coverage in each region ranges from 0.3 to 1.2 per cent of the population. In total, social salary policies reached about 75,000 families. Although the programmes achieved some goals and were a first step towards protecting the most deprived, the population covered was relatively small and heterogeneous. Their main limitations include the lack of central coordination, the limited funding, and the difficulty of reaching marginal populations, such as the elderly poor, the homeless, immigrants, drug-users and so on.

Policies or interventions to reduce health inequalities have not been formulated as one of the main goals of the national and regional health strategies (26). This omission is a major concern in regard to the reduction of socioeconomic inequalities in health. However, a number of structural socioeconomic interventions having the potential to reduce such inequalities need to be considered. Social protection encompasses interventions from public or private bodies intended to relieve households and individuals of the burden of a defined set of risks or needs, such as unemployment, healthcare, housing or social exclusion, among others. In Spain the degree of social protection is substantially lower than the EU average, and there are major differences when it comes to relative importance by group of functions. Although the share of social protection devoted to unemployment, old age, healthcare and disability is relatively high, percentages are much lower regarding family/children, housing and social exclusion. In addition, policies on poverty at the regional level, and interventions on health-related behaviours targeting populations living in areas with extreme socioeconomic conditions, have been implemented.

Spain's healthcare system is divided into several regional systems managed by the corresponding regional government, making the establishment and coordination of national health policies very difficult. Examples of this are shown by differences between regions in schedules for the provision of dental care, financing of drugs, and other health-related services. Moreover, the new model of primary care has been only partly implemented (24). Another problem is the lack of an adequate formula for funding healthcare in the regions. The global budget for health is approved annually by the Spanish parliament and then allocated to the regional health authorities. Financing is based mostly on population size in each region, but barely takes into account demography, population density, or morbidity and mortality. Furthermore, the final allocation of funding for each regional system is decided at the national level, and depends on alliances between regional and national political parties. The net result is that the funding mechanisms for the different regional systems generate substantial inequality (24). Catalonia, for example, one of the most affluent regions in Spain, receives 10 per cent more funding per person annually. At present, healthcare is the main public health policy concern, and the debate on interventions to tackle health inequalities or even public health issues has been replaced by one that centres on funding and access to services. The low use of non-hospital health services by the most advantaged groups has important policy implications. If a wide sector of the advantaged classes does not use publicly funded services, such services are likely to receive less political priority and funding in the future (20).

Information on policies and interventions at the local level related to the reduction of health inequalities is difficult to trace. Many interventions are not published officially, reports are few, and their potential impact is mainly unknown. Most interventions are not designed to decrease health inequalities between groups but to improve quality of life or health among the general population. The best example of interventions aimed specifically at reducing health inequalities is found in Barcelona (see Chapter 5).

Possible lessons to be learned

Research has found consistent evidence of socioeconomic inequalities in health in Spain. In spite of the progress achieved in understanding health inequalities, the number of groups focusing on research and funding resources are still very limited, and nationally sponsored research does not currently exist. Regular airing of health inequalities has produced little reaction with regard to health policies and interventions. The main reasons for the lack of official reaction include both the weakness of public health groups, social organizations, trade unions and other social movements, and the lack of political will of the conservative government. In Spain, no national or regional policies seeking to reduce health inequalities with the specific goal of reducing socioeconomic inequalities in health have been formulated: only vague, non-specific targets may be found in health plans at the regional level. Today, most policy-makers are stuck in a 'denial/indifference' phase. If socioeconomic inequalities in health are to be reduced, it is essential to carry out a wide range of interventions and policies, implemented and evaluated at all levels. A crucial policy issue is to put both health inequalities research and policy on the national, regional and local government agenda.

Acknowledgements

We are grateful to Carlos Alvarez-Dardet and Carles Muntaner for their comments in preparing this chapter.

References

1. Almeda E, Sarasa S. Spain: growth to diversity. In: George V, Taylor-Gooby P, eds. *European Welfare Policy*. London: Macmillan, 1996: 155–76.
2. Salmon K. *The Modern Spanish Economy. Transformation and Integration into Europe*, 2nd edn. London: Pinter, 1995.
3. Garde JA, ed. *Políticas sociales y estado de bienestar en España. Informe 1999* (Social Policies and Welfare State in Spain. 1999 Report). Madrid: Fundación Hogar del Empleado-Trotta, 1999.
4. Benach J, Borrell C, García MD, Chamizo H. Desigualdades sociales en mortalidad en áreas pequeñas de España (Social inequalities in mortality in small areas in Spain). In: Catalá F, de Manuel E, eds. *Informe SESPAS 1998: La salud pública y el futuro del estado del bienestar* (SESPAS Report 1998: public health and the future of the welfare state). SESPAS (Spanish Society of Public Health and Health Management). Granada: Escuela Andaluza de Salud Pública, 1998: 141–75.
5. Borrell C, Pasarín MI. The study of social inequalities in health in Spain: where are we? *J Epidemiol Commun Health* 1999: 53: 388–9.
6. Regidor E, Gutiérrez-Fisac JL, Rodríguez C. Increased socioeconomic differences in mortality in eight Spanish provinces. *Soc Sci Med* 1995: 41: 801–7.
7. Benach J, Yasui Y. Geographical patterns of excess mortality in Spain explained by two indices of deprivation. *J Epidemiol Commun Health* 1999: 53: 423–31.
8. Benach J, Yasui Y, Borrell C, Sáez M, Pasarín MI. Material deprivation and leading causes of death by gender: evidence from a nationwide small area study. *J Epidemiol Community Health* 2001: 55(4): 239–45.
9. Benach J, Yasui Y, Borrell C, Pasarín MI, Daponte A. The public health burden of material deprivation: excess mortality in leading causes of death in Spain (submitted).
10. Urbanos RM. Análisis y evaluación de la equidad horizontal interpersonal en la prestación pública de servicios sanitarios. Un estudio del caso español para el período 1987–95 (Analysis and evaluation of horizontal equity in public provision of health services. A case study of Spain in 1987–95). Madrid: Ph.D. Dissertation, Universidad Complutense, 1999.
11. Regidor E, Gutiérrez-Fisac JL, Rodríguez C, De Mateo S, Alonso I. Las desigualdades sociales y la salud en España (Social inequalities and health in Spain). In: Navarro C, Cabasés JM, Tormo MJ, eds. *Informe SESPAS 1995:*

La salud y el sistema sanitario en España (SESPAS Report 1995: health and health system in Spain). SESPAS (Spanish Society of Public Health and Health Management). Barcelona: SG Editores, 1995: 19–44.

12. Regidor E, Navarro P, Dominguez V, Rodriguez C. Inequalities in income and long-term disability in Spain: analysis of recent hypotheses using cross sectional study based on individual data. *Br Med J* 1997: 315: 1130–5.

13. Gutierrez-Fisac JL, Regidor E, Rodríguez C. Trends in obesity differences by educational level in Spain. *J Clin Epidemiol* 1996: 49: 351–4.

14. Navarro V, Benach J and the Scientific Commission for the study of health inequalities in Spain. *Desigualdades sociales en salud en España* (Social Inequalities in Health in Spain). Madrid: Ministerio de Sanidad y Consumo, 1996.

15. Borrell C. Rué M, Pasarín MI, Rohlfs I, Ferrando J, Fernández E. Trends in social class inequalities in health status, health-related behaviors and health services utilization in a Southern European urban area (1983–94). *Prev Med* 2000: 31: 691–701.

16. Fernández E, Schiaffino A, García M, Borràs JM. Widening social inequalities in smoking cessation in Spain, 1987–97 *J Epidemiol Community Health* 2001: 55(10): 729–30.

17. Alvarez-Dardet C, Montahud C, Ruiz MT. The widening social class gap of preventive health behaviours in Spain. *Eur J Public Health* 2001: 11(2): 225–6.

18. Fernández de la Hoz K, Leon AD. Self-perceived health status and inequalities in use of health services in Spain. *Int J Epidemiol* 1996: 25: 593–603.

19. Regidor E, de Mateo S, Gutierrez-Fisac JL, Fernández de la Hoz K, Rodriguez C. Diferencias socioeconómicas en la utilización y accesibilidad de los servicios sanitarios en España (Socioeconomic differences in the use and access of health services in Spain). *Med Clin (Barc)* 1996: 107: 285–8.

20. Borrell C, Fernandez E, Schiaffino A, Benach J, Rajmil LL, Villalbí JR, Segura A. Social class inequalities in the use of and access to health services in Catalonia (Spain): what is the influence of a supplemental private health insurance? *Int J Quality Healthcare* (in press).

21. Benach J. Análisis bibliométrico de las desigualdades en salud en España (1980–94) (Bibliometric analysis of health inequalities in Spain). *Gac Sanit* 1995: 251–64.

22. Navarro V. Topics of our times: 'The Black Report' of Spain – The Commission on Social Inequalities in Health. *Am J Public Health* 1997: 87: 334–5.

23. Elola J. Sistema Nacional de Salud: *Evaluación de su eficiencia y alternativas de reforma* (National Health System: Evaluation of its Efficiency and Alternatives for Reform). Barcelona: SG Editores, 1994.

24. Reverte-Cejudo D, Sánchez-Bayle M. Devolving health services to Spain's autonomous regions. *Br Med J* 1999: 318: 1204–5.

25. Argentaria. *Las desigualdades en España. Síntesis estadística* (Inequalities in Spain. Statistical Synthesis). Madrid: Argentaria, 1995.

26. Benach J, Urbanos RM. Desigualdades en salud (Equity in health). In: Alvarez-Dardet C, Peiró S, eds. *Informe SESPAS 2000: La salud pública ante los desafíos de un nuevo siglo*. (SESPAS Report 2000: Public Health before the Challenges of a New Century). SESPAS (Spanish Society of Public Health and Health Management). Granada: Escuela Andaluza de Salud Pública, 2000: 51–7.

19 Sweden

Bo Burström, Finn Diderichsen,
Piroska Östlin and Per-Olof Östergren

Introduction

Sweden is an example of a country which for many years has pursued active
equality-orientated social and labour market policies. In international comparison, employment rates are high among both men and women, and poverty
rates are low. Health indicators are favourable in terms of infant mortality
rates and life expectancy. However, there are still socioeconomic inequalities
in health, and other health divides are emerging. A new multisectoral public
health policy has recently been developed with a broad political consensus,
and emphasizes actions directed at the determinants of disease.

The socioeconomic situation

From the 1930s onward Sweden has pursued active equality-orientated policies regarding family and child welfare, education, housing and the labour
market (1). Since the Second World War, Sweden has had a universal and
highly decommodifying welfare state (2) which has been able to combine
generous welfare state entitlements with rapid economic growth, low unemployment and very high levels of labour force participation, particularly
among women (3). A guiding principle has been that everyone able to do so
should work to support himself or herself, and that the state should provide
reasonable social security benefits for those unable to work. A precondition
for the maintenance of the benefits of the welfare state has been high employment rates. Through employment protection laws and active labour
market policies (including sheltered employment) the state has striven to
maximize labour market participation, including among vulnerable groups
such as the chronically ill and disabled (4).

The extent of income inequality is smaller in Sweden than in many other
countries. In the period 1991–7 the Gini coefficient remained at around 0.25.
By international comparison, the prevalence of poverty (income < 50 per cent
of mean income) is low and evenly distributed across socioeconomic groups, as
defined by occupational status. In 1992–5 the prevalence of poverty among
men ranged from 2.3 per cent in the higher non-manual occupational groups

to 3.6 per cent in the unqualified manual group, and from 1.8 per cent to 4.1 per cent, respectively, among women (5). Compared with the prevalence of child poverty before and after government intervention in 19 countries, Sweden and Finland had the lowest percentage (3 per cent) (6). Hence, public transfers appear to have been successful in redistributing income in Sweden.

The extent of socioeconomic inequalities in health

Socioeconomic inequalities in health have been considered to be smaller in Sweden than elsewhere. However, a recent study found similar relative inequalities in Sweden as in other European countries (7). The size and public health importance of socioeconomic inequalities in health depend on the measure used. Another analysis showed that Sweden had the lowest levels of absolute mortality among the countries studied, among both manual and non-manual occupational groups (8).

In recent years there has been evidence of increasing inequalities in health (9). From 1981 to 1995 there was a decline in mortality in all socioeconomic groups, among both men and women. However, the decline was faster among higher non-manual than among manual occupational groups. In absolute terms the risk difference between non-manual and manual groups has remained fairly constant from 1981 to 1995. The socioeconomic inequalities in health are present in all age groups. Perinatal mortality has been reported to be higher among immigrant women in Malmö (the third largest city in Sweden) (10). The children of the higher non-manual groups have the lowest mortality rates, whereas those of unqualified manual workers have the highest mortality rates. Children of lone mothers and immigrant children have higher rates of injury mortality than do other children. The risk of dying before 65 years of age is higher for individuals in manual than in non-manual occupational groups (50 per cent for men, 20 per cent for women). The risk of death from ischaemic heart disease is nearly twice as high among men in manual occupations as among those in non-manual ones. Socioeconomic inequalities in alcohol-related mortality are even greater (9).

There are regional differences in health, to the advantage of the population in urban areas. This may be due in part to labour market characteristics and to health selection: for example the migration of younger, healthy and well educated persons to cities with better employment opportunities, leaving older, less healthy and less educated persons behind. Within urban areas those in attractive inner-city neighbourhoods and in detached housing areas are healthier than the population in the public housing areas in the suburbs (11). In Stockholm and Malmö considerable differences in life expectancy (4–6 years) are still reported between deprived and affluent areas. Similarly, rates of sickness absence and early retirement due to sickness are higher, and smoking, physical inactivity, overweight, economic problems, unemployment and exposure to violence are more common in deprived than in affluent areas (9, 12, 13). There are growing health inequalities among

Table 19.1 Odds ratios for socioeconomic inequalities in morbidity in Sweden (men and women 25–64 years)

Socioeconomic category	Long-standing illness	With slightly reduced working capacity	With greatly reduced working capacity and not in the workforce
Professional	1.0	1.0	1.0
Intermediate non-manual	1.1	1.4	1.8
Routine non-manual	1.5	2.2	3.8
Skilled manual	1.7	3.3	6.0
Unskilled manual	1.8	3.2	6.2
Percentage of the population 25–64 years	39.7	20.8	6.0

Source: National Public Health Commission

immigrants compared to Swedish-born persons, particularly in certain urban areas (14). The socioeconomic inequalities in morbidity in the general population vary with the measure used, and are greater if the social consequences of disease are also included (Table 19.1).

The consumption of alcohol is lower in Sweden than in most other European countries: in 1995 the average consumption of pure alcohol per person aged 15 years and over was 6 litres (9). The proportion of persons with high consumption was previously higher in the higher non-manual occupational groups, but in a recent study no significant differences between socioeconomic groups were found (12). However, alcohol-related mortality is still two to three times higher among manual workers than among individuals in higher and intermediate non-manual occupations (9).

There are growing socioeconomic inequalities in the utilization of healthcare in Sweden (15). Although morbidity is higher in the lower socioeconomic groups, the odds ratio for having visited a doctor in the last 3 months was lower among those in the lowest income quintile. The odds ratio for having needed but not sought medical attention was higher among people in the lowest than in the highest income quintile (16).

Research

Health inequality was a hot political issue in Sweden in the 1930s, not least because of inequalities in infant mortality between rich and poor, which were seen as unjust, and resulted in the implementation of health and welfare policies previously described. Health was seen as a basic human right that also influenced access to other human rights, such as full participation in society. However, with the implementation of welfare policies and provisions for maternal and child health, health inequalities were not seen as a major problem until the 1970s (17).

The major source of inspiration behind the growing political and scientific concern with socioeconomic inequalities in health and its causes was the publication of the Black Report in the United Kingdom (UK) (see Chapter 2). A cross-national comparison showed that socioeconomic inequalities in health also existed in Sweden, although they appeared smaller than those in the UK (18). The explanations behind the British situation were, however, not convicingly plausible in the Swedish context, given the universal welfare state, the low level of poverty, low unemployment rate and high standard of housing. The research community in Sweden was puzzled by these findings and was greatly inspired to study more systematically socioeconomic inequalities in health and, for the Swedish context, plausible explanations for them.

In the mid-1980s, the Swedish parliament passed a bill with a major policy objective of reducing inequalities, stipulating also that reports on health and socioeconomic inequalities should be presented to parliament every 3 years. In 1991, another bill proposed the establishment of a National Institute of Public Health, whose focus would be equality in health. The Conservative–Liberal coalition elected in 1991 accorded less priority to equality issues. When the Social Democrats returned to power, following a severe recession in the early 1990s with high unemployment rates, a parliamentary committee was established to define national objectives for health development, emphasizing the reduction of class- and gender-related inequalities in health. In December 1996 a national research policy bill was passed, which included the establishment of a programme of health inequalities research (17, 19). By 1997 the Social Research Council, the Medical Research Council and the National Institute of Public Health had been commissioned to draw up and monitor the national programme. The emphasis was on social justice, the incorporation of a gender perspective, and the consideration of the importance of wider structural policies to inequalities in health (17).

Research on inequalities in health is currently considered important and is also high on the political agenda in Sweden. The main funding agency has been the Swedish Social Research Council. The council recently allocated SEK 4 million (€0.43 million) towards creating a multidisciplinary centre in Stockholm for research into health inequalities, and additional funds for a number of research positions elsewhere in the country. Since 1996 the National Institute of Public Health has also funded a number of research positions on inequalities in health, and maintains a national network of researchers. An increasing number of research groups are engaging in studies of inequalities in health, and the National Institute of Public Health has recently restated its emphasis on such inequalities.

Policies

A new national health policy has recently been presented with a strong focus on equality, supported by scientific evidence. The instructions to the

Box 19.1   Proposed National Public Health Strategy for Sweden (Socialdepartementet, 1999)

Visions and strategic intents for a health-friendly society

Vision for a health-friendly society:

A health-friendly society gives everyone equal opportunity to influence individual and shared causes and consequences of sickness and disease. In such a society, everyone has the opportunity to manage challenges of life and take personal responsibility for those aspects of health that can be influenced by the individual. Factors in the surrounding environment that cause physical and mental illness, such as inequitable living conditions and unsanitary environments, have been eliminated to a significant extent.

Strategic intents for a health-friendly society

1. Strengthen the social cohesion and solidarity in society.
2. Increase opportunities for integration into the labour market and reduce social exclusion.
3. Increase influence and security for people in the workplace.
4. Give priorities to families with children, economically and with respect to time for being together.
5. Give children and youth equal life chances by reducing segregation and implementing compensatory measures.
6. Give senior citizens and people with long-term illnesses or disabilities opportunities to shape their lives according to their needs.
7. Create opportunities for sustainable enhancement of health.
8. Increase solidarity with those who are vulnerable to lifestyle risks.

Commission included a focus on inequalities in health between socioeconomic groups, ethnic groups, geographical areas and the sexes (20). Developed by a commission consisting of a parliamentary group and a number of scientific experts and advisers from national authorities, universities, trade unions and non-governmental organizations, the strategy has taken its starting point in ethical considerations based on the thinking of Rawls (21) and Sen (22), and emphasized actions directed at the causal determinants of disease, as summarized in Box 19.1 (23). The commission has worked for over three years and the proposal has been referred for consideration and comments to nearly 500 organizations, authorities, academic institutions, non-governmental organizations and others. The decision to propose health targets primarily in terms of reduced exposure to determinants of disease and injuries, and not in terms of reduced mortality and morbidity, is a result of the understanding that exposures can clearly be related to their causal roles for the level and distribution of different diseases and their consequences, and has been based on a concurrent analysis of determinants of disease and ill-health. The proposal includes action by a wide range of sectors in society. Quantitative targets were proposed in previous versions of the strategy, but are now to be further elaborated by the National Institute of Public Health and other relevant authorities. It is the Commission's hope that the targets and strategies proposed will guide society in promoting health and preventing diseases and injuries and their consequences in terms of disability and mortality, and contribute to the reduction of inequalities in health between socioeconomic groups, women and men, ethnic groups, and between geographical regions of the country.

Labour market policies

Employment rates are high and poverty rates are low among men and women in most social groups in Sweden, and also among those with chronic illness (24). However, following the economic recession in the early 1990s, the workforce has declined by about 10 per cent. Employment rates are lower among foreign citizens and in the youngest age group, and increasing numbers are now outside the benefit system. The collapse in demand for unqualified labour which has hit the OECD (Organization for Economic Cooperation and Development) countries for more than three decades was felt strongly in most countries. However, in international comparison the Swedish labour market policies seem to have had a buffering effect in this respect, particularly for vulnerable and lower socioeconomic groups. A comparative study of employment rates and rates of exclusion from the labour market across socioeconomic groups among men with and without limiting long-standing illness in Sweden and Britain during the period 1979–95, showed that Swedish men with limiting long-standing illness had higher rates of employment and lower rates of exclusion from the labour market than their British counterparts. Furthermore, the differences in employment rates and rates of exclusion from the labour market across socioeconomic groups were considerably smaller in Sweden than in Britain. It appeared from the study that Swedish policies (strong employment protection and active labour market policies) were beneficial to men with a limiting long-standing illness, equally across socioeconomic groups. Furthermore, the burden of unemployment was distributed across the population in Sweden, whereas in Britain it fell more disproportionately on the less-skilled members of society and those in poorer health (24).

Social policy measures for lone mothers

Many of the policies that constitute the Swedish welfare state were instituted to create equal opportunities for all, not least for children and their families.

Lone mothers are a vulnerable group in most societies, as they are in Sweden (25), and a number of general social policy measures exist to alleviate their situation. The provision of subsidized public childcare has allowed such women to work outside the home. Sweden's proportion of lone mothers is similar to many other European countries, but it has fewer teenage mothers than, for instance, Britain. This may be related to the introduction of active sex education programmes in schools since 1956, and the subsequent development of services providing free counselling and contraceptives for teenagers and young adults (26).

The parental insurance scheme allows parents full sick leave benefits for 15 months with the birth of each child. The compensation levels have varied between 75 and 90 per cent of earnings. Until the child reaches 12 years of age, parents are allowed to stay at home for a maximum of 60 days per year with sick pay. The stigma associated with being a lone mother has declined in most countries, as in Sweden. Lone mothers are expected to work and support themselves and their children, and policies exist to promote their active participation in paid employment. Public childcare is heavily subsidized and fees are often income-related. The children of lone mothers have priority in public childcare (26). Swedish mothers receive child maintenance support from the government, which claims the money from the father. The employment rate among Swedish lone mothers was about 72 per cent in 1992–5. The poverty rate among lone mothers was 10 per cent over the same period. In comparison, the employment rate among British lone mothers in 1992–5 was 42 per cent and 70 per cent were poor. The health inequalities between lone and couple mothers were similar in Sweden and Britain, but the factors explaining these inequalities were different. Poverty and joblessness explained 50 per cent of the difference in Britain, but only between 3 and 13 per cent in Sweden (26).

The comparative study found indications of a stronger health impact of poverty in Britain than in Sweden. Whereas the rate differences of limiting long-standing illness between employed and unemployed mothers were similar among couple mothers in both Britain and Sweden (about 8.5 per cent), the rate difference of such illness between poor and non-poor mothers was about twice as great among British (about 6 per cent) as among Swedish mothers (about 3 per cent), and similar between lone and couple mothers. The greater rate difference between poor and not poor mothers in Britain suggested that poverty was more strongly related to health in Britain than in Sweden – that something in the British social context made the experience of being poor worse for mothers in terms of its impact on health.

The difference in relative terms refers to the health disadvantage of lone to couple mothers in the two countries – this was similar in both Britain and Sweden. The absolute rate differences of the impact of poverty on health showed a difference in terms of the social contexts of Sweden and Britain, on the experience of being poor and its relation to health. For instance, it might be 'easier' to be poor in Sweden than in Britain, as there may be more 'public goods' in Sweden that do not need to be purchased (for example, virtually all housing is of good quality; childcare fees are waived or reduced for those on lower incomes; there is not the same geographical concentration of families living in poverty in Sweden as in Britain; public transport may be better organized in Sweden, etc.). These are of course just speculations, not empirically tested in our studies.

Another study comparing relative deprivation in Britain and Sweden found that deprivation and poverty were more prevalent in Britain (27). Britons were more deprived according to British standards than Swedes according to Swedish standards. The mechanisms that generate deprivation and poverty were similar in both countries. In Sweden there were no differences in deprivation between men and women, whereas British women were more deprived than British men. The study concluded that 'The fact that deprivation is less severe in Sweden can be seen as a confirmation of the success of the "Swedish model".' Active labour market policies, low unemployment, an extensive redistribution of income and an income maintenance system covering the major part of the population have clearly succeeded when it comes to the prevention and alleviation of deprivation and poverty' (27).

Possible lessons to be learned

For many years Sweden has pursued deliberate equality-orientated health and social policies, active labour market policies and family-friendly policies which have resulted in higher levels of workforce participation, less income inequality, lower poverty rates and smaller socioeconomic inequalities in the distribution of poverty than in most other countries. Certain vulnerable groups (for example, lone mothers) have considerably lower rates of poverty than corresponding groups in other countries, people with a chronic illness can remain in the labour market, and the health impact of poverty seems to be smaller in Sweden. Compared to many other countries, Sweden has low mortality levels, high life expectancy and favourable health indicators across all socioeconomic groups. However, there are still considerable relative socioeconomic inequalities in health, and some indications that these inequalities are now increasing. Other health divides are also emerging, not least between immigrants and those born in Sweden.

From this review, it might be concluded that within the action spectrum described by Whitehead (17), Sweden is in the 'more structured developments' stage.

References

1. Höjer KJ. *Den svenska socialpolitiken. En översikt* (Swedish Social Policy. An Overview). Stockholm: Nordstedts, 1969.
2. Esping-Andersen G. *The Three Worlds of Welfare Capitalism*. Oxford: Polity Press, 1990.

3. Stephens JD. Decline or renewal in the advanced welfare states? In: Esping-Andersen G, ed. *Welfare States in Transition*. London: Sage, 1996: 32–65.
4. van den Berg A., Furåker B., Johansson L. *Labour Market Regimes and Patterns of Flexibility. A Sweden–Canada Comparison*. Lund: Arkiv förlag, 1997.
5. Burström B, Diderichsen F. Income-related policies in Sweden 1990–8. In: Mackenbach JP, Droomers M, eds. *Interventions and Policies to Reduce Socioeconomic Inequalities in Health*. Rotterdam: Department of Public Health, Erasmus University, 1999: 135–42.
6. Smeeding TM. Financial poverty in developed countries: the evidence from LIS. Luxembourg Income Study, Working Paper no. 155, April 1997.
7. Mackenbach JP, Kunst AE, Cavelaars AEMJ, Groenhof F, Geurts JJM, the EU Working Group on Socioeconomic Inequalities in Health. Socioeconomic inequalities in morbidity and mortality in Western Europe. *Lancet* 1997: 349: 1655–9.
8. Vågerö D, Erikson R. Socioeconomic inequalities in morbidity and mortality in Western Europe (Letter). *Lancet* 1997: 350: 516.
9. Socialstyrelsen. *Folkhälsorapport 1997* (Public Health Report). Stockholm: National Board of Health and Welfare, 1997.
10. Essén B, Hanson BS, Östergren P-O, Lindquist P, Gudmundsson S. Increased perinatal mortality among sub-Saharan immigrant women in a city-population in Sweden. *Acta Obstet Gynecol Scand* 2000: 107: 1507–12.
11. Ministry of Health and Social Affairs. *Hur står det till med folkhälsan i Sverige? Första steget mot nationella folkhälsomål. Delbetänkande av Nationella folkhälsokommittén* (Public Health in Sweden – the First Step towards National Targets for Public Health). SOU 1998: 43. Stockholm: Ministry of Health and Social Affairs, 1998.
12. Stockholms läns landsting. *Folkhälsorapport 1999. Om hälsoutvecklingen i Stockholms län* (Public Health Report for Stockholm County 1999). Stockholm: Socialmedicin, SLL, 1999.
13. Lindström M, Rosvall M, Hanson BS. *Hur mår Malmö? Folkhälsorapport 1996* (Public Health Report for Malmö 1996). Malmö: City of Malmö, 1996.
14. Ministry of Health and Social Affairs. *Hälsa på lika villkor – andra steget mot nationella folkhälsomål. Delbetänkande av Nationella folkhälsokommittén* (Health on Equal Terms – the Second Step towards National Targets for Public Health). SOU 1999: 137. Stockholm: Ministry of Health and Social Affairs, 1999.
15. Whitehead M, Evandrou M, Haglund B, Diderichsen F. As the health divide widens in Sweden and Britain, what's happening to access to care? *Br Med J* 1997: 315: 1006–9.
16. Diderichsen F. Ska inkomster eller sjukdom beskattas – fördelningseffekter av patientavgifter (Tax on income or disease – distributive effects of user fees). In: *Socialstyrelsen. Patientavgifter och vårdefterfrågan*. SoS Rapport 2000: 8. Stockholm: National Board of Health and Welfare, 2000.
17. Whitehead M. Diffusion of ideas on social inequalities in health: a European perspective. *Milbank Q* 1998: 76: 469–92.
18. Lundberg O. Class and health: comparing Britain and Sweden. *Soc Sci Med* 1986: 23: 511–17.
19. Arve-Parès B, ed. *Promoting Research on Inequality in Health* (Proceedings from an international expert meeting in Stockholm 24–25 September, 1997). Stockholm: Swedish Council for Social Research, 1998.

20. Ministry of Health and Social Affairs. *Hälsa på lika villkor – nationella mål för folkhälsan. Slutbetänkande av nationella folkhälsokommittén* (Health on Equal Terms – Final Proposal on National Targets for Public Health). SOU 2000: 91. Stockholm: Ministry of Health and Social Affairs, 2000.

21. Rawls JA. *A Theory of Justice.* Cambridge, MA: Harvard University Press, 1971.

22. Sen. A. *Inequality re-examined.* Cambridge, MA: Harvard University Press, 1992.

23. Östlin P, Diderichsen F. *Equity-oriented National Strategy for Public Health in Sweden.* WHO Policy Learning Curve Series number 1, May 2000.

24. Burström B, Whitehead M, Diderichsen F. Inequality in the social consequences of illness: how well do people with long-term illness fare on the labour markets of Britain and Sweden? *Int J Health Serv* 2000: 30: 435–51.

25. Burström B, Diderichsen F, Shouls S, Whitehead M. Lone mothers in Sweden: trends in health and socioeconomic circumstances, 1979–95. *J Epidemiol Commun Health* 1999: 53: 750–6.

26. Whitehead M, Burström B, Diderichsen F. Social policies and the pathways to inequalities in health: a comparative analysis of lone mothers in Britain and Sweden. *Soc Sci Med* 2000: 50: 255–70.

27. Halleröd B. Poor Swedes, poor Britons: A comparative analysis of relative deprivation. In: Andress, HJ, ed. *Empirical Poverty Research in a Comparative Perspective.* Aldershot: Ashgate, 1998: 283–311.

Part IV
Evaluation issues

20 Health impact assessment

An approach to promote intersectoral policies to reduce socioeconomic inequalities in health

Anna Ritsatakis, Ruth Barnes,
Margaret Douglas and Alex Scott-Samuel

Introduction

Recognizing that social and economic development and the circumstances in which people live, work and play are the main determinants of health, the 51 countries of the World Health Organization (WHO) European Region have, since the early 1980s, advocated intersectoral policies for health development (1). Implementing such policies has, however, proved more difficult than anticipated (2) and, over 20 years later, lasting cross-sector partnerships for health are still not generally in place.

Recent events, particularly in Eastern Europe, have refocused attention on increasing health gaps between and within countries, and on the need to raise awareness of the socioeconomic determinants of health inequalities (3), including the role of issues such as relative poverty and social cohesion (4). The new European Union (EU) public health strategy consequently aims at tackling the determinants of health (5), and in 1999 the European Council called for procedures to 'monitor the impact of Community policies and activities, especially those relating to the internal market, on public health and healthcare' (6). From 2001, 'proposals with a particular relevance to health will include an explanation of how health requirements have been addressed, normally by including a statement in the proposal's explanatory memorandum . . . a priority task will be to develop criteria and methodologies, such as appraisal guidelines and checklists, for evaluating policy proposals and their implementation. In addition, certain Community actions or policies could be singled out for a thorough impact assessment' (7).

At the national level, in Sweden for example, the government has recently set targets addressing the determinants of a 'health-friendly society' (8) and health impact assessment (HIA) is being developed to support this. The Netherlands screens legislation going to parliament for its possible impact on health (9). In the United Kingdom (UK) the Acheson report (10) recommended that 'all policies likely to have a direct or indirect effect on health should be evaluated in terms of their impact on health inequalities', and this has already been done, for example, for regeneration policy and fuel poverty (11).

So far, attempts to carry out HIA have focused more on selected pilot projects and on issues with a strong environmental link, rather than on broad social or economic policies. HIA was not established specifically to reduce socioeconomic inequalities in health, but the developing methodology does offer an exciting opportunity to systematically identify potential health inequalities that may arise as a result of a proposed policy, and to recommend alternative actions that could promote greater equality in health.

What is health impact assessment?

Most of the definitions of HIA used in different countries are similar to that adopted by Health Canada: 'any combination of procedures or methods by which a proposed policy or program may be judged as to the effect(s) it may have on the health of a population' (12). Since early 1999, WHO's European Centre for Health Policy (ECHP), together with partners across Europe, has initiated a project to clarify appropriate principles and approaches to HIA. In the framework of this project it was agreed that a commitment to promoting equality in health should be explicitly reflected in HIA. Based on an e-mail consultation and an international workshop (13), a consensus paper (14) defines HIA as 'a combination of procedures, methods and tools by which a policy, programme or project may be judged as to its potential effects on the health of a population, *and the distribution of those effects within the population*'.

As will be seen in Chapter 21, whereas the term 'evaluation' is used when examining the impact of policies that have health improvements among their primary objectives, HIA more usually deals with the unintended health impact of policies designed with non-health primary objectives in mind. The consensus paper clarifies that HIA is usually prospective and is concerned with the impact on the population of a particular area, in terms of gender, age, ethnic background and socioeconomic status.

The inclusion of distributional effects in the HIA definition represents an aspiration rather than a current reality. There is not as yet sufficient consensus on HIA methods and procedures to ensure that all current assessments focus routinely on equality. This is partly due to HIA's origins in environmental impact assessment and healthy public policy. Whereas environmental impact assessment has been in existence for over 30 years, environmental equality (also known as environmental justice) only became a consideration in the last decade of the twentieth century, and thus equality is less routinely considered than in public health policy.

There is considerable confusion concerning concepts and definitions. Equality is both a *value* which should underpin HIA, and also a *health determinant* (and thus a potential health impact of policies or projects). For equality to consistently form part of HIA there is a need for consensus on whether HIA should address differences in health status or the ethical concept of unfair and avoidable health inequalities (15); deprivation or distribution (that is, disadvantage or inequalities); relative or absolute disadvantage/inequality.

The recommendation of the UK Acheson report referred to earlier resulted in some exponents arguing for a separate health inequalities impact assessment tool. This notion was tested at an international seminar (16) in Manchester in June 2000, where 'equality-focused HIA' and 'health inequalities impact assessment' methods – focusing respectively on deprived groups alone and on the total distribution – were applied to the same projects to test which approach was preferable. The conclusion of the seminar was that *all* HIA methods and procedures should incorporate a focus on equality, explicitly addressing both impacts on disadvantaged groups and the distribution of impacts across the population.

According to the Gothenburg consensus paper, HIA includes consideration of evidence about the anticipated relationships between a proposed policy or project and the health of a population and of the opinions, experience and expectations of those who may be affected. It aims to provide more informed understanding by decision-makers and the public regarding the effects of the proposed policy, and to propose adjustments/options to maximize positive and minimize negative health impacts.

The first stage in HIA is to select which policies or programmes could have an impact on health and what kind of impact (screening process), and to determine what further work should be carried out, by whom and how (scoping process). If screening and scoping indicate that further work should be done, then the consensus paper suggests that one of three broad categories of action are usually taken. These are shown graphically in Figure 20.1: rapid health impact appraisal based on existing knowledge; a more in-depth health impact analysis examining potential impacts and opportunities for adjustment of the proposal, requiring the compilation and analysis of new information; and thirdly, in the case of broad policies, or clusters of programmes that make an in-depth analysis infeasible, a broad-brush health impact review (17). Whatever type of approach is agreed, this will be followed by a report of the findings (including recommendations to adjust the proposed policy or project); appraisal of the report; and, finally, by appropriate action to enhance potential positive and reduce possible negative impacts on health and socioeconomic inequalities in health.

What is the added value of using HIA as a tool to promote socioeconomic equality in health?

First, HIA is largely used prospectively. In contrast to interventions designed to deal with health inequalities after they have arisen, HIA offers a powerful

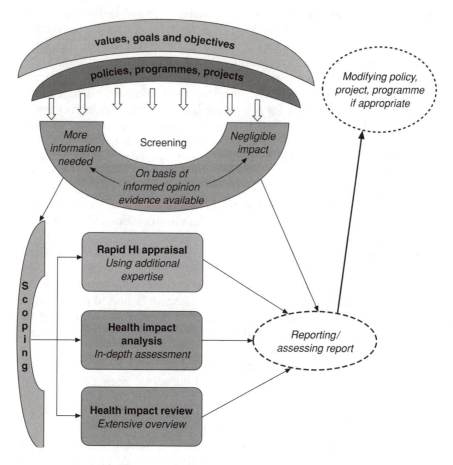

Figure 20.1 An approach to health impact assessment

process for avoiding the creation of new, or the exacerbation of existing, inequalities. It does this by flagging up the possible creation of inequalities and making recommendations for their avoidance, but also by considering the enhancement of potential health-promoting factors.

The values underpinning HIA strengthen its potential for promoting equality in health: *democracy*, emphasizing the right to participate in a transparent process for the assessment of policies that affect life circumstances, which, if fully implemented, could empower disadvantaged groups; *sustainable development*, emphasizing that both short- and long-term, as well as more and less direct, impacts are taken into consideration; and *ethical use of evidence*, emphasizing the rigorous use of quantitative and qualitative evidence based on various scientific disciplines and methodologies, thus giving a more comprehensive assessment of possible impacts.

If the insight, information, skills and opportunities for partnership building developed through the HIA process were embedded firmly in the overall policy development process, there would be added value on a number of levels. In the policy formulation stage in any sector, the essential situation analysis would be enhanced by a health profile of the population. Prospective HIA would allow an assessment of unintended health impacts of the proposed policy on different population groups. Decision-makers in other sectors, together with those in the health sector, could then explicitly take account of the health impacts on different groups when weighing possible policy options.

The qualitative assessments frequently made through HIA highlight potential outcomes and options that might otherwise be missed. The HIA process would strengthen the participation of vulnerable groups and the development of a transparent civic society. The knowledge and partnerships created during HIA would inform and strengthen the policy implementation process.

Information gathered on changes in the health status of different population groups could be included in the monitoring and evaluation stage of a policy. Retrospective HIA of existing policies and assessment of the quality of previous prospective HIAs could inform the policy reformulation process. The quantitative and qualitative measures developed, the skills and capacities gained and the participatory mechanisms developed during HIA processes should improve overall monitoring and evaluation processes for policy-making in general.

To summarize, fully integrating HIA in the policy-making process could give the following added value:

- As a minimum, HIA helps ensure that health consequences and effects of future decisions on different population groups are not overlooked.
- HIA's prospective nature helps prevent the increase of socioeconomic inequalities in health by limiting unintended negative consequences of a wide range of policies.
- Concomitantly, HIA focuses on enhancing the potential positive impact of a wide range of policies in order to promote equality in health.
- HIA encourages transparency in decision-making by requiring participatory processes and public reporting.
- HIA facilitiates the consideration of alternative policy proposals and weighing of trade-offs.
- HIA can force a focus on values, for example by requiring a definition of the population to be considered (local, national, global) and the time-frame (next year, next five years, next generation, etc.) and a discussion of acceptable or unacceptable trade-offs.
- By including the main stakeholders in the process, HIA empowers vulnerable groups and could generally improve participation in decision-making.

Applications of HIA

Applications are not easily found through the usual literature search. A quick check of more than twenty HIAs compiled during our project showed that although most made at least a token reference to inequality in health, either explicitly or implicitly, there was less indication of how this dimension was tackled in practice. The following are examples with a clearly defined equality focus, selected to highlight some of the issues we have referred to.

Health impact assessment of the City of Edinburgh Council's urban transport strategy

The objective of this application (18) was to compare the health impacts of three different transport scenarios, based on different levels of available funding. It was carried out in Edinburgh, a city with 450,000 people, more affluent than the Scottish average but with deprived housing estates on its outskirts. The HIA was to inform a transport strategy for the City of Edinburgh Council to reduce traffic congestion.

The study gathered information, including a literature review, analysis of local data and the views of a group of key informants. The main areas of health impact identified were accidents; pollution; access to amenities, jobs and social contacts; opportunities for healthy sustainable physical activity in walking and cycling; and impacts on community networks.

The study took a distributional approach, comparing impacts borne by different population groups. Two main groups were described: middle-class, affluent, predominantly car-owning; and disadvantaged, predominantly non-car-owning. Within these groups a number of subgroups were identified (young families, adolescents, the elderly, working people, unemployed people).

Six grids were constructed and used to record the health impacts for each group within each of the three scenarios. Table 20.1 summarizes the health impacts under scenario 1 (low spend) and scenario 3 (high spend). Data were not available to quantify the impacts for each subgroup. The 'scores' shown in Table 20.1 were only a visual summary of likely impacts, based on literature evidence and key informant views. The grids aided comparison of impacts borne by different population groups under the three funding assumptions.

Most detrimental impacts were concentrated in more disadvantaged communities. Pollution affected all groups, but people who spend a lot of time in cars (young families and working people) were at higher risk because urban car occupants are exposed to poorer air quality than those using other modes of transport (19, 20). The scenario with the greatest funding was recommended as producing the greatest health gain. Scenarios with lower funding would have adverse effects on overall health and health inequalities.

Table 20.1 Health impacts on different population groups under scenarios 1 (low spend) and 3 (high spend)

	Accidents		Pollution		Physical activity		Access to goods and services		Community network	
	1	3	1	3	1	3	1	3	1	3
Young families										
Affluent	+	+	--	+	-	+	-	+	-	++
Deprived	--	+	-	+	--	+	--	+	-	++
Adolescents										
Affluent	-	++	--	+	-	+	--	++	--	++
Deprived	--	+	-	+	-	++	--	++	--	++
Elderly										
Affluent	-	++	-	+	--	++	-	+	-	++
Deprived	--	+	-	+	--	++	--	++	-	++
Working People										
Affluent	0	+	--	+	-	+	-	++	-	+
Deprived	-	+	-	+	-	++	--	++	-	++
Unemployed										
Deprived	-	+	-	+	-	+	--	++	--	++

This HIA described explicitly the distribution of impacts, demonstrating that transport policy affects different population groups differently in ways that are both avoidable and unjust and therefore inequitable. It also raised important issues related to a focus on socioeconomic inequalities:

- It was not possible to obtain quantitative estimates for impacts on different groups, but qualitative estimates can also aid decision-making.
- To be relevant to a transport policy, population groups were defined predominantly by car ownership, which might bring additional problems in obtaining appropriate health data.
- Identifying the groups potentially disadvantaged by a proposal may be difficult at the start of an assessment.
- Some impacts fall on 'external' populations (for example, commuters into Edinburgh, who were excluded from the assessment). Defining the populations for the HIA is thus an ethical issue.
- It proved impossible to achieve meaningful, representative participation of so many different groups of people in a city population.
- The recommendations supported the high-spend scenario, which would benefit all groups and especially the disadvantaged. Should the funding not be available, there should also be recommendations to mitigate the identified adverse impacts on vulnerable groups.
- Overall, the approach demonstrated that HIA can make explicit any potential future health inequalities that may arise from a policy, and thereby prevent them arising.

Health impact assessment of the regeneration project on the Ferrier estate, Greenwich, London

This was a large regeneration project in Greenwich, south London (21), intended to radically transform local housing on the Ferrier estate, one of the most disadvantaged areas of the borough and home to 6,800 people. It was part of a single regeneration budget programme aiming to tackle social exclusion and promote opportunities for employment and education; to address crime and raise the level of public safety; and to transform housing stock and local infrastructure.

Three options were being developed for consideration by the local author-ity and Single Regeneration Budget Partnership Board for the redevelopment of the Ferrier estate: refurbishment, demolition, or partial demolition with refurbishment of the remaining parts of the estate. A prospective, in-depth assessment was made of the health impact on residents of the three options, paying particular attention to impacts on health inequalities.

The HIA was timed for a strategic planning stage where its recommenda-tions could be most effective, both in informing the options for the future development of the estate and in assessing the health impacts of the transi-tional phase of the changes.

The HIA was undertaken by a multidisciplinary team including an inde-pendent public health consultant, representatives of the health authority public health directorate, the local authority regeneration, housing, educa-tion and environmental health departments, the health and local authority Joint Health Unit and the South Greenwich Forum, an umbrella group for local community organizations. It was funded jointly by local and national authorities as one of a series of national pilots.

The active involvement of key stakeholders was crucial to the process. In structured interviews, individuals and community groups were asked to help identify current health issues they saw as important; long-term positive and negative health impacts of the refurbishment and demolition options; and shorter-term transitional health impacts during the period of change. A framework based on the Merseyside Guidelines for HIA (22) was used for this purpose. Key issues defined were then explored in more detail and evidence collated relating to the current situation described in a detailed community profile, the interviews and a residents' survey. Both published and 'grey' literature provided evidence for the links between these key issues and health.

A series of recommendations was then developed, together with sugges-tions as to how their implementation could be facilitated.

The key issues and areas of concern that emerged were poverty, unem-ployment, education and training; recreation and leisure; social networks – belonging to the local community; housing; management by the council; the local environment; and crime and the fear of crime. These potential impacts were summarized in tabular form and, from an analysis of the findings, it was possible to identify opportunities to maximize the positive and minimize the negative health impacts, as well as the constraints likely to be imposed by each option.

Potentially substantial benefits included a decrease in accident rates resulting from better designed and better quality housing; lower rates of respiratory disease, stress and anxiety as a result of more appropriate central heating systems and the elimination of infestation in their homes; improvements to diet and other health-related choices as a result of increasing opportunities for paid employment and higher income levels; and better psychological health and well-being as a result of improved security measures and a reduction in levels and fears of crime. Significant 'health warnings' also emerged which would need to be addressed as a matter of urgency at an early stage.

The key areas recommended for action related to: support for existing communities; management of the redevelopment process; asbestos; sustainability; and health inequalities. In relation to health inequalities the biggest single issue was the need to be clear about the target population – whether it was the current population of the estate that was the focus of the redevelopment, or the geographical area itself. The HIA was explicit in focusing on the current population, and in doing so identified issues that needed to be addressed to ensure that the benefits of redevelopment went to the more vulnerable members of society and that socially excluded people were not moved to other, equally deprived areas, transferring the problem rather than attempting to solve it.

Additional recommendations related to poverty and income; women and young children; elderly people; and people from black and minority ethnic groups. It was important to identify such equality issues specifically during the course of the HIA to ensure that interventions were targeted appropriately. Otherwise, the recommendations would have been more general and might have resulted in implementation programmes that widened the gap between the various groups of 'beneficiaries'.

The value of wide consultation, including the residents' survey, was clearly demonstrated. Without this, the identification of some of the most vulnerable groups might have been missed, as the estate was home to a large number of residents whose voices were not normally heard and who felt they had no vested interest in the area. Its benefits are now bearing fruit in terms of how the findings and recommendations are being taken on board in considering the options for the future of the estate.

The counties and local authorities in Sweden

The HIA system set up by the Federation of Swedish County Councils was designed to 'establish whether there are particular groups whose health has been affected by, or is already exposed to, many and serious health hazards, and whether there are other groups whose health trends may become problematic' (23). This effort was linked to the overall public health

	Prioritized group		Entire population	
	Long term	Short term	Long term	Short term
Democracy/opportunity to exert influence/equality				
Financial security				
Employment/meaningful pursuits/education				
Social network				
Access to healthcare and welfare services				
Belief in the future/life goals and meaning				
Physical environment				
Living habits				

Figure 20.2 The health matrix

programme that listed 'prioritized groups' such as children and young people, women, immigrants and weak socioeconomic groups. The system suggests that such groups should be adjusted according to local circumstances and the policy proposal in question.

Figure 20.2 shows the matrix proposed for checking (with plus or minus signs) the potential positive or negative impact that a policy may have on a prioritized group or on the entire population. Cells related to other determinants of health are to be added as necessary.

The matrix, other advice, guidelines and examples are available on the website and counties are invited to share their experiences through a network site on the web. Attention has been given to training local decision-makers for HIA and a large number of such assessments are currently being carried out by local authorities throughout the country.

One example, for instance, is that the Southwestern Health District of Stockholm County Council in 1998 decided to test the HIA concept. Since September 1999 HIA has been carried out on all of the proposals referred to the Medical Services Board. The instrument, that is, the Health Question and the Health Matrix, is continually being revised to meet current practices and needs. One practical example is the use of the Health Matrix on a proposal for an agreement about research and development of migration, psychiatry, labour market and health. The result of the HIA is that for immigrants in the long term there would be a positive impact on economic security, employment/education, social network, belief in the future and living habits. Access to healthcare would, on the other hand, be influenced on a long- and short-term basis for immigrants, and in the long term for the entire population. According to the HIA one can expect further development of health-promoting work for different ethnic groups.

The reaction from the local politicians so far has been quite positive. They stress that HIA is an attitude or approach, not the mechanistic application of any formula; that tools should not be too complicated and that they should be developed in a constantly ongoing process.

Conclusions

There is increased interest in HIA at international, national and local levels. There is also increased concern in some countries with growing health gaps. This offers a unique opportunity for taking a strategic position to ensure that HIA achieves its potential to:

- make equality in health a central value against which to test policy proposals in all sectors;
- identify population groups that may be disadvantaged by policy proposals in other sectors;
- achieve greater transparency regarding the potential impacts of decision-making;
- empower people who participate in HIA, particularly the disadvantaged or vulnerable;
- identify alternative policy proposals to reduce health gaps;
- monitor the impacts that arise after proposals are implemented.

It is recommended that policy-makers should be quickly informed about the main challenges and opportunities HIA presents. It is essential they are made aware of the ethical issues involved, and understand that although HIA is a political process, unavoidable value judgements can be made in a more transparent, democratic manner.

The research community will need to quickly improve two basic types of knowledge: what could be termed 'quantified risk assessment', and more qualitative measures frequently more appropriate for HIA, but which must be equally credible and reliable. The availability of data on subgroups of the population needs to be greatly improved. Some groups are doubly disadvantaged, having not only higher exposure to harmful impacts but greater susceptibility to them; furthermore, they are frequently the victims of multiple disadvantages. Disentangling these various strands also presents a challenge. If HIA can meet these challenges, it will contribute to strengthening the evidence base for policy-making.

The knowledge base for HIA needs to be quickly shared. Much of the existing knowledge is available only in the grey literature or through pains-taking networking between HIA exponents. Mechanisms need to be set up to allow countries across Europe to share relevant knowledge. This would not only improve the HIA process, but also enhance policy-relevant know-ledge in general.

There are insufficient people available to carry out HIA in most countries in Europe. There is an urgent need to develop capacity through training and the sharing of skills and experiences.

HIA can only become an effective tool for the promotion of equality in health if it is seen to be feasible and effective, not unduly resource-consuming, and if stakeholders, including the most vulnerable, have ownership of the process. This will require ethical discussions related to the balancing of resources and time needed for democratic processes and the challenge of involving vulnerable groups. The HIA process must be reasonably rapid and effective, and integrated in the overall policy development process.

This will require ingenuity and resourcefulness in breaking away from some of the old ways of doing things, and properly funded, staffed and organized structures and processes. It will also mean exploring more fully the possibilities offered by new communications technology.

References

1. WHO. *Health 21 – The Health for All Policy Framework for the WHO European Region*. European Health for All Series no. 6. Copenhagen: WHO Regional Office, 1990.
2. Ritstakis A, Barnes R, Dekker E, Harrington P, Kokko S, Makara P, eds. *Exploring Health Policy Development in Europe*. European Series no 86. Copenhagen: WHO Regional Office, 2000.
3. Marmot M, Wilkinson RG, eds. *Social Determinants of Health*. New York: Oxford University Press, 1999.
4. Wilkinson RG. *Unhealthy Societies – the Afflictions of Inequality*. New York: Routledge, 1996.
5. Commission of the European Communities. *Communication from the Commission to the Council, the European Parliament, the Economic and Social Committee and the Committee of the Regions on the Health Strategy of the European Community*. Brussels: COM (2000) 285, 2000.
6. Council resolution of 8 June 1999 on the future Community action in the field of public health. *Official Journal* C200, 15/07/1999, 0001–0002.
7. *Ibid.* pp. 19–20.
8. Ostlin P, Diderichsen F. *Equity-oriented National Strategy for Public Health in Sweden*. Policy Learning Curve Series no 1. Brussels: WHO European Centre for Health Policy, 2000.
9. Roscam-Abbing EW, van Zoest FF, Put GV. Health impact assessment and intersectoral policy at national level in The Netherlands. In: *Health Impact Assessment: from Theory to Practice. Report on the Leo Kaprio Workshop.*

Gothenburg: WHO European Centre for Health Policy and Nordic School of Public Health, 2001.

10. Acheson Sir D (Chair) *Independent Inquiry into Inequalities in Health. Report.* London: The Stationery Office, 1998.

11. Department of Health. *Reducing Health Inequalities: an Action Report.* London: The Stationery Office, 1999.

12. Frankish CJ, Green LW, Ratner PA, Chomik T, Larsen C. *Health Impact Assessment as a Tool for Population Health Promotion and Public Policy. A Report Submitted to the Health Promotion Development Division of Health Canada.* British Columbia: Institute of Health Promotion, Research University of British Columbia, 1996.

13. *Health Impact Assessment: from Theory to Practice. Report on the Leo Kaprio Workshop.* Gothenburg: WHO European Centre for Health Policy and Nordic School of Public Health, 2001.

14. *Health Impact Assessment: Main Concepts and Suggested Approach.* Consensus paper. Brussels: WHO European Centre for Health Policy. Website: http://www.who.dk/hs/EHCP.index.htm.

15. Whitehead M. *The Concepts and Principles of Equity and Health.* Copenhagen: WHO Regional Office, 1990.

16. Barnes R, ed. *Equity and Health Impact Assessment Seminar* (Manchester 16–17 June 2000: Report). Liverpool: Public Health Observatory, 2000. Website: www.liv.ac.uk/Public Health/obs/OBS.HTM.

17. Goran NP, Whitehead M, eds. *Health Impact Assessment of the EU Common Agricultural Policy.* Stockholm: Swedish National Institute of Public Health, 1996.

18. Scottish Needs Assessment Programme. *Health Impact Assessment of the City of Edinburgh Council's Urban Transport Strategy.* Glasgow: Scottish Needs Assessment Programme, 2000.

19. British Medical Association. *Road Transport and Health.* London: BMA, 1997.

20. Jefferis P, Rowell A, Fergusson M. *The Exposure of Car Drivers and Passengers to Vehicle Emissions: Comparative Pollution Levels inside and outside Vehicles. A Report for Greenpeace by Earth Resources Research.* London: Greenpeace 1992.

21. The full report and a summary of this HIA are currently in press.

22. Scott-Samuel A, Birley M, Ardern K. *The Merseyside Guidelines for Health Impact Assessment.* Liverpool: Public Health Observatory, 1998.

23. *Focusing on Health: How can the Health Impact of Policy Decisions be Assessed?* Stockholm: Federation of Swedish County Councils, Association of Swedish Local Authorities, 1998. Website: http://www.lf.se.

21 Theory-based evaluation

New approaches to evaluating complex community-based initiatives

Ken Judge and Mhairi Mackenzie

Introduction

A growing number of European countries acknowledge the importance of socioeconomic inequalities in health. Many of them are now committed to identifying and promoting policies that will reduce avoidable deaths and diseases associated with material and social disadvantage, but the evidence base to guide positive action is relatively weak. A recent review of policy recommendations for tackling inequalities in the United Kingdom (UK), for example, concludes that the goal of evidence-based public policy is currently an aspiration rather than a reality (1). This knowledge gap poses a challenge to the scientific community to make the most effective use of what is already known, but it also requires the development of new approaches to learning about effective methods of intervening to promote a more equitable distribution of health opportunities.

It is useful to distinguish between two main strands of action that can be taken to tackle socioeconomic inequalities in health: broadly based public policies and actions, and more focused health promotion initiatives. The first relates to those policies with primary goals that are not directly health-related. Such policies might include anti-poverty strategies, welfare to work schemes, and the economic and physical regeneration of disadvantaged neighbourhoods. The challenge in these areas is to assess the health-related impact of policies and practices that may have a multiplicity of other objectives. This is very much the territory that health impact assessment seeks to evaluate and which was considered in detail in Chapter 20.

The second area of action is concerned with interventions, policies, practices and processes that have improvements in health, for either the population as a whole or for subgroups within it, among their primary objectives. The challenge here is to consider what evaluation methods are most appropriate to the generation of effective learning about how best to promote health for particular communities. In part the answer will be a very familiar one. Over many years the scientific community has developed reliable methods for evaluating the cost-effectiveness of interventions that lend themselves to experimental evaluation at the individual level. These approaches are particularly applicable to assessing the impact on the health of individuals of particular drugs or other kinds of therapeutic interventions. Carefully designed studies with well defined interventions can generate very powerful learning about the health consequences of different courses of action. However, there are a host of other forms of health-promoting interventions that combine a number of mechanisms within complex contexts. These are aimed as much at groups or communities as they are at individuals, and as Davey Smith *et al.* point out (2), 'The sort of evidence gathered on the benefits of interventions aimed at individuals may not help in guiding policies directed towards reducing health inequalities' (p. 184).

As a result, there is a growing body of opinion that broadly based approaches to health promotion require rather different methods of evaluation (3). Moreover, it is not only in the fields of health promotion and public health, where there is an increasing emphasis on building comprehensive intervention strategies through partnerships with multiple agencies and communities, that the challenge of evaluation in the face of complexity is acknowledged. For example, there is a growing recognition among health services researchers that many common healthcare interventions – such as stroke units or hospital at home schemes – have their own forms of complexity that demand new approaches to evaluation (4). But we are concerned with initiatives that are not only complex in terms of their interconnecting parts but which are very wide-ranging in their scope and are about achieving social change in a rapidly changing world.

The aim of this chapter is to outline one approach that lends itself particularly well to the evaluation of those kinds of complex community-based health promotion initiatives that are likely to be most suited to tackling inequalities in health. Such schemes vary considerably in their scope and detail, but typically they tend to have a number of features in common.

Connell and Kubisch (5), for example, describe the aim of Comprehensive Community Initiatives (CCIs) as being: to promote positive changes in individual, family and community institutions; to develop a variety of mechanisms to improve social, economic and physical circumstances, services and conditions in disadvantaged communities; and to place a strong emphasis on community building and neighbourhood empowerment.

These characteristics pose a number of challenges for evaluation because:

- Such initiatives have multiple, broad goals.
- They are highly complex learning enterprises with multiple strands of activity operating at many different levels.
- Objectives are defined and strategies chosen to achieve goals that often change over time – for example, interventions that aim to be locally driven need to respond to community needs, and these cannot necessarily be defined at the outset.
- Many activities and intended outcomes are difficult to measure, because units of action are complex, open systems in which it is

> virtually impossible to control all the variables that may influence the conduct and outcome of evaluation.

- The saturation of a given community with a particular intervention limits further the potential for traditional experimental designs.
- Improving health outcomes which are socially determined takes longer than the lifespan of an evaluation.

So, as Schorr (cited in (6)) argues, comprehensive interventions are both the most promising in terms of impact and the least likely to be understood using traditionally credible methods.

These considerations point to the pressing need to review more flexible evaluation frameworks, as simply to ignore investments in highly complex programmes or initiatives would be to seriously reduce the potential for learning about how best to tackle many intractable social problems, including socioeconomic inequalities in health.

What is required is an approach that can help to modify or clarify the design and implementation of initiatives in ways that lend themselves to evaluation. This is where theory-driven approaches have a crucial role to play, although it is important not to place excessive weight on the use of the term 'theory'. For example, a discussion document drafted by members of the Health Services and Public Health Research Board of the Medical Research Council in the UK (4) recommends that investigators should:

> incorporate a theoretical phase to the development of their evaluation of a complex intervention. In this way investigators force themselves to consider underlying assumptions being made, whether at the physiological, psychological, organizational or whatever level regarding postulated mechanisms and processes in the intervention being examined. The use of the term 'theoretical' is intended to refer to formal studies of evidence where they exist, but ... for many areas fields may not have been developed to a stage of providing clearly delineated bodies of evidence, 'theory' may be too grand a term for the body of evidence or the field may be fluid and the choice of relevant theory very unclear for any given research problem. In some cases, the relevant body of evidence may be less formal 'theory' and more accumulating wisdom from empirical evidence. (p. 6)

Theory-based evaluation

Definition

The concept of theory-based evaluation has evolved over the past 25 years or so in response to the kinds of difficulties outlined earlier. For example, Wholey (7, 8) developed the concept of *evaluability assessment*, which implies 'that prior to the start of a formal study, the evaluator should analyse the logical reasoning that connected programme inputs to desired outcomes to see whether there was a reasonable likelihood that goals could be achieved'. Since then a number of contributors (9, 10) have made significant advances to thinking about how best to evaluate complex public policy programmes and the results have manifested themselves in a variety of ways in a number of countries, including Australia, Canada, the UK and the United States (USA).

One of the most comprehensive and persuasive approaches to evaluation that follows the logic of theory-based evaluation and which seems especially applicable to learning about community-based initiatives that aim to reduce health inequalities is described by the Aspen Institute in the USA (11, 12) as 'theories of change'.

The theory of change approach to evaluation has been developed over a number of years through the work of the Aspen Institute's Roundtable on Comprehensive Community Initiatives. It was developed in an effort to find ways of evaluating processes and outcomes in community-based programmes that were not adequately addressed by existing approaches, and is defined as 'a systematic and cumulative study of the links between activities, outcomes and contexts of the initiative' (5). The approach aims to gain clarity around the overall vision or theory of change of the initiative, meaning the long-term outcomes and the strategies that are intended to produce them. In generating this theory, steps are taken to link the original problem or con-text in which the programme began with the activities planned to address the problem and the medium- and longer-term outcomes intended. This framework has much in common with the development in the UK of 'real-istic evaluation' (13).

Advantages

Connell and Kubisch (5) provide a number of convincing reasons why this approach to evaluating complex and evolving initiatives is an attractive one.

First, a theory of change can sharpen the planning and implementation of an initiative. An emphasis on programme logic or theory during the design phase can increase the probability that stakeholders will clearly specify the intended outcomes of an initiative, the activities that need to be imple-mented in order to achieve them, and the contextual factors that are likely to influence them. Secondly, with a theory of change approach the measure-ment and data collection elements of the evaluation process will be facili-tated. It requires stakeholders to be as clear as possible about not only the final outcomes and effects they hope to achieve, but also the means by which they expect to achieve them. This knowledge is used to focus scarce evaluation resources on what and how to measure. Finally, and most import-antly, articulating a theory of change early in the life of an initiative, and gaining agreement about it by all the stakeholders, helps to reduce problems associated with causal attribution of impact.

Problems associated with attribution, causation and generalization are common to most health promotion initiatives. A theory of change approach explicitly addresses these issues. It involves the specification of how activities will lead to intermediate and long-term outcomes and an identification of the contextual conditions that may affect them. This helps strengthen the scientific case for attributing subsequent change in outcomes to the activities included in the initiative. Of course, it is important to acknowledge that using the theory of change approach to evaluation cannot eliminate all alternative explanations for a particular outcome. What it can do is to provide key stakeholders with evidence grounded in their own assumptions and experiences that will be convincing to them. Indeed, at the most general level the theory of change approach assumes that the more the events predicted by theory actually occur over the lifetime of an initiative, the more confidence evaluators and others should have that the initiative's theory is right.

We acknowledge that not everyone feels comfortable about this assumption: it is counterintuitive for many people who are more familiar with traditional approaches to evaluation. The important point to emphasize, however, is that we are not asserting that prospective, theory-based approaches to evaluation are superior to other methods: what we do believe is that in some circumstances a theory of change approach can usefully complement quasi-experimental designs.

Illustrations

To illustrate the ways in which more traditional methods can be embedded within a theory-based approach we consider the examples of Starting Well and Have a Heart Paisley, two of four recently established Scottish Health Demonstration Projects. These projects are topic-based interventions operating at an individual and a community level with a common goal of tackling health inequalities. Starting Well, based in Glasgow, focuses on mechanisms for reducing early childhood inequalities, whereas Have a Heart Paisley aims to address coronary health inequalities. A similar evaluation framework has been developed for both interventions and can be characterized as follows:

- Understanding the theory, context and process of the intervention
- Assessing the impact of the intervention
- Drawing policy lessons from the pilot projects.

The first component of the evaluation will include the development of a theoretical understanding of the intervention and its intended outcomes, an exploration of the social context within which the project is located, and an in-depth investigation of participants' views of the utility of the initiative.

The second element of the evaluation will consist of a more traditional, quasi-experimental approach utilizing outcome data from the intervention and control areas. However, given the scale of the health and social problems with which these pilot projects will be operating, changes in outcome over a 3-year period are likely to be small. We believe that setting the quasi-experimental design within the theory-based approach should augment the learning of policy lessons about the realistic impacts of initiatives on both process and outcome.

This point assumes even greater importance when the scope for introducing an experimental component to the evaluation of an initiative is severely limited. For example, with the widespread introduction of Health Action Zones (HAZs) (see Chapter 12 and Box 21.1) to localities containing more than a quarter of the English population, the possibility of finding satisfactory control areas was seriously limited. In this case a theory-based approach may offer the only realistic way of introducing an element of structure and discipline to the process of designing and learning from 'messy' initiatives in 'real world' situations. We are in no doubt that theory-based approaches can and do improve the quality of learning, and strengthen the kinds of inferences that can be made about cause and effect mechanisms in complex social change processes, even in the absence of more traditional evaluation designs.

Theories of change in Health Action Zones

Choice of evaluation method

A theory-based approach informs the national evaluation of Health Action Zones (see Box 21.1) in England (14–16). Figure 21.1 illustrates the approach being adopted. The starting point is the context within which HAZs operate – the resources available in the communities and the challenges that they face. Once this is established, the key challenge is for HAZs to articulate a logical way of achieving social change and to specify targets for each of their interventions that satisfy two requirements. First, they should be articulated in advance of the expected consequences of actions. Second, these actions and their associated milestones or targets should form part of a logical pathway that leads towards strategic goals or outcomes.

Initial work with HAZs is yielding valuable lessons about the type of information needed if any serious attempt is to be made to learn from their activities. Knowledge is required regarding the ways in which different configurations of contexts, strategies, interventions and their associated consequences contribute to improving health and healthcare for disadvantaged communities. This type of knowledge can be gained only on a continuous basis, through an approach to evaluation that recognizes the evolving nature of HAZ plans and activities. Promoting and achieving change in pursuit of ambitious goals will be possible only if HAZs are encouraged to invest in the planning process, to take risks, and to adapt to changing circumstances.

Box 21.1 Health Action Zones

In the first few months of office New Labour announced their intention to set up Health Action Zones (HAZs) in selected areas as 7-year pilot projects 'to explore mechanisms for breaking through current organizational boundaries to tackle inequalities and to deliver better services'. Local partnerships between health and local authorities were invited to bid for HAZ status. Forty-one bids were received; 11 areas were successful in achieving HAZ status in April 1998, and a further 15 in April 1999. Together these areas cover 13 million people in England and include some of the most disadvantaged areas of the country.

Tackling inequalities in health is central to HAZs' agenda, with Ministers frequently describing them as being in the 'vanguard' or 'frontline of the war on health inequalities'. Although HAZs have been given modest additional funding to adopt new and innovative projects to modernize services or reduce health inequalities, the key to their success is that they act as a catalyst to reorientate mainstream activities in their zone to work in new more effective ways. The foundation of this new way of working is a partnership between health and local authorities, voluntary and community groups and, in some places, other agencies. The way in which these partnerships are formed and work together to assess their needs, develop their strategies and deliver their services is fundamental to the success of the HAZ initiative. Crucially, they must develop a strategy to achieve their goal of improving health and reducing health inequalities, and ways of monitoring and learning from what they achieve.

What are HAZs doing about health inequalities?

A review of HAZs' plans shows that their goals to reduce health inequalities range along a spectrum. At one end are those HAZs with high deprivation and mortality rates, whose goals focus on reducing inequalities between them and an external reference point, for example the national average. At the other extreme are those zones whose levels of health status and deprivation are nearer to the national average and have focused almost entirely on reducing inequalities within their zone. The kind of activities that HAZs have funded varies considerably. Some have chosen to focus very specifically on reducing inequalities in access to health services, because it is something they feel they can achieve in the short term. Others have very much taken a lifestyle/settings approach, whereas others have focused on some of the social and economic determinants of health such as unemployment, low incomes, social isolation and poor neighbourhood infrastructures.

Early lessons from HAZ

Early interviews with key stakeholders in HAZs showed incredible enthusiasm and commitment to really making a difference to the lives of their populations. HAZs have introduced some innovative plans to address some of the key determinants of health, as well as tackling some of the obstacles to effective access to health services. However, progress has been frustratingly slow for a number of reasons. First, establishing effective partnership arrangements and actively involving communities in decision-making takes time. Secondly, in addition to being HAZs, many of these areas are the subject of a range of other partnership initiatives, each with their own structures and goals. Some areas feel paralysed by partnerships, rather than liberated through them to work in new ways. Thirdly, many HAZs failed to develop coherent strategies. To varying degrees their plans were strong on identifying problems and articulating long-term objectives, but much less effective on filling in the gap between the two. Early interventions were often 'leaps of faith' rather than clear and logical steps in the pathway between their problems and desired outcomes. This problem is not unique to HAZs, but common to many complex community initiatives. Nevertheless, HAZs have made significant progress since then in clarifying their strategies and strengthening their partnership foundations. Given sufficient time and space they have a real opportunity to make a difference to the health of their populations and to generate real policy learning about how to reduce inequalities in health in the future.

Source: Judge *et al.* (14)

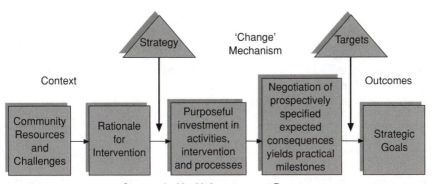

Community Health Improvement Process

Figure 21.1 Realistic evaluation and theories of change

Practical examples

All HAZs start with a vision statement of some kind that embraces their primary goals. In each HAZ a set of strategic goals or 'aspirational' targets is closely related to the vision. These objectives are then pursued through a series of work-streams or programmes that comprise a large number of projects. Each of these activities is expected to generate a range of outcomes in the short, medium and longer term. At each stage in this process – the project, the programme and the overall initiative in each HAZ – it is possible and desirable to develop a theory of change. In practice, it has proved easier for the zones to start to develop theories of change for individual projects than at the most general level; for an example of a logic model relating to smoking cessation services see 16. A key challenge is to develop convincing and acceptable theory of change models for HAZs as whole systems. For the moment we provide an illustration of the kind of progress that is being made and the difficulties being encountered.

Developing a logic model

In practice, developing models of logical pathways is typically a complex business. It is clear that many social goals, such as reducing health inequalities, require multiple interventions that interact in a variety of ways, some of which can be quite subtle. As a result it becomes even more important to work prospectively with key stakeholders to:

- clarify the nature of, and rationale for, interventions;
- map the outcomes that are expected to materialize at different points in time so that they can be monitored;
- use evidence about impact to review the underlying theory and to modify it if necessary.

Our experience to date is that this is a demanding set of requirements. Health Action Zones are making determined attempts to develop logical pathways in many complex areas. However, given the resources and time at their disposal, questions arise as to their capacity to make effective progress.

We can illustrate the state of development with a reasonably typical example taken from the annual progress report of one HAZ.

Table 21.1 extracts some key information about strategies, intermediate outcomes and ultimate purposes or goals associated with a typical example of a local intervention that forms part of a determined attempt to reduce health inequalities. Our purpose in using this example is to illustrate the degree to which HAZs still have a great deal of work to do if they are to develop clear and plausible pathways of change that stand any chance of delivering the ambitious goals that they have set for themselves.

Table 21.1 An embryonic logic model

Strategies	Intermediate outcomes	Purposes and goal
Develop accessible, appropriate health information for young people	Health education modules incorporated into all government training schemes by April 2000	**General purpose:** to improve the health of children and young people through coordinated efforts of communities and organizations in partnership with young people
Reduce number of young people involved in risk-taking behaviour	2,000 young people contacted by peer educators on sexual health	**Specific objective:** to reduce the incidence of teenage conceptions
	40 at event on boys and sexual health	**Related goal:** rate of conceptions under 16 reduced by at least one-third by 2005 against a 1989 baseline
	500 pupils benefit from peer education in a baby doll project	

This particular example relates to one HAZ goal of reducing pregnancies in girls under the age of 16 by one-third within a specified time-frame as part of an overall purpose of improving the health of children and young people. Our purpose is to examine the extent to which the example satisfies the principal criteria of a logic model, that it should be plausible, doable, testable and meaningful (17).

Problems encountered

The first thing to note is that the specific objective of reducing teenage conceptions as part of a general policy of improving the health of children and young people is a testable one. A very clear target is specified: to reduce conceptions in those under the age of 16 by at least one-third by 2005 compared with a 1989 baseline. However, one aspect of the general purpose is not so clear: it is not obvious from the information contained in the plan how success will be assessed in relation to the goal of improving health through a strategy that involves coordinated efforts of communities and organizations in partnership with young people. Furthermore, there is virtually no information about intervention strategies to pursue this goal, or indicators of intermediate outcomes that would demonstrate progress towards the partnership goal. More generally, even in the specific case of reducing teenage conceptions, where there is at least an indication of the nature of strategic interventions and how they might be developed in practice, there is a huge plausibility gap between actual activities and the ambitious nature of the long-term target. The progress associated with specific activities in the *intermediate outcomes* column of Table 21.1 is all very well in itself, but it is not obvious why they should be sufficient to achieve the level of reduction in conceptions that is sought. The pathways of expected change are simply not specified in sufficient detail for it to be possible to make a reasonable judgement about whether the target is feasible. Part of the reason for this, we suspect, is that agencies are cajoled into setting themselves unrealistic targets for political reasons. The overemphasis in the modern world on aspirational goals leaves organizations floundering in search of effective change strategies. A more realistic approach would be to set targets only in terms of the genuinely expected consequences of well specified interventions. But given the existing state of knowledge about how best to reduce social problems, such an approach might look very modest and rather piecemeal to politicians, who are always tempted to promise that they can change the world before the next election.

Although the details vary, these kinds of questions arise in relation to almost all of the logical pathways that we have looked at. Partly this is a function of the difficulty of specifying change where it is likely to be synergistic. A more general problem is that even when an initial change pathway has been agreed at the local level, stakeholders fail to identify or reach agreement about which precise indicators demonstrate the success of a project, programme or initiative.

Nevertheless, the teenage pregnancy example captures the importance of theory-based evaluation as a means of improving the planning of an intervention (and the articulation of that planning). When it is used properly it helps to make explicit the assumptions about expected outcomes associated with purposeful interventions. More generally, it provides a means of identifying priorities for monitoring and evaluation by bringing to the surface potentially testable theories about complex processes of social change. Unfortunately, local stakeholders are rarely given sufficient time and technical assistance to pursue these objectives.

Conclusions

Satisfying the needs of policy-makers for clear guidance about how best to reduce health inequalities is not straightforward. There are conflicting views, for example, in the scientific community about what constitutes good evidence and how such knowledge should be acquired (1, 2).

Some commentators argue that simple observation might be a more practical tool than the evaluation of experiments, which in any event can be seen as relatively trivial in relation to the problems they are intended to address. Nevertheless, whatever their merits might be, it is clear that many governments are wedded to the process of developing, and trying to learn from, targeted initiatives that are intended to contribute to the reduction of health inequalities. In these circumstances, maximizing clarity about the aims and methods of such interventions is a critical requirement.

Our experience of working with Health Action Zones is that there will be more scope for productive action and learning if a theory-based approach to design, implementation and evaluation is adopted at the earliest possible stage (18). As Carol Weiss (19) has persuasively written, 'there is nothing as practical as good theory'.

But no matter how creative researchers and practitioners prove to be in devising and learning about new approaches to tackling intractable social problems, there are real limitations. 'Politicians and civil servants need to be aware that in many fields there are no unequivocal answers to the question "what works?"' (1). Nevertheless, strenuous efforts to expand the scope of knowledge about what works and for whom and in what circumstances are worthwhile.

There are two key challenges for the future. One prerequisite is to find better ways of empowering demonstration projects, pathfinder initiatives and pilot schemes to fulfil their potential by helping them to develop and implement more explicit theories of change from which new knowledge can be generated and disseminated. The second requirement is to educate policymakers about the pros and cons of different kinds of evidence, the length of time that it takes to learn worthwhile lessons, and the value of employing mixed methods to strengthen the inferences that can be obtained from the evaluation of complex community-based interventions.

References

1. Macintyre S, Chalmers I, Horton R, Smith R. Using evidence to inform health policy: case study. *Br Med J* 2001: 322: 222–5.
2. Davey Smith G, Ebrahim S, Frankel S. How policy informs the evidence. *Br Med J* 2001: 322: 184–5.
3. Gillies P. *Evidence Base 2000: Evidence into Practice*. London: Health Education Authority, 1999.
4. Campbell M, Fitzpatrick R, Haines A, Kinmouth AL, Sandercock P, Spiegelhalter, D *et al*. Framework for design and evaluation of complex interventions to improve health. *Br Med J* 2001: 321: 694–6.
5. Connell JP, Kubisch AC. Applying a theory of change approach to the evaluation of comprehensive community initiatives: progress, prospects, and problems. In: Fulbright-Anderson K, Kubisch AC, Connell JP, eds. *New Approaches to Evaluating Community Initiatives. Volume 2 Theory, Measurement, and Analysis.* Washington DC: The Aspen Institute, 1998.
6. The Brookings Institution Governmental Studies Program. *Learning what Works: Evaluating Complex Social Interventions, Report on the Symposium.* 1998.
7. Wholey JS. *Evaluation and Effective Public Management.* Boston: Little, Brown, 1983.
8. Weiss C. Theory-based evaluation: past, present and future. *New Directions for Evaluation* 1997: 76: 41–55.
9. Chen H. *Theory-driven Evaluation.* California: Thousand Oaks, 1990.
10. Weiss C. How can theory-based evaluation make greater headway? *Evaluation Rev* 1997: 21(4): 501–8.
11. Connell JP, Kubisch AC, Schorr LB, Weiss CH, eds. *New Approaches to Evaluating Community Initiatives: Concepts, Methods and Contexts.* Washington DC: The Aspen Institute, 1995.

12. Fulbright-Anderson K, Kubisch AC, Connell, JP, eds. *New Approaches to Evaluating Community Initiatives. Volume 2 Theory, Measurement, and Analysis.* Washington DC: The Aspen Institute, 1998.

13. Pawson R, Tilley N. *Realistic Evaluation.* London: Sage, 1997.

14. Judge K, Barnes M, Bauld L, Benzeval M, Killoran A, Robinson R *et al. Health Action Zones: Learning to Make a Difference.* PSSRU Discussion Paper 1546. Canterbury: University of Kent at Canterbury, 1999. Website: http://www.ukc.ac.uk/pssru/download.html.

15. Judge K. Testing the limits of evaluation: Health Action Zones in England. *J Health Serv Res Policy* 2000: 5(1): 3–5.

16. Judge K, Bauld L. Strong theory, flexible methods: evaluating complex community-based initiatives. *Critical Public Health* 2001: 11(1): 19–38.

17. Connell JP, Klem AM. *You Can Get there from here: Using a Theory of Change Approach to Plan Urban Education Reform.* Philadelphia, PA: Institute for Research and Reform in Education, 1999.

18. Adams C, Bauld L, Judge K. No smoking without fire: smoking cessation in Health Action Zones. *Health Serv J* 2000: 28–31.

19. Weiss C. Nothing as practical as good theory. Exploring theory-based evaluation for comprehensive community initiatives for children and families. In: Connell JP, Kubisch AC, Schorr LB, Weiss CH, eds. *New Approaches to Evaluating Community Initiatives. Vol 1.* Washington DC: The Aspen Institute, 1995.

Part V

Reflections

22 Gender perspective on socioeconomic inequalities in health

Piroska Östlin

Introduction

The aim of this chapter is to provide evidence that could justify the need for gender-sensitive policies and interventions to more effectively reduce socioeconomic inequalities in health among women and among men. We discuss why it is important to consider the interaction of socioeconomic position and gender in health equality studies, and summarize what we know about the extent of socioeconomic inequalities in health among men and women. Then we discuss why policies and interventions may not have the same effect on men and women. Furthermore, the policies described in other chapters will be reviewed through a gender lens. Finally, two examples of interventions, from Sweden and Scotland, will be given that may have important bearings on reducing socioeconomic inequalities between men and women, as well as within different groups of women and different groups of men.

Why is gender an important issue in relation to socioeconomic inequalities in health?

The growing interest in socioeconomic inequalities in health has not yet spilled over effectively into a consideration of gender. Similarly, the accumulating literature on gender inequalities in health has not fully recognized that neither women nor men are homogeneous categories in terms of socioeconomic background. This is probably due to the common fallacy that conflates gender with biological difference (1). It is important for both research and policy to recognize the analytical distinction between *sex* and *gender*. *Sex* refers to the biologically recognized differences between men and women, pertaining to the ability to reproduce; *gender* is a social category that defines the social and cultural construction of femininity and masculinity. Moreover, gender, as a key form of social stratification, has a paramount importance in relation to the hierarchical ordering of society in terms of wealth, power and prestige, which in turn generates inequalities in the distribution of resources, benefits and responsibilities. As health-damaging gender relations are socially and culturally constructed, these could be changed through active measures (2).

Gender, interacting with socioeconomic group, is profoundly and consistently related to health, mainly because these fundamental factors structure over the life course the likelihood of women's and men's differential risks, exposures and susceptibility to disease, their access to health protective resources, as well as differential consequences of ill health (3, 4). Health inequalities between women and men within any given socioeconomic group can be significant: even though socioeconomic group may be the main determinant of health inequalities, significant differences in health outcomes by gender still remain within each class level (5, 6). The interaction between gender and socioeconomic group may be either additive or multiplicative: factors related to socioeconomic position can deepen or counteract the effect of gender on health outcomes (1). The interface between gender and social position should therefore be a significant issue in research on socioeconomic inequalities in health, and for policy implications.

The extent of socioeconomic inequalities in health among men and women

High socioeconomic status is consistently associated with better health among both women and men in all societies, regardless of how we measure social position or health outcome. There are, however, a few examples of specific diseases where health status is inversely related to social status. For example, breast cancer incidence is associated with higher socioeconomic status in women, and lung cancer is more common in higher social classes in countries where smoking is more prevalent among these classes. Such associations can be explained by particular causal factors (7).

In countries where analyses of the magnitude of socioeconomic inequalities in total mortality among both women and men have been performed, apparently smaller socioeconomic inequalities were reported for women (8–11). A number of potential mechanisms behind this commonly observed pattern have been suggested (8): choice of indicator used to measure socioeconomic position; the confounding influence of various sociodemographic variables; and differences in the distribution of causes of death among men and women. Although the choice of socioeconomic indicator does affect the relative magnitude of inequalities among both men and women, these inequalities, regardless of the measures used, still appear to be smaller among women. However, in a study of Finnish men and women, Koskinen and Martelin (8) found that this general observation applied only to married individuals. The socioeconomic mortality gradient was just as steep in relative terms among single, divorced or widowed women as among men.

Those studies where larger socioeconomic inequalities among men rather than women were reported suggest that the pattern may be partly the result of the distribution of causes of death among men and women (8, 9, 11, 12).

At the level of total mortality, it has been shown that the causes of death with large inequalities tend to be common among men, whereas those for which socioeconomic inequalities in mortality are small or even reversed (for example, breast cancer) are often common among women (13). An international study of differences by sex in the magnitude of socioeconomic inequalities in cause-specific mortality in seven countries (USA, Finland, Norway, Italy, Czech Republic, Hungary and Estonia) revealed large male/female contrasts for mortality from lung cancer, respiratory diseases and external causes (11). Inequalities for these causes of death were very large among men and almost absent among women. However, relative inequalities were larger in most countries among women than among men for cardiovascular diseases, and particularly for ischaemic heart disease. Similar results have also been observed in Sweden (9).

Regarding morbidity, the general observation is that socioeconomic inequalities are more obvious among men than among women (14, 15). A study by Stronks and colleagues (14) found that inequalities in chronic conditions and perceived general health were clearly evident among men, but there were hardly any differences among women. There is, however, a growing body of evidence that indicates the complexity of these findings. Again, the choice of indicator used to measure socioeconomic position appears to have a great relevance: for instance, when studying rates of self-perceived health, educational qualifications showed a sharper gradient than occupational class among women (16). Age seems to have a confounding influence as well: among 18-year-olds West (17) found steep occupational class gradients in various self-reported health measures for men but not for women. However, when socioeconomic gradient in self-assessed health among 33-year-olds was analysed, no difference could be observed between men and women (18). Moreover, the magnitude of socioeconomic inequalities in morbidity is influenced differently in men and women also by country (19), health measure (16) and working conditions (20).

In spite of these gender associations in socioeconomic inequalities in health, the general belief that the socioeconomic gradient among women is systematically less steep than among men might be one reason why women have been relatively invisible in both research and policy discussions of socioeconomic inequalities in health.

Interventions and policies

Why should policies and interventions to reduce inequalities in health among men and women have a different focus?

Gender differences in cause-specific mortality and morbidity suggest that interventions to reduce inequalities in health among women should have a (partly) different focus. This is confirmed by analyses of inequalities in risk factors among women compared to men, which show that the explanation of inequalities in health may be different among women than among men. Whereas most factors that contribute to socioeconomic inequalities in health among men (for example, material disadvantage, employment status, marital status, childhood conditions, work environmental factors and health-related behaviours) also contribute to inequalities among women, there may be important gender differences in regard to the social patterning of these determinants of health.

One example is the social patterning of harmful exposures at work, which are strongly associated with socioeconomic status and vary greatly by gender because of gender-segregated labour. In most industrialized countries more men than women are exposed to noise, vibrations, unfavourable climate, organic solvents and most other types of physical and chemical risk. Consequently, solvent-related illnesses, hearing loss, vibration injuries and occupational accidents are more common among men. These exposures and related illnesses are considerably more prevalent in low socioeconomic groups. Women, on the other hand, are more often than men exposed to repetitive working movements, monotonous work, the risk of being subjected to violence and negative stress, 'the combination of high mental strain at work and low decision latitude' (21, 22). Consequently, feelings of fatigue, repetitive strain injury and other work-related musculoskeletal disorders, and psychosocial health problems are more common among women than among men. Thus, interventions to eliminate heavy lifting at work would be an effective measure to reduce socioeconomic inequalities in musculoskeletal disorders among men. More effective interventions to reduce such inequalities among women would be the elimination of repetitive working movements and stress. This different focus of intervention is needed simply because of the gender differences in the work-related aetiology of musculoskeletal disorders.

Another example is the social patterning of those health-related behaviours that are assumed to make a major contribution to mortality from lung cancer, respiratory diseases and external causes, for example, smoking behaviour and heavy drinking, proved in a number of studies to be stronger among men than among women. The currently observed larger inequality among men in lung cancer and respiratory disease mortality reflects the social patterning of smoking around the 1960s, when smoking was more prevalent among men in the lower socioeconomic groups. At the same time, the reverse pattern can be seen among women. As socioeconomic inequalities in current cigarette smoking are larger among women (for example, in Sweden) than among men, we can expect that the importance of smoking behaviour for socioeconomic inequalities in health in the future will increase among women and decrease among men.

Because inequalities in ischaemic heart disease mortality tend to be larger among women than among men, the social patterning of related risk factors, such as diet, lack of physical activity and obesity, is assumed to be stronger among women than among men. This is confirmed by an international study showing that inequalities in the prevalence of obesity were clearly larger among women (23). According to studies carried out in Britain and Sweden the highest body mass index is found in lower socioeconomic groups, whereas men show a reverse pattern (24). Thus, interventions to prevent obesity should be directed particularly towards the socially less advantaged women, whereas among men such interventions should focus on those in higher socioeconomic positions.

It is important to note that even if women are exposed to a particular health-damaging factor to the same degree as men, they may experience worse effects because of both biological and social factors. For example, because women have a higher proportion of fat tissue than men, they are at greater risk of harm from fat-soluble chemicals (25). Women's greater vulnerability to a particular risk may also be a result of socially and culturally determined factors. Swedish research has shown that ten hours' overtime a week increased the risk of heart attacks in women, whereas male subjects working a similar amount of overtime actually had a lower incidence than expected (26). The different consequences of overtime for women's and men's health, also within the same socioeconomic group, may reflect the higher level of stress put on women because of the conflict that can arise between their greater responsibility for household duties and gainful employment. As exposure to overtime work varies with socioeconomic group, it may contribute to socioeconomic inequalities in myocardial infarction in women, but may probably be unimportant in relation to the inequalities among men. The extent to which women in various social classes have the chance or the resources to balance themselves between the private sphere of family life and the public sphere of gainful employment, is probably significant in relation to socioeconomic inequalities in health among women, and increasingly also among men. Thus, policies that limit the extent of overtime working would probably have a greater positive health effect on women than on men.

The gender perspective in this book

A review of the policies and interventions described in other chapters included in the sections on 'Interventions and policies to reduce socioeconomic inequalities in health' through a gender lens show clearly the lack of gender perspective in most interventions. Generally, there seems to be an assumption that interventions to reduce socioeconomic inequalities in health will be just as effective for men as for women. Many interventions are gender blind and label those who are their subjects in such a way that it is not possible to decide whether men or women or both were included. Gender-neutral expressions, such as bus driver or hospital orderly (Chapter 6), homeless and immigrant (Chapter 5), children, students and adolescents (Chapter 9) or patients (Chapter 11) are frequently used. Mielck and colleagues in Chapter 9, however, remind us that it was not possible to distinguish between boys and girls in the statistics presented because such information was not available; moreover, there are hardly any gender-specific interventions, despite good scientific arguments for such interventions.

An example of a gender-sensitive intervention, described by Platt and colleagues in Chapter 8, is the Women, Low Income and Smoking Initiative, which paid attention to issues concerning smoking in ways that were more sensitive to women's needs and their daily lives. This initiative is an example of good practice also from a gender perspective. It would be instructive to design a similar intervention among men that took into account their needs and everyday life, and to compare how these interventions differ from those applied among women.

It is obvious that even though knowledge of gender differences in relation to socioeconomic inequalities in health is increasingly available, it does not always translate easily into political realities of health planning and programme implementation.

'Focus – development of the workplace from a gender perspective', Sweden

In a Swedish study 31 per cent of women and 11 per cent of men among skilled manual workers were exposed to negative stress at work, defined as low decision latitude combined with high mental demand (27). Among professionals the corresponding figures were 18 per cent for women and 12 per cent for men. Thus, the gender gap was considerably larger in the lower socioeconomic group. From other studies it is well known that negative stress is associated with a risk of myocardial infarction, mental health and musculoskeletal disorders (28). Most studies have concluded that the lack of potential to influence working conditions in particular had the strongest association with negative health effects.

Because the majority of women in the skilled manual working group in Sweden are assistant nurses, the Federation of County Councils, together with two county councils, in 1996 initiated an intervention programme called 'Focus – development of the workplace from a gender perspective', aimed at improving working conditions within the healthcare sector, with a special emphasis on the possibilities for work control (29). The intervention took place locally in two counties, with four particular workplaces as arenas. The implementation was advanced by participatory models that effectively engaged men and women in all personnel categories (including administrators), from physician to assistant nurse. The methods for improving working conditions included different forms of organizational change related to working hours; improving communications between men and women and between personnel categories; strengthening social networks in the workplace; introducing mentor programmes; improvements in professional competence and ability to use existing tools (for example, trade unions) more effectively to improve working conditions; and increasing the knowledge of staff regarding gender equality in the workplace. The intervention was performed from September 1996 until July 1997.

The evaluation of the Focus programme included a questionnaire survey before and after the intervention at the selected workplaces. On both occasions the questionnaire was also given to control groups at three workplaces not included in the programme. The survey included questions regarding gender equality in different respects at work, the possibility of influencing decisions, job satisfaction, the atmosphere at work, the possibility of learning new things at work, communication between men and women, and the time available for patients. No significant changes in these conditions could be shown for the control groups between the two surveys, but in the four workplaces where the intervention took place, significant positive changes could be measured in all personnel categories. However, there were some notable differences between these categories. For example, women in general reported more positive changes than did men: 30 per cent of the women (compared to none of the men) reported that their chance of influencing decisions at work had increased. Registered nurses reported the greatest increase (33 per cent) and assistant nurses the least (14 per cent); 48 per cent of the assistant nurses reported increased possibilities to learn new things at work, compared to 28 per cent of registered nurses and zero per cent among physicians; 57 per cent of all men and 36 per cent of all women reported that the communication between men and women had improved as a result of the programme.

Following the success of Focus, the Federation of County Councils arranges courses and seminars to teach project leaders about its implementation. The programme can easily be adjusted for any kind of work setting.

Glasgow Women's Health Policy, Scotland

A participatory approach is also encouraged in the Glasgow Women's Health Policy (30). Glasgow was the first city in the United Kingdom to adopt a multi-agency women's health policy from the perspective of a social, rather than a medical, model of health. As such, it aims to address three inter-related determinants of women's health: women's complex reproductive system; sex differences in the aetiology, presentation and treatment of different forms of illness; and the impact of gender inequality in society. Although the policy seeks to promote and improve the health of women and girls overall, it explicitly recognizes that some health needs within the female population are affected by other forms of inequality, for example, social class, race, disability and sexuality.

The policy was produced by a working group of the World Health Organization (WHO) Glasgow Healthy City Project in 1992 (revised in 1996) and adopted by the key partner agencies in the city – health authority, local government, non-governmental organizations and universities. Its objectives are designed to facilitate changes in the policy and planning processes of these organizations so that they are sensitive to both health and gender.

The impact of the policy can be seen in six main areas:

1. the development of structures within the partner organizations with the responsibility for considering women's health;
2. improvements in certain health and social services which have made them more sensitive to women;
3. the production of information and resource materials for women and professionals to raise awareness of women's health;
4. improvements in links between policy-makers and practitioners and local communities of women;
5. the development and funding of a model project (Centre for Women's Health) which identifies and responds to women's unmet health needs, provides training on women's health issues, and works with other agencies to help them shape their response to women's health; and
6. the development of a strategic approach to tackling violence against women, including its health consequences.

Conclusions

The aim of this chapter was to demonstrate the need for gender-sensitive policies and interventions to reduce socioeconomic inequalities in health. Evidence from studies on socioeconomic inequalities in mortality and morbidity suggest that the determinants of these inequalities may not be the same for men and women or, if they are the same, they may affect inequalities differently among women and men. Thus, interventions and policies should ensure that men and women will be treated equally where they share common needs and, where their needs are different for biological or social reasons, these differences will be addressed in an equitable manner. If research and policy address the interaction between socioeconomic position and gender in the social patterning of health more systematically and symmetrically, we could go a fair way towards effectively reducing health inequalities between men and women.

Acknowledgements

I wish to thank Dr Alex Scott-Samuel, Dr Sue Laughlin, Mrs Monica Stenberg, Mrs Christina Norlin Mistander and Dr Karien Stronks for documents they have kindly provided.

References

1. Sen G, George A, Östlin P. Engendering health equality: a review of research and policy. In: Sen G, George A, Östlin P, eds. *Engendering International Health: the Challenge of Equality*. Cambridge: MIT Press, 2002 (in press).

2. Annandale E, Hunt K. Gender inequalities in health: research at the crossroads. In: Annandale E, Hunt K, eds. *Gender Inequalities in Health*. Philadelphia: Open University Press, 2000.

3. Macintyre S, Hunt K. Socioeconomic position, gender and health. how do they interact? *J Health Psychol* 1997: 3: 315–34.

4. Lynch J, Kaplan G. Socioeconomic position. In: Berkman L, Kawachi I, eds. *Social Epidemiology*. Oxford: Oxford University Press, 2000.

5. Krieger NN, Rowley AA, Avery B, Phillips MT. Racism, sexism, and social class: implications for studies of health, disease, and well-being. *Am J Preventive Med* 1993: 9: 82–122.

6. Östlin P, George A, Sen G. Gender, health and equity: the intersections. In: Evans T, Whitehead M, Diderichsen F, Bhuiya A, Wirth M, eds. *Challenging Inequities in Health: From Ethics to Action*. New York: Oxford University Press, 2001.

7. Breen N. *Social Class and Health. Understanding Gender and its Interaction with Other Social Determinants*. Working Paper Series, Volume 10, No 3. Cambridge: Harvard Center for Population and Development Studies, Harvard School of Public Health, 2000.

8. Koskinen S, Martelin T. Why are socioeconomic mortality differences smaller among women than among men? *Soc Sci Med* 1994: 38: 1385–96.

9. Vågerö D, Lundberg O. Socioeconomic mortality differentials among adults in Sweden. In: Lopez A, Caselli G, Valkonen T, eds. *Adult Mortality in Developed Countries*. Oxford: Clarendon Press, 1995: 223–42.

10. Kaplan GA, Pamuk ER, Lynch JW, Cohen RD, Balfour JL. Inequality in income and mortality in the United States: analyses of mortality and potential pathways. *Br Med J* 1996: 312: 999–1003.

11. Mackenbach JP *et al.* Socioeconomic inequalities in mortality among women and among men: an international study. *Am J Public Health* 1999: 12: 1800–6.

12. Martikainen P. Socioeconomic mortality differentials in men and women according to own and spouse's characteristics in Finland. *Soc Health Illness* 1995: 17: 353–75.

13. Hemström Ö. Biological and social conditions: hypotheses regarding mortality differentials between men and women. In: Östlin P, Danielsson M, Diderichsen F, Härenstam A, Lindberg G, eds. *Gender Inequalities in Health: a Swedish Perspective*. Cambridge: Harvard Center for Development and Population Studies, Harvard University Press, 2001.

14. Stronks K, van de Mheen H, van den Bos J, Mackenbach JP. Smaller socioeconomic inequalities in health among women: the role of employment status. *Int J Epidemiol* 1995: 24: 559–68.

15. Matthews S, Manor O, Power C. Social inequalities in health: are there gender differences? *Soc Sci Med* 1999: 48: 49–60.

16. Arber S. Comparing inequalities in women's and men's health: Britain in the 1990s. *Soc Sci Med* 1997: 44: 773–87.

17. West P. Health inequalities in the early years: is there an equalisation in youth? *Soc Sci Med* 1997: 44: 833–58.

18. Power C, Matthews S, Manor O. Inequalities in self-rated health in the 1958 birth cohort: lifetime social circumstances or social mobility? *Br Med J* 1996: 313: 449–53.

19. Kunst AE, Genrts JJM, van den Berg J. International variation in socioeconomic inequalities in self reported health. *J Epidemiol Commun Health* 1995: 49: 117–23.

20. Wamala PS, Mittleman MA, Horsten M, Schenck-Gustafsson K, Orth-Gomér K. Job stress and the occupational gradient in coronary heart disease risk in women. The Stockholm Female Coronary Risk Study. *Soc Sci Med* 2000: 51: 481–9.

21. Östlin P. *Gender Inequalities in Occupational Health*. Cambridge: Harvard Center for Population and Development Studies, Working Paper Series, Volume 10, Number 9, September 2000.

22. Joint Work Environment Council for the Government Sector. *Reflections on Women in Working Life*. Stockholm: SAN, 1997.

23. Cavelaars AEJM, Kunst AE, Mackenbach JP. Socioeconomic differences in risk factors for morbidity and mortality in the European Community: an international comparison. *J Health Psychol* 1997: 2: 353–72.

24. Marmot MG, Davey Smith G, Stansfeld S, Patel C, North F, Head J *et al.* Health inequalities among British civil cervants: The Whitehall II study. *Lancet* 1991: 337: 1387–93.

25. Meding B. Work-related skin disease. In: Kilbom Å, Messing K, Bildt Thorbjörnsson C, eds. *Women's Health at Work*. Solna: National Institute of Working Life, 1998.

26. Alfredsson L, Spetz C-L, Theorell T. Type of occupation and near-future hospitalization for myocardial infarction and some other diagnoses. *Int J Epidemiol* 1985: 14: 378–88.

27. Szulkin R, Tåhlin M. Arbetets utveckling (The development of work) (in Swedish). In: Fritzell J, Lundberg O. *Vardagens villkor – levnadsförhållanden i Sverige under tre decennier*. Stockholm: Brobergs, 1994.

28. Karasek R, Theorell T. *Healthy Work*. New York: Basic Books, 1990.

29. Larsson B, Svenhammar K. *Focus-arbetsplatsutveckling med ett genusperspectiv*. Stockholm: Landstingsförbundet, 1998.

30. Laughlin S. From theory to practice: the Glasgow experience. In: Doyal L, ed. *Women and Health Services: An agenda for Action*. Open University Press, 1998.

23 Room for a view

A non-European perspective on European policies to minimize socioeconomic inequalities in health

*Philippa Howden-Chapman and
Ichiro Kawachi*

Introduction

This book, written largely by Europeans, provides an important overview of recent European research and policy developments to reduce socioeconomic inequalities in health. However, the purpose of this chapter is different: written by two non-Europeans, it aims explicitly to provide an outside view. We reflect on European policies to reduce socioeconomic inequalities in health and compare the approaches and policies outlined in this book with our Australasian and American experiences. From this perspective, we consider the strengths and weaknesses of European policy development and implementation and the possibilities for international cross-fertilization.

This cross-national European Union (EU) initiative is impressive and unique in its scope. After earlier, more limited international reviews by Gepkens and Gunning-Schepers (1), the World Health Organization (WHO) (2), the Acheson report (3) and the King's Fund report (4), this book appears to be the first effort to cluster information at the European level and to move on from the ubiquitous and somewhat depressing descriptions of socioeconomic inequalities in health, to systematically analyse the relative effectiveness of population-level interventions in different countries for the express purpose of ameliorating those inequalities. This is a hopeful and more uplifting enterprise, which is a critical step in linking research with policy development and implementation.

Observations on the European experience

Until the 1990s, few European countries, apart from the United Kingdom (UK), where publication of the Black Report had been infamously delayed, had undertaken any systematic research examining socioeconomic inequalities in health (5). During the 1990s, European national efforts gradually increased and were usefully documented in the international literature (3, 4,

6–8). Countries such as France had produced statistical series demonstrating gradients in morbidity and mortality by social class, but there was little analysis of the underlying social and economic determinants of health, or any overview.

Policies and interventions

Health inequalities are not immutable but are amenable to change through the development of government policies and regional and local initiatives. Yet when reviewing the interventions that the European countries have proposed, it is evident to the outsider that, despite the innovations, in most cases only a limited range of the policy levers available to governments have been deployed. In part, this seems to depend on the political complexion of the particular government in power: for example, in the UK and Spain conservative political parties dropped existing social inequalities and health programmes.

Some countries, such as Sweden and Finland, have consistently adopted a broad social policy approach, which has to some extent been successful in minimizing health inequalities by focusing on comprehensive policies, including employment, occupation, accident compensation, income, tax, social security, education, childcare, food, nutrition, risk behaviours and primary care. However, most countries have restricted their activities to less broad packages. Moreover, few have consistent long-term policies related to socioeconomic inequalities that are coordinated or effective at all levels of government, national, regional and local. Positive examples are the recent initiatives in England to address social exclusion, as well as the systematic attempt to identify intersectoral policies to abate socioeconomic inequalities in health represented by the recent Acheson report (3).

Looking at the EU research and policies in this area, it is something of a paradox that the European countries with smaller income inequalities, such as The Netherlands, Finland and Sweden, have had the most active research programmes and policy initiatives (although even in these relatively egalitarian countries health inequalities between social groups are still significant). For example, in The Netherlands the difference in healthy life expectancy between men from different social groups is still 12 years, and people from lower socioeconomic groups are three times as likely to rate their health as very bad.

Governments also have powers to set up organizational structures. It is apparent, for example, that long-standing government committees may be one way of developing and maintaining a policy to reduce health inequalities, regardless of government stability, for instance The Netherlands versus Lithuania. In addition to funding research, government agencies in The Netherlands and the UK have designated academics to disseminate the results of the research to policy-makers as well as to the research community.

Healthcare reforms

In Europe, as in many other Organization for Economic Cooperation and Development (OECD) countries, health sector institutional reforms have been accorded greater priority than the broader social and economic determinants of health that require intersectoral action. National governments have concentrated primarily on policies involving health services, such as improving access and increasing funding. Notwithstanding the evidence that health services have less of an impact on health inequalities than do structural factors, their organization can nevertheless have an important impact on inequalities in health. For example, there is clear evidence of socioeconomic inequalities in access to healthcare. In terms of co-payments, which are widespread in Europe, there is evidence that 50 per cent of co-payments are borne by 5 per cent of the population, and that chronically ill patients pay a substantially higher proportion than the acutely ill. However, this situation is still more equitable than in the United States (USA), where 47 million people, or about 17 per cent of the population, are either underinsured or uninsured, or in New Zealand, where about half the adult population pays the full cost of primary care consultations (9).

Redistributive policies

In contrast to health sector reforms, redistributive policies, which are considered by some to have a side-effect of weakening work and saving incentives, are far more politically contentious. Nonetheless, in countries such as Sweden and Finland, where such policies are integral to the welfare state and where income inequality is monitored, they help to sustain a political consensus that is part of the socially inclusive Nordic model, which is associated with keeping the inequalities in income largely unchanged during economic cycles. This was the case during the recession in the early 1990s in Finland, which was deeper than the 1930s depression but which, because of social and income policies, had no discernible impact on health inequalities.

Comparison of the European situation with New Zealand/ Australia and the USA

There appear to have been two reasons for the historical lack of attention to socioeconomic inequalities in health. In countries that pride themselves on being egalitarian, such as the Scandinavian countries, the social gradient of health was until recently thought to be either non-existent owing to the comprehensive nature of the welfare state, or at least of minimal importance. In less egalitarian countries there has been a lack of political will to focus on population health inequalities that might highlight the health impacts of very economically stratified societies.

In more individualistic pro-market societies, such as the United States, Australia and New Zealand, the lack of public discourse about inequalities can be attributed to a popular belief in social mobility and individual responsibility, as well as to the reluctance of politicians and business groups to acknowledge the social costs of inequality (even though the same groups are quick to extol the virtues of inequality for motivating workers) (10, 11). Indeed, when issues of inequality are discussed the problem is usually framed in terms of 'the health of the poor', a device that then enables the majority to dismiss the issue as being a minority problem, with the result that the 'war on poverty' becomes a 'war on the poor' (12). To some extent there is a parallel in New Zealand and Australia, where issues of health inequality are framed in terms of 'the health of Maori and Aborigines'.

In this book, national efforts are identified and clearly referenced. The setting up of a new organization, the European Network on Interventions and Policies to Reduce Socioeconomic Inequalities in Health, facilitated considerable cross-fertilization of research and some policy initiatives within Europe. The scope and rigour of this work has also had a major influence on national frameworks outside Europe, such as New Zealand (13, 14) and Australia (15).

Why is it that this initiative took off in Europe? Our view is that in Europe there is a greater historical consciousness of the need for and place of collective effort to address socioeconomic issues, at both national and EU level. From the point of view of outsiders, this supranational effort appears more extensive than any other regional initiative, and builds on systematic national efforts in countries such as the UK, Sweden and The Netherlands. In contrast, countries such as the USA and New Zealand may be more open to social or technological innovations that apparently enhance individual opportunities, but are less interested in 'social engineering' for collective benefits. For example, in the USA there is a federal overview of socioeconomic status and health (16), but this is really the exception. Also, it is only in the past year that an effort has been made to set up an equivalent Australasian initiative.

What are the institutional catalysts to this collective action? Most importantly, since the early 1980s the WHO European Office has played a pivotal role in promoting health equality, at critical points providing opportunities for collaboration, as well as strongly advocating and supporting the monitoring of health inequalities as an important public policy at national level. The EU also requires an annual report on the health implications of all EU policies, and more latterly has identified inequalities in health as a priority for its public health programmes (8). These combined initiatives have provided an important stimulus in raising the priority given to social and economic inequalities in Europe, primarily by diffusing the systematic efforts of countries such as the UK and The Netherlands to other European countries.

The impetus for sustained policies to reduce social and economic inequalities in health is reduced in countries which are highly politically divided, but also in those that are largely indifferent to class divisions. In the UK, where class differences are party-politicized, the consequence has been predominantly short-term programmes which to date have not had a major impact on health inequalities. In the USA, where class differences have not been so institutionalized in political parties, preferences for redistribution, as gauged by popular opinion surveys, are remarkably low, even among the poorest segments of the population (10). Thus, the USA, which maintains one of the most deplorable degrees of inequality among the ranks of rich nations, paradoxically appears to be the one least inclined to change.

Monitoring

Monitoring health inequalities is an essential prerequisite to action. In countries such as the USA, the government's ability to do so has been severely hampered by the absence of socioeconomic data on official and routine sources of data collection, such as the state vital records and cancer registries (17). Consequently, official US statistics tend to report health inequalities by race rather than socioeconomic status, resulting in a fallacious tendency to ascribe health inequalities to biological or cultural causes.

The social indicators movement offers valuable lessons with regard to monitoring of health inequalities. As Miringoff and colleagues (18) have pointed out, the USA is much more attuned to indicators of *economic* performance – for example, minute-by-minute updates of stock market performance, or quarterly reports of employment and consumer confidence – than to indicators of *social* performance, and this is also likely to be true in Europe. Efforts have been initiated in the USA to redress this imbalance, for instance, in the form of a National Index of Social Health, issued annually by the Fordham Institute on Innovation in Social Policy (which includes indicators such as infant mortality, homicide, teenage pregnancies and drug abuse). Even so, the USA lags considerably behind the levels of official support and public awareness that economic indicators currently enjoy.

From an outsider's perspective the selection of particular measures for social and economic determinants of health inequalities is evidently culturally determined at a national level. For example, in the UK social class is generally the key determinant; in the USA this is black or white race; and in New Zealand Maori or non-Maori. Thus in New Zealand the government's initiative Closing the Gaps referred to reducing inequalities in health and other social policy areas between Maoris, Pacific peoples and non-Maoris, although under recent political pressure the focus has broadened to include the non-Maori poor. For the reverse reasons, countries with a colonial history, whose former subjects frequently now have citizenship of the 'home' country, often pay particular attention to the vulnerability of migrants' health.

Targets

The adoption of government goals and targets that include the reduction of inequalities, such as in Sweden and the United Kingdom, is one way in which the political community can highlight and monitor the health impacts of policies. New Zealand has recently adopted such targets as high-level goals and objectives, but the priority population health objectives are still focused on health risks for particular diseases (19). In the USA the Surgeon General's Healthy People 2010 health objectives include 'the elimination of racial disparities in health' by the year 2010; however, there is as yet no comparable goal to reduce socioeconomic inequalities in health. Once again, the issue of health inequalities in the USA tends to be based on ethnicity, partly because there is no other means of monitoring progress towards eliminating social class inequalities. Cross-national comparisons of the effectiveness of different approaches to setting goals and targets to reduce health inequalities are needed.

Health promotion

As well as legislating and operating institutionally, governments can also use educational methods to promote health, though this is generally thought to be the least effective intervention. For certain risk factors, such as smoking, major health promotion initiatives have been targeted in all countries. Smoking is a key example of a risk that is not evenly spread over all strata of society, but the usual patterning of socioeconomic characteristics, whereby people in the lower strata are more at risk, varies according to the stage of the smoking epidemic in a particular country. In New Zealand smoking rates are highest among Maori people, particularly young women, who are among the most socially and economically deprived groups. As in Europe, targeted approaches have been implemented to complement broad taxation policies, but so far this has not been particularly effective (20).

Subjugated people

There are historical patterns of conquest and reconquest of cultural groups which appear to have left an imprint in terms of poorer health status, which are not explored in this book. Why do the peoples of Scotland, Ireland and Wales still have poorer health than those in England? Why do people in Denmark have noticeably poorer health than those in Sweden? To non-Europeans living in countries that were long settled by indigenous people before they were colonized, it appears that these patterns of health inequality need to be addressed. The expropriation of land assets and the stripping away of cultural capital by the dominant society, which then establishes institutional structures that favour its own culture, seems to have been a major factor throughout the British and other European empires in explaining the poorer health of the subjugated people.

This book does not address the impact of these historical patterns of power and settlement, which are one of the social and economic determinants of health inequalities that, in other parts of the world, loom large. In the USA, for example, race/ethnicity clearly marks out the descendants of Afro-American slaves. Similarly, in Australia the indigenous Aboriginal people, who were not classified as citizens until the 1970s, live on average 20 years less than the European immigrant population, and in New Zealand a similar but smaller gap exists, despite a colonial treaty that binds contemporary governments legally and morally to maintain health equality between the indigenous peoples and others. In all three of these countries, the emphasis on the poorer health status of the indigenous or subjugated people has been associated until recently with a convenient lack of emphasis on the broader socioeconomic inequalities in health.

Conclusions

Socioeconomic inequalities in health are evidently difficult to eliminate because they are integral to the entrenched distributions of material resources controlled by powerful elites. However, as the distinguished British economist Atkinson (21) commented recently on the *Acheson Report*, governments have an important role in reducing inequalities through their budgets and their influence on social judgements that affect the labour market. Governments working with researchers, policy-makers and the public can help to generate and support the social concern for an inclusive society, where growing inequalities in health become politically unacceptable.

Research/policy links are crucial for understanding the connections between causal factors and health outcomes, which can then effectively influence the formulation and implementation of policies to minimize socioeconomic inequalities in health. European Union initiatives are important benchmarks for areas outside Europe, for example, New Zealand and Australia, although it remains to be seen how important or valid it is to extrapolate from one country to another, or whether nationalism and the specific local context means that it is necessary to produce corroborating local national evidence before policies are adopted.

In terms of developing good practice, generalizability is a key issue. How does the socioeconomic context of the country (for example, the history and political system, the extent of the social security system and the present level of socioeconomic inequalities) shape the acceptability and possibility of implementing policy or programme initiatives that have been identified as minimizing socioeconomic inequalities in health? This is an important issue, not just in Europe, but outside as well. For example, this has been a key issue in the debate about how to generate and maintain social capital. In *Making Democracy Work: Civic Traditions in Modern Italy*, Putnam *et al.*

(22) imply that the roots of democracy go back to the Middle Ages and earlier, so that modern social capital is embedded in long-standing institutional rules. It is unclear whether European initiatives would work in the USA, Australia or New Zealand.

The exploration in this book of key interventions to reduce socioeconomic inequalities in health is timely and innovative, and provides useful policy examples that are likely to stimulate replication or imitation outside Europe. Hopefully, in turn, some of the innovations being tried outside Europe, such as devolution of the control of population and health services to disadvantaged populations in New Zealand, and family support programmes to enhance educational achievement such as Head Start in the USA and Family Start in New Zealand, will also be taken up within Europe.

References

1. Gepkens A, Gunning-Schepers LJ. Interventions to reduce socioeconomic health differences. *Eur J Public Health* 1996: 6: 2218–26.
2. Dahlgren G, Whitehead M. *Policies and Strategies to Promote Equity in Health.* Copenhagen: World Health Organization, 1992.
3. *Independent Inquiry into Inequalities in Health.* Report. London: The Stationery Office, 1998.
4. Benzeval M, Judge K, Whitehead M. *Tackling Inequalities in Health: an Agenda for Action.* London: King's Fund, 1995.
5. Townsend P, Whitehead M, Davidson M. *Inequalities in Health: the Black Report and the Health Divide.* London: Penguin Books, 1992.
6. Mackenbach J. Socioeconomic inequalities in health in The Netherlands: impact of a five year research programme. *Br Med J* 1994: 309: 1487–91.
7. Mackenbach JP, Kunst AE, Cavelaars AE *et al.* Socioeconomic inequalities in morbidity and mortality in Western Europe. The EU Working Group on Socioeconomic Inequalities in Health. *Lancet* 1997: 349: 1255–69.
8. Whitehead M. Diffusion of ideas on social inequalities in health: a European perspective. *Millbank Quarterly* 1998: 76: 469–92.
9. Scott KM, Marwick JC, Crampton PR. Utilisation of general practitioner services in New Zealand and its relationship with income, ethnicity. *Soc Sci Med* (in press).
10. Lipset SM. *American Exceptionalism: a Double-edged Sword.* New York: WW Norton, 1997.
11. Marks G, Lipset SM. *It Didn't Happen Here: Why Socialism Failed in the United States.* New York: WW Norton, 2000.
12. Katz MB. *The Undeserving Poor: from the War on Poverty to the War on Welfare.* New York: Pantheon Books, 1990.
13. Howden-Chapman P, Tobias M, eds. *Social Inequalities in Health; New Zealand in 1999.* Wellington: Ministry of Health, 2000.
14. National Health Committee. *The Social, Cultural and Economic Determinants of Health in New Zealand: Action to Improve Health. A Report from the National Advisory Committee on Health and Disability.* Wellington, 1998.

15. Turrell G, Oldenburg B, McGuffog I, Dent R. *Socioeconomic Determinants of Health: towards a National Research Program and a Policy and Intervention Agenda.* Canberra: Queensland University of Technology, School of Public Health, Ausinfo, 1999.
16. Pamuk E, Makuc D, Heck K, Reuben C, Lochner K. *Socioeconomic Status and Health Chartbook. Health, United States*, 1998. Hyattsville, Maryland: National Center for Health Statistics, 1998.
17. Krieger N, Williams DR, Moss NE. Measuring social class in US public health research: concepts, methodologies, and guidelines. *Annu Rev Public Health* 1997: 18: 341–78.
18. Miringoff ML, Miringoff ML, Opdycke S. *The Social Health of the Nation: how America is Really Doing.* New York: Oxford University Press, 1999.
19. King A. *The New Zealand Health Strategy.* Wellington: Ministry of Health, 2000.
20. Crampton P, Salmond C, Woodward A, Reid P. Socioeconomic deprivation and ethnicity are both important for anti-tobacco health promotion. *Health Educ Behav* 2000: 27: 317–27.
21. Atkinson AB. Income inequality in the UK. *Health Econ* 1999: 8: 283–8.
22. Putnam R, Leonardi R, Nanetti RY. *Making Democracy Work: Civic Traditions in Modern Italy.* Princeton: Princeton University Press, 1993.

Part VI
Key messages

24 By way of conclusion
Key messages for policy-makers

Introduction

This final chapter is a collaborative effort of all authors who contributed to this book and is edited by Martijntje Bakker and Johan Mackenbach. This book set out to collect and analyse European experiences in the field of policies and interventions to reduce socioeconomic inequalities in health. These experiences were ordered in two ways: by policy area and by country. What did we learn?

Policies and interventions

The evidence base

As others have noted before, the available evidence on the effectiveness of policies and interventions to reduce socioeconomic inequalities in health is very limited. Until recently most of the research in this field has been devoted to describing and explaining such inequalities, and there has understandably been a relative scarcity of studies evaluating the effect of interventions or policies. Now that our understanding of the problem has reached the point where we can identify entry points for policies and interventions, the time has come to increase our investment in evaluation studies.

It is important that rigorous evaluation takes place, but although traditional forms of evaluation certainly have a role to play, some of the more complex interventions and most policy measures cannot be evaluated properly in, for example, controlled experiments. Opportunities for learning should not be forgone only on the basis of the impossibility of a traditional research design. Other rigorous methods are available, and these should be applied when appropriate. Examples include international comparative studies of the effects of national policies, and theory-based evaluation.

Accessibility of the results of evaluation studies is another important prerequisite for policy-making. One problem we have encountered is that it is difficult to find such studies in the literature databases, because keyword systems do not adequately identify these studies, and because some of them are not included in conventional databases. Another problem is that some studies are not reported in the international scientific literature, but only in national journals or 'grey reports'. We therefore need a special effort to increase the accessibility of evaluation results, for example in the form of special documentation centres. These may, on the basis of carefully designed search strategies and an international reporting system to collect information on ongoing and recently completed evaluation studies, increase the accessibility for policy-makers to relevant information.

Still another problem that we encountered related to the methodological evaluation of the evidence presented in the literature. Because of the difficulties in applying traditional research methods, many studies use alternative designs, which are sometimes difficult to evaluate. It would therefore be useful to have a sort of Cochrane collaboration for interventions and policies tackling inequalities in health.

Effective interventions and policies

The preceding chapters have revealed a number of effective interventions and policies to reduce socioeconomic inequalities in health. Quite clearly, these do not cover all entry points or all possible ways to use those entry points. Nevertheless, we think that our inventory has yielded some encouraging results.

Tackling health inequalities requires a broad response from many policy sectors, but sectors all have their own goals, and reducing health inequalities is only one of a number of legitimate policy objectives. Health impact assessment, if given an equality focus, will help in raising awareness of and commitment to health inequalities among policy-makers in other areas. It offers the opportunity for adapting proposed policies so that they enhance potential positive impacts on health inequalities, and reduce potentially negative impacts.

'Upstream' interventions and policies are potentially powerful ways to reduce socioeconomic inequalities in health. Changes in poverty and income inequality can be achieved through a variety of employment policies, but improving living standards through the social security system is essential if substantial inroads are to be made into the numbers on low incomes.

A broad universal social welfare system (welfare state) is likely to buffer against widening health inequalities during adverse economic development. Despite a severe economic recession, health inequalities in Finland remained stable during the late 1980s and early 1990s, probably due to such a buffering effect.

The link between the political context and the policies devised is important. If we wish to understand the health policy process in a realistic manner, political ideology and economic interests of key players in the health decision-making process cannot be avoided.

In addition to 'upstream' interventions and policies, 'midstream' and 'downstream' measures are also necessary. Reducing unfavourable physical and psychosocial working conditions is a very important entry point for reducing socioeconomic inequalities in health. National chemical hazards hygiene standards have contributed enormously to reducing chemical hazards, and thereby socioeconomic inequalities in occupational cancer and certain other occupational disorders. Further health gains can be achieved by focusing on reducing heavy physical work and preventing work-related accidents.

It is less likely that legislation will be effective against adverse psychosocial working conditions. On the other hand, work environment interventions are continuously carried out by employers to increase efficiency. Although few of these have as their main aim the improvement of health, optimizing the psychosocial working environment could lead to health improvements as well. There is a need to link these two fields.

Reducing smoking in lower socioeconomic groups is an important entry point for reducing socioeconomic inequalities in health. Smoking cessation interventions which are probably effective in disadvantaged groups include free/cheap prescriptions for nicotine replacement therapy, increasing prices by raising tobacco taxes, and smoking restrictions in the workplace (these restrictions need to be accompanied by health education and information). Governments should emphasize equality of outcomes in the development, implementation and evaluation of all interventions to reduce the level of smoking in the population. Governments should strive to create societal conditions that are conducive to less inequality in smoking, for instance, by increasing financial security for disadvantaged/excluded groups.

In the field of nutrition, carefully tailored 'selectivist' measures that are sensitive to the cultural, social and economic conditions of the target group may improve the diet of that group. Examples of effective measures are food and nutrition programmes that enable people to purchase more healthy foods (such programmes have shown success in providing food assistance to low-income groups).

In the long run, however, such selectivist measures may reproduce inequalities. 'Universalist' measures which increase the likelihood of healthier food choices among large population groups, such as interventions dealing with dietary and other behavioural changes (school meal programmes, community interventions) and changes in the content of cheap and fast food (reduction of trans-fatty acid content in cheap margarines), may also reduce nutritional inequalities and may in the longer term be more effective.

Childhood health inequalities are still a major problem in Europe, and may contribute to the perpetuation of adult health inequalities in the future. Some interventions have been shown to effectively reduce childhood health inequalities, such as targeted vaccination programmes, safety education, screening programmes, early educational interventions, and the provision of social security benefits, supplemental security income payments and housing subsidies.

Finally, the health service also has a role to play, both in ensuring equality of access to its services and in leading and shaping the wider agenda.

Healthcare interventions that have been shown to be effective include screening programmes, which pay specific attention to increasing the attendance rates of lower socioeconomic groups, home visitation programmes and easily accessible special clinics.

Since the 1980s, patient cost sharing has been introduced on a large scale in many European countries as a cost containment measure. Although this has reduced the demand for healthcare services, it is unsuitable for making qualitative adjustments to patient demand behaviour and it raises the financial accessibility threshold of healthcare for those most in need. Therefore, patient cost sharing may lead to increased socioeconomic inequalities in health and should be avoided as a policy measure.

Simultaneously with national policy action, local intersectoral partnerships can work together to address particular local issues. Health Action Zones (HAZs) in the United Kingdom are complex, partner-based entities that have set themselves ambitious goals to transform the health and well-being of disadvantaged communities and groups. Early interviews with key stakeholders in HAZs showed incredible enthusiasm and commitment to really making a difference to the lives of their populations. HAZs have introduced some innovative plans to address some of the key determinants of health, as well as tackling some of the obstacles to effective access to health services.

In addition to national governments, local governments also have an important role to play, as the example of Barcelona shows. Various interventions carried out in this city (a mother and child health programme, tuberculosis control among the homeless and intravenous drug users, a drug abuse programme, and a reform of primary healthcare) have probably been followed by health improvements in the target groups. Although this experience cannot be directly translated to other cities in Europe, it does show that local governments can help to reduce socioeconomic inequalities in health.

As there may be different explanations behind socioeconomic health inequalities between women and men (determinants of inequalities may not be the same for men and women, or may affect inequalities differently among men and women), interventions aiming at reducing such inequalities should be gender-sensitive. Gender differences have been highlighted in relation to working life and health-related behaviours. Because the strongly gender-segregated labour market substantially contributes to women's inferior position in society, the workplace is a fruitful starting point for identifying health-damaging and health-promoting factors in women's and men's work, and for understanding gender differences in socioeconomic inequalities in health.

National experiences

National policy-makers in the countries described in this book are in different phases of awareness of, and willingness to take action on, socioeconomic inequalities in health. Margaret Whitehead has proposed a schematic 'action spectrum' to characterize the stage of diffusion of ideas on socioeconomic inequalities in health. Starting with a primordial stage in which socioeconomic inequalities in health are not even measured, the spectrum covers the stages of 'measurement', 'recognition', 'awareness', 'denial/indifference', 'concern', 'will to take action', 'isolated initiatives', 'more structured developments' and 'comprehensive coordinated policy' (1). The action spectrum should not be regarded as a linear progress and countries will not necessarily go through all stages of it.

Based on the descriptions of the national experiences presented in this book, we conclude that whereas Greece still seems to be in the measurement stage, Spain currently finds itself in the 'denial/indifference' stage, and France and Italy are in the 'concern' stage. Lithuania, on the other hand, has rapidly reached the 'will to take action' stage, The Netherlands and Sweden are in the 'more structured developments' stage, and Britain may recently have entered the 'comprehensive coordinated policy' stage. The descriptions of these national experiences also suggest factors that may have been influential in promoting or blocking progression on the action spectrum.

In many countries the initiation of the process (raising awareness and concern among policy-makers) has been facilitated by the availability of convincing data. The existence of health information systems which are able to monitor socioeconomic inequalities is a fundamental prerequisite: in countries in early stages of the action spectrum, such as Greece, the creation of relevant databases should be a priority. Another factor is research: in many countries researchers from various disciplines have actively promoted the issue of socioeconomic inequalities in health on the basis of research findings. In the later stages of the action spectrum, the quality and policy relevance of these findings are heavily dependent on contributions by and cooperation between different disciplines (medical, social, economic, etc., perhaps with epidemiology as a common language). Research programmes in Britain, The Netherlands, Finland and Sweden clearly illustrate the importance of a multidisciplinary approach.

The presence or absence of political will is another obvious and important influence. At least the most sensitive political parties or social forces should recognize the importance of knowing, taking action and evaluating policies to reduce socioeconomic inequalities in health. The contrasting experiences of Britain and Spain, and within Spain, between Barcelona and the national policy level, demonstrate this. After more than a decade of blocked progression on the action spectrum, the election of a Labour government has quickly brought Britain into the most active stage of the countries described in this book. On the other hand, the publication of the 'Spanish Black Report' and other regular airing of data on health inequalities has produced little reaction at the national level in Spain. In Barcelona, however, where a succession of coalitions led by the Socialist Party has governed the city for many years, the study of socioeconomic inequalities in health has been a priority of the Municipal Public Health Institute since the 1980s, and programmes have been developed and implemented to tackle these inequalities, mainly in the inner city.

As is evident from these examples, some countries have seen a strong degree of party-politicization of this subject. This is not always the case, however. In The Netherlands, for instance, deliberate efforts by those promoting the issue have led to a broad consensus among left, centre and right-wing parties that socioeconomic inequalities in health have to be addressed, at least by national research programmes. Similarly, the new national health policy in Sweden has been developed with a broad political consensus. In order to guarantee continuity of policy development to reduce socioeconomic inequalities in health, it is important that these inequalities be recognized as a priority regardless of political signature, but this may come at the price of continuous compromises.

Lithuania is a clear example of the powerful influence of international agencies such as the World Health Organization. As it had done during the late 1980s and early 1990s for countries in Western Europe, WHO's European office has actively supported the development of a health inequalities focus in national health policy in Lithuania. Lithuania also secured cross-political party support through the involvement from the beginning of the Parliamentary Health Committee.

Further work

As this book has shown, knowledge of effective interventions and policies to reduce socioeconomic inequalities in health is still very fragmentary. There seem to be many entry points, but for only some of these have policies and interventions been devised, only some of them have been evaluated, and not all of the results have been made available to policy-makers around Europe. Further development and evaluation of policies and interventions therefore is urgently needed.

Although this will have to be primarily at the national level (and support from national governments is essential), international efforts are also important. As the example of the European Network on Interventions and Policies to Reduce Socioeconomic Inequalities in Health shows, international exchange of experiences and evaluation results can be very fruitful. We have identified a wide range of experiences and have uncovered evaluation studies which had not reached the international scientific literature. Continuation of such international exchange can therefore be expected to maintain a higher learning speed around Europe.

Reference

1.   Whitehead M. Diffusion of ideas on social inequalities in health: a European perspective. *Millbank Quarterly* 1998: 76: 469–92.

Appendix
Review search strategy

For the chapters on work-related policies and interventions (Chapter 6), food and nutrition policies and interventions (Chapter 7), smoking policies (Chapter 8), children, an important target group for the reduction of socio-economic inequalities in health (Chapter 9), and equality of access to healthcare (Chapter 10), a review was conducted of examples of policies and interventions to reduce socioeconomic inequalities in health.

For this review the following search strategies were used:

Articles were selected in Medline (1966–August 2000) by means of the following search strategy:

1. Exp socioeconomic factors*
2. Randomized controlled trial or RCT
3. Community intervention trial or CIT
4. Exp program evaluation
5. Combine 2 or 3 or 4
6. Combine 5 and 1
7. 6 and human

By putting an asterisk (*) after 'socioeconomic factors', Medline incorporates the following words for socioeconomic factors:

Career mobility
Poverty (poverty areas)
Social class (social mobility)
Educational status
Employment (unemployment)
Family characteristics
Income (pensions, salaries and fringe benefits)
Medical indigency
Occupations
Social change (urbanization)
Social conditions

This search strategy resulted in 593 references. Abstracts were checked for relevance based on the following criteria:

- Intervention aimed at low socioeconomic status groups, reported to be effective
- Intervention aimed at low socioeconomic status groups, reported to be non-effective
- Intervention aimed at general population, reported to be at least as effective in low as in high socioeconomic groups
- Intervention aimed at general population, reported to be less effective in low than in high socioeconomic groups.

In addition, relevant references which were included in the review of Gepkens and Gunning-Schepers (1), were added to the list as well as references selected in the database of the Socioeconomic Health Differences (SEHD) Documentation Centre of the Institute of Public Health, Erasmus University Rotterdam.

There are some individual differences in the reviews of the different topics. In Chapters 7, 8 and 10 all relevant interventions were included, regardless of country of origin. In Chapter 9, however, only interventions from Europe have been included to keep the numbers in the table feasible (with regard to interventions aimed at children very many references were found). Furthermore, in Chapter 9 interventions were also included if the objective of the intervention was relevant to low socioeconomic groups but results were not specified by socioeconomic group.

In the review for Chapter 7 references were also included about nutrition interventions which were selected for a report of the Dutch Ministry of Health about nutrition interventions which have the possibility to reduce socioeconomic inequalities in health (2).

The review just described did not result in any relevant interventions or policies for Chapter 6 about work-related policies and interventions. Therefore, the authors have included a table with several review articles which described interventions aimed for instance at the reduction of work-related stress.

References

1. Gepkens A, Gunning-Schepers LJ. Interventions to reduce socioeconomic health differences: a review of the international literature. *Eur J Public Health* 1996: 6: 218–26.
2. Stasse-Wolthuis M, Wiegersma W. *Goede voeding voor iedereen?! Advies op basis van platformdiscussie over effectieve voedingsinterventies gericht op achterstandsgroepen d.d 8 februari 2000* (Healthy Nutrition for Everyone?! Advice Based on a Platform Discussion about Effective Nutrition Interventions Aimed at Minority Groups, 8th February 2000). Den Haag: Voedingscentrum, 2000.

Glossary

Absolute difference   Difference expressed in absolute terms (that is, in the original units in which the observations were made, such as number of deaths per 1,000 population). Usually obtained by subtracting the values of different observations. See also: relative differences; rate difference.

Confounding   A situation in which the association between a factor under investigation (such as socioeconomic status) and a health outcome (such as mortality) is biased, because there is a third variable (such as age) that is not part of the causal pathway between the factor under investigation and the health outcome, or is not equally distributed across the factor under investigation and influences the health outcome. Such a third variable is called a confounder or confounding variable.

Cross-sectional study   A study that examines the relationship between a factor under investigation (such as socioeconomic status) and a health outcome (such as morbidity) at one particular time. The temporal sequence of cause and effect cannot be determined in a cross-sectional study.

Effectiveness   A measure of the extent to which a specific intervention, procedure, regimen, or service, when deployed in the field in routine circumstances, does what it is intended to do for a specified population.

Equity   Principle of being fair to all, with reference to a defined and recognized set of values.

GDP (Gross Domestic Product)   A measure of the total production and consumption of goods and services. The gross domestic product (GDP) is the most important economic indicator. It represents a broad measure of economic activity and signals the direction of overall aggregate economic activity.

Gini coefficient   An indicator of income inequality reflecting the distribution of income throughout the population. If income is distributed equally across the population, the coefficient is equal to 0, and if a few individuals predominantly hold the wealth, the coefficient is closer to 1.

Health   Health is usually defined as the absence of disease. However, in this book health is considered to be more than the absence of disease. Therefore, we have included the definition used by the World Health

Organization. Health is a state of complete physical, mental and social well-being and not merely the absence of disease or infirmity. Health is a resource for everyday life, not the object of living. It is a positive concept emphasizing social and personal resources as well as physical capabilities.

Incidence   The number of new events (such as new cases of disease) occurring in a defined population during a specified period of time. See also: prevalence; rate.

Intervention   An activity or set of activities aimed at modifying a process, course of action or sequence of events, in order to change one or several of their characteristics such as performance or expected outcome.

Observational study   Epidemiological study that does not involve any intervention, experimental or otherwise. Such a study may be one in which nature is allowed to take its course, with changes in one characteristic being studied in relation to changes in other characteristics. Analytic epidemiological methods, such as case-control and cohort study designs, are properly called observational epidemiology because the investigator is observing without intervention other than to record, classify, count and statistically analyse results.

Odds ratio   An odds ratio indicates how much more likely an individual with a given characteristic is to have a specific outcome than someone without the characteristic.

Prevalence   The number of persons sick or portraying a certain condition in a stated population at a particular time (point prevalence), or during a stated period of time (period prevalence), regardless of when that illness or condition began. See also: incidence; rate.

Purchasing power parity (PPP)   The PPP represents the relationship between the amounts of national currency needed to purchase a comparable, representative basket of goods in the countries concerned. The use of figures expressed in ECUs introduces disadvantages, since the exchange rate is mainly determined by the currency's supply and demand and by factors such as capital flows, speculation and the country's social and economic situation. The use of PPP reduces the discrepancies related to the exchange rate and allows better comparison among countries, mainly based on the consideration of each country's real purchasing power.

Quasi-experiment   A situation in which the investigator lacks full control over the allocation or timing of intervention but nonetheless conducts the study as if it were an experiment, allocating subjects to groups. Inability to allocate subjects randomly is a common situation that may be best described as a quasi-experiment.

Randomized controlled trial (RCT)   An epidemiologic experiment in which subjects in a population are randomly allocated into groups, usually called study and control groups, to receive or not to receive an experimental preventive or therapeutic procedure, manoeuvre, or intervention. The results are assessed by rigorous comparison of rates of disease, death, recovery, or other appropriate outcome in the study and control groups. Randomized controlled trials are generally regarded as the most scientifically rigorous method of hypothesis testing available in epidemiology.

Rate The frequency with which an event occurs. The incidence rate is the frequency with which new cases of disease occur (numerator) during a certain number of person-years at risk (denominator). The prevalence rate is the frequency with which (existing) cases of the disease are present (numerator) in a certain number of people (denominator).

Rate ratio The ratio of two rates. Used to measure relative differences. See also: relative differences; relative risk.

Rate difference The (absolute) difference between two rates. Used to measure absolute differences. See also: absolute difference.

Record linkage study A method for assembling the information contained in two or more records and a procedure to ensure that the same individual is counted only once. This procedure incorporates a unique identifying system such as a personal identification number or birth name(s) of the individual's mother. Record linkage makes it possible to relate significant health events that are remote from one another in time and place or to bring together records of different individuals, for instance members of a family. The resulting information is generally stored and retrieved by computer, which can be programmed to tabulate and analyse the data.

Relative differences Difference expressed in relative terms (that is, as a proportion or percentage of the value obtained for a reference category). Usually obtained by calculating the ratio of two figures. See also: rate ratio; absolute difference.

Social group Any set of persons within society that differs from other sets due to demographic, economic or social characteristics such as age, sex, education level, race, religion, income level, lifestyle, beliefs, and so on.

Social stratification A concept describing the perception of societies as consisting of strata in a hierarchy, with the more favoured at the top and the less privileged at the bottom. In modern societies, social stratification principally occurs on the basis of socio-economic characteristics, such as occupation.

Socioeconomic inequalities in health Systematic differences in morbidity and mortality rates between individual people of higher and lower socioeconomic status to the extent that these are perceived to be unfair.

Socioeconomic status A person's relative position in the social stratification of a society. Frequently used indicators of socioeconomic status are income level, level of education and occupational class or occupational prestige.

Variations in health Systematic differences in morbidity and mortality rates between individual people of higher and lower socioeconomic status.

Index